Infections in Older Adults

Editors

ROBIN L.P. JUMP
DAVID H. CANADAY

INFECTIOUS DISEASE CLINICS OF NORTH AMERICA

www.id.theclinics.com

Consulting Editor
HELEN W. BOUCHER

December 2017 • Volume 31 • Number 4

ELSEVIER

1600 John F. Kennedy Boulevard ● Suite 1800 ● Philadelphia, Pennsylvania, 19103-2899.

http://www.theclinics.com

INFECTIOUS DISEASE CLINICS OF NORTH AMERICA Volume 31, Number 4
December 2017 ISSN 0891–5520, ISBN-13: 978-0-323-55280-6

Editor: Kerry Holland
Developmental Editor: Donald Mumford

Infectious Disease Clinics of North America (ISSN 0891–5520) is published in March, June, September, and December by Elsevier Inc., 360 Park Avenue South, New York, New York 10010-1710. Periodicals postage paid at New York, NY and additional mailing offices. Subscription prices are $301.00 per year for US individuals, $588.00 per year for US institutions, $100.00 per year for US students, $357.00 per year for Canadian individuals, $734.00 per year for Canadian institutions, $428.00 per year for international individuals, $734.00 per year for international institutions, and $200.00 per year for Canadian and international students. To receive student rate, orders must be accompanied by name of affiliated institution, date of term, and the *signature* of program/residency coordinator on institution letterhead. Orders will be billed at individual rate until proof of status is received. Foreign air speed delivery is included in all *Clinics* subscription prices. All prices are subject to change without notice. **POSTMASTER**: Send address changes to *Infectious Disease Clinics of North America*, Elsevier Health Sciences Division, Subcription Customer Service, 3251 Riverport Lane, Maryland Heights, MO 63043. **Customer Service: 1-800-654-2452 (US). From outside of the US and Canada, call 1-314-447-8871. Fax: 1-314-447-8029. E-mail: JournalsCustomerService-usa@elsevier.com (print support) or JournalsOnlineSupport-usa@elsevier.com (online support).**

Infectious Disease Clinics of North America is also published in Spanish by Editorial Inter-Médica, Junin 917, 1er A 1113, Buenos Aires, Argentina.

Reprints. For copies of 100 or more, of articles in this publication, please contact the Commercial Reprints Department, Elsevier Inc., 360 Park Avenue South, New York, New York 10010-1710. Tel. 212-633-3874, Fax: 212-633-3820, E-mail: reprints@elsevier.com.

Infectious Disease Clinics of North America is covered in *MEDLINE/PubMed (Index Medicus), Current Contents/Clinical Medicine, Science Citation Alert, SCISEARCH,* and *Research Alert.*

Contributors

CONSULTING EDITOR

HELEN W. BOUCHER, MD, FIDSA, FACP
Director, Infectious Diseases Fellowship Program, Division of Geographic Medicine and
Infectious Diseases, Tufts Medical Center, Associate Professor of Medicine, Tufts
University School of Medicine, Boston, Massachusetts, USA

EDITORS

ROBIN L.P. JUMP, MD, PhD
Assistant Professor of Medicine, Division of Infectious Diseases and HIV Medicine,
Department of Medicine, Case Western Reserve University, Geriatric Research Education
and Clinical Center (GRECC), Specialty Care Center of Innovation, Louis Stokes Cleveland
Veterans Affairs Medical Center, Cleveland, Ohio, USA

DAVID H. CANADAY, MD
Associate Professor of Medicine, Division of Infectious Diseases and HIV Medicine,
Department of Medicine, Case Western Reserve University, Geriatric Research Education
and Clinical Center (GRECC), Louis Stokes Cleveland Veterans Affairs Medical Center,
Cleveland, Ohio, USA

AUTHORS

ADAM BAGHBAN, MD
Infectious Diseases Fellow, Section of Infectious Diseases, Department of Internal
Medicine, Yale School of Medicine, New Haven, Connecticut, USA

JOHN M. BENSON, PharmD
Director of Pharmacy, Promise Hospital of Salt Lake, Adjunct Associate Professor,
College of Pharmacy, The University of Utah, Salt Lake City, Utah, USA

ROBERT A. BONOMO, MD
Geriatric Research Education and Clinical Center (GRECC), Infectious Disease Section,
Medical Division, Research Services and Specialty Care Center of Innovation, Louis
Stokes Cleveland VA Medical Center, Division of Infectious Diseases and HIV Medicine,
Department of Medicine and Departments of Pathology, Pharmacology, Molecular
Biology and Microbiology, and Biochemistry, Case Western Reserve University School of
Medicine, Cleveland, Ohio, USA

WESTYN BRANCH-ELLIMAN, MD, MMSc
Medical Service, Section of Infectious Diseases, VA Boston Healthcare System,
Harvard Medical School, Boston, Massachusetts, USA

DAVID H. CANADAY, MD
Associate Professor of Medicine, Division of Infectious Diseases and HIV Medicine, Department of Medicine, Case Western Reserve University, Geriatric Research Education and Clinical Center (GRECC), Louis Stokes Cleveland Veterans Affairs Medical Center, Cleveland, Ohio, USA

CRISTINA V. CARDEMIL, MD, MPH
Viral Gastroenteritis Branch (proposed), Division of Viral Diseases, Centers for Disease Control and Prevention, Atlanta, Georgia, USA

NICOLAS W. CORTES-PENFIELD, MD
Clinical Fellow, Section of Infectious Diseases, Department of Medicine, Baylor College of Medicine, Houston, Texas, USA

CHRISTOPHER J. CRNICH, MD, PhD
University of Wisconsin-Madison School of Medicine and Public Health, University of Wisconsin Hospital and Clinics, William S. Middleton Veterans Affairs Hospital, Madison, Wisconsin, USA

CURTIS J. DONSKEY, MD
Geriatric Research Education and Clinical Center (GRECC), Louis Stokes Cleveland VA Medical Center, Professor, Department of Medicine, Case Western Reserve University School of Medicine, Cleveland, Ohio, USA

NADIM G. EL CHAKHTOURA, MD, MPH
Geriatric Research Education and Clinical Center (GRECC), Louis Stokes Cleveland VA Medical Center, Division of Infectious Diseases and HIV Medicine, Department of Medicine, Case Western Reserve University, Cleveland, Ohio, USA

ARON J. HALL, DVM, MSPH
Viral Gastroenteritis Branch (proposed), Division of Viral Diseases, Centers for Disease Control and Prevention, Atlanta, Georgia, USA

ORYAN HENIG, MD
Division of Infectious Diseases, Department of Medicine, University of Michigan, Ann Arbor, Michigan, USA

AMRITA R. JOHN, MBBS
Division of Infectious Diseases and HIV Medicine, Department of Medicine, Case Western Reserve University, Cleveland, Ohio, USA

ROBIN L.P. JUMP, MD, PhD
Assistant Professor of Medicine, Division of Infectious Diseases and HIV Medicine, Department of Medicine, Case Western Reserve University, Geriatric Research Education and Clinical Center (GRECC), Specialty Care Center of Innovation, Louis Stokes Cleveland Veterans Affairs Medical Center, Cleveland, Ohio, USA

MANISHA JUTHANI-MEHTA, MD
Associate Professor, Section of Infectious Diseases, Department of Internal Medicine, Yale School of Medicine, New Haven, Connecticut, USA

ROBERT C. KALAYJIAN, MD
Associate Professor, Division of Infectious Diseases, Department of Medicine, Case Western Reserve University School of Medicine, Geriatric Research, Education, and Clinical Center (GRECC), Louis Stokes Cleveland VA Medical Center, The MetroHealth System, Cleveland, Ohio, USA

KEITH S. KAYE, MD, MPH
Professor of Internal Medicine, Director of Clinical Research, Division of Infectious Diseases, Department of Medicine, University of Michigan, Ann Arbor, Michigan, USA

FUMIHIRO KODAMA, MD
Department of Infectious Diseases, Sapporo City General Hospital, Sapporo, Hokkaido, Japan

MIRANDA MCELLIGOTT, RN, MS
University of Wisconsin-Madison School of Medicine and Public Health, Madison, Wisconsin, USA

JUNE M. MCKOY, MD, MPH, JD, MBA
Associate Professor, Department of Medicine and Preventive Medicine, Program Director, Geriatric Medicine Fellowship, Director of Geriatric Oncology, Northwestern University Feinberg School of Medicine, Chicago, Illinois, USA

DAVID A. NACE, MD, MPH
Division of Geriatric Medicine, Department of Medicine, University of Pittsburgh, Pittsburgh, Pennsylvania, USA

RAJESHWARI NAIR, PhD, MBBS
Postdoctoral Research Scholar, Department of Internal Medicine, University of Iowa Carver College of Medicine, Comprehensive Access & Delivery Research & Evaluation (CADRE), Iowa City VA Health Care System, Iowa City, Iowa, USA

UMESH D. PARASHAR, MBBS, MPH
Viral Gastroenteritis Branch (proposed), Division of Viral Diseases, Centers for Disease Control and Prevention, Atlanta, Georgia, USA

AURORA POP-VICAS, MD
University of Wisconsin-Madison School of Medicine and Public Health, Madison, Wisconsin, USA

JENNIFER C. PRICE, MD, PhD
Assistant Professor, Department of Medicine, University of California San Francisco, San Francisco, California, USA

MICHAEL REID, MD, MPH
Post-Doctoral Fellow, Department of Medicine, University of California San Francisco, San Francisco, California, USA

THERESA A. ROWE, DO, MS
Assistant Professor, Department of Medicine, General Internal Medicine and Geriatrics, Northwestern University Feinberg School of Medicine, Chicago, Illinois, USA

GREGORY SCHRANK, MD
Department of Medicine, Division of Infectious Diseases, Beth Israel Deaconess Medical Center, Harvard Medical School, Boston, Massachusetts, USA

MARIN L. SCHWEIZER, PhD
Assistant Professor, Department of Internal Medicine, University of Iowa Carver College of Medicine, Comprehensive Access & Delivery Research & Evaluation (CADRE), Iowa City VA Health Care System, Iowa City, Iowa, USA

NAMRATA SINGH, MD, MSCI
Clinical Assistant Professor, Department of Internal Medicine, University of Iowa Carver College of Medicine, Comprehensive Access & Delivery Research & Evaluation (CADRE), Iowa City VA Health Care System, Iowa City, Iowa, USA

H. KEIPP TALBOT, MD, MPH, FIDSA
Associate Professor, Departments of Medicine and Health Policy, Vanderbilt University Medical Center, Nashville, Tennessee, USA

LYNDSAY TAYLOR, MD
University of Wisconsin Hospitals and Clinics, Madison, Wisconsin, USA

PHYLLIS C. TIEN, MD, MSc
Professor, Department of Medicine, University of California San Francisco, Medical Service, Department of Veteran Affairs Medical Center, San Francisco, California, USA

BARBARA W. TRAUTNER, MD, PhD
Associate Professor, Section of Infectious Diseases, Department of Medicine, Baylor College of Medicine, Center for Innovations in Quality, Effectiveness, and Safety, Michael E. DeBakey VA Medical Center, Houston, Texas, USA

PUJA VAN EPPS, MD
Assistant Professor, Division of Infectious Diseases, Department of Medicine, Case Western Reserve University School of Medicine, Geriatric Research, Education, and Clinical Center (GRECC), Louis Stokes Cleveland VA Medical Center, Cleveland, Ohio, USA

GRACE WELHAM, PharmD, PhD
University of Wisconsin-Madison School of Medicine and Public Health, Madison, Wisconsin, USA

Contents

In older adults, pathophysiologic, clinical, and environmental factors all affect the presentation of infections. We explore how age-related changes influence the manifestation and evaluation of infections in this population. Specific topics include immunosenescence, age-related organ-specific physiologic changes, and frailty. We also describe clinical factors influencing infection risk and presentation in older adults, including temperature regulation, cognitive decline, and malnutrition. Finally, we discuss the influence of the setting in which older adults reside on the clinical evaluation of infection. Understanding the influence of all these changes may facilitate the prevention, early recognition, and treatment of infections in older adults.

Antimicrobial use in older adults requires working knowledge of the pharmacokinetics and pharmacodynamics of these drugs, and the alterations known to occur with these models as patients age. A summary of pharmacokinetic principles relevant to antimicrobials and an overview of published medical literature describing pharmacokinetic changes known to correlate with age are presented. Pharmacodynamic models that apply to antibacterial agents are reviewed, as are likely effects of aging on these models. The understanding of how older adults respond in terms of efficacy and toxicity is increasing but limited. Further research into the effects of aging on the actions of antimicrobials in the elderly is needed.

Misuse and overuse of antibiotic therapy is a frequent cause of resident harm in nursing facilities. As a result, newly released policy and regulatory initiatives will require antibiotic stewardship programs (ASPs) in nursing facilities. Although implementing ASPs can be challenging, improving the quality of antibiotic prescribing is achievable in this setting. The authors review the determinants of antibiotic prescribing in nursing facilities, strategies to improve antibiotic prescribing in this setting, current status of ASPs in nursing facilities, and steps that facilities can take to enhance existing ASP structure and process.

At least one-third of patients at the end of life (EOL) receive interventions that are without benefit, and a similar proportion of patients die in the intensive care unit. Here, the authors discuss the role of antimicrobials in patients at the EOL, including the patient populations and scenarios in which antimicrobials may or may not have benefit. They also review adverse outcomes associated with antimicrobial use at the EOL, including societal harms. Finally, an algorithm to aid management of suspected infections at the EOL is proposed.

Device-related infections (DRIs) are a significant cause of morbidity and mortality among older adults. Indwelling devices (urinary catheters, percutaneous feeding tubes, and central venous catheters) are frequently used in this vulnerable population. Indwelling devices provide a portal of entry for pathogenic organisms to invade a susceptible host and cause infection and are an important target for infection prevention and antimicrobial stewardship efforts. Within the "Chain of Infection" that leads to DRIs in older adults, multiple opportunities exist to implement interventions that "break the links" and reduce colonization with multidrug-resistant organisms, reduce infections, and improve antimicrobial use.

Urinary tract infections (UTIs) are a significant cause of morbidity among older adults. However, antibiotic prescriptions for clinically suspected UTIs are often inappropriate. Health care providers frequently struggle to differentiate UTI from asymptomatic bacteriuria, particularly in patients presenting with nonspecific symptoms. Patients with baseline cognitive impairments that limit history-taking can be particularly challenging. This article reviews the epidemiology and pathogenesis of UTI in older adults. It discusses an approach to diagnosis and treatment focused on recognizing patients who would likely benefit from antibiotic treatment and on identifying patients for whom empiric antibiotic therapy should not be given.

The incidence of pneumonia increases with age, and is particularly high in patients who reside in long-term care facilities (LTCFs). Mortality rates for pneumonia in older adults are high and have not decreased in the past decade. Atypical symptoms and exacerbation of underlying illnesses should trigger clinical suspicion of pneumonia. Risk factors for multidrug-resistant organisms are more common in older adults, particularly among LTCF residents, and should be considered when making empiric treatment decisions. Monitoring of clinical stability and underlying comorbid conditions, potential drug–drug interactions, and drug-related adverse events are important factors in managing elderly patients with pneumonia.

Rajeshwari Nair, Marin L. Schweizer, and Namrata Singh

Older adults are at increased risk for septic arthritis and prosthetic joint infections (PJIs), owing at least in part to comorbid conditions and frailty. An increasing number of older adults undergo total joint arthroplasty to improve their quality of life. Infections in older adults differ from younger populations by the causative organisms, a great proportion of which are *staphylococcal* infections. Targeting important modifiable and nonmodifiable risk factors may prevent or reduce the burden of joint infections in older adults. This article summarizes the epidemiology, pathogenesis, clinical manifestations, diagnosis, management, and prevention of septic arthritis and PJIs in older adults.

Theresa A. Rowe and June M. McKoy

Sepsis disproportionally affects older adults, with more than 60% of sepsis diagnoses attributed to adults aged 65 years and older. Identifying, diagnosing, and treating sepsis in older individuals remain a challenge for clinicians, and few studies focus specifically on older adults with multiple medical comorbidities. Principles guiding management of sepsis for older adults are generally the same as in younger adults; however, unique considerations particularly pertinent to the care of older adults include antimicrobial selection and dosing, delirium management, and goals of care discussions. Other factors, such as medical comorbidities, cognitive impairment, and functional status, impact outcomes more than age alone.

Curtis J. Donskey

Recent increases in the incidence of *Clostridium difficile* infection (CDI) have been observed in all age groups, but the elderly have been disproportionately affected and long-term care facilities (LTCFs) have borne a significant proportion of the increasing burden. Recurrences are common in older adults and may have significant adverse effects on quality of life. Ensuring appropriate diagnostic testing and management is challenging for older adults in the community and in LTCFs. This article focuses on current concepts related to the epidemiology, diagnosis, and management of CDI in older adults.

H. Keipp Talbot

Annually, influenza viruses cause significant disease in older adults, varying with the virulence of the circulating strain, prior exposure to circulating strain, and influenza vaccine effectiveness. Older adults often present atypically (eg, without fever) and with complications of influenza infection, such as chronic obstructive pulmonary disease and congestive heart failure exacerbations. Prevention methods include antiviral medications and vaccines. Current influenza vaccines have moderate effectiveness for the prevention of hospitalization, but newer more immunogenic vaccines designed for adults 65 and older have been licensed.

Respiratory viral infections may cause serious complications for older adults, including residents of long-term care facilities (LTCFs). Although influenza is the most common cause of viral respiratory infections among older adults, several other respiratory viruses also cause significant morbidity and mortality, most notably respiratory syncytial virus. Other noninfluenza respiratory viral pathogens include human metapneumovirus, parainfluenza virus, rhinovirus, coronavirus, and adenovirus. All of these may cause outbreaks among LTCF residents. Recently developed rapid diagnostic molecular tests may clarify the epidemiology of these viruses and have potential, through early identification, to limit the severity of outbreaks among older adults living in LTCFs.

Persons living with human immunodeficiency virus (HIV) infection (PLWH) have accentuated risks for age-associated comorbidities. Compared with the general population, PLWH have a twofold higher risk of cardiovascular disease, a threefold increased risk of fracture, and a risk of kidney disease that is comparable to that in diabetes. Some comorbidities may present at younger ages than among the general population, suggesting the possibility of accelerated aging with HIV infection.

Herpes zoster (HZ) is the result of reactivation of latent varicella zoster virus and occurs most frequently in older adults. Classically, HZ presents as a unilateral, self-limited, dermatomal rash. Postherpetic neuralgia (PHN) is a common sequela, presenting as severe pain that persists after the rash has resolved. In the elderly, PHN can be debilitating and requires a prompt diagnosis, treatment with antivirals, and adequate pain control. A longer-term pain management strategy is required if PHN occurs. A modestly effective vaccine exists and is recommended for older individuals.

Hepatitis C virus (HCV) is the most common blood-borne infection in the United States and is of concern in older adults. HCV infection is associated with not only hepatic but also extrahepatic comorbidities common to the aging patient, including diabetes, kidney and cardiovascular diseases, and neurocognitive impairment. The effect of direct-acting antiviral agents to treat HCV on these outcomes is limited. This article summarizes the literature regarding the epidemiology and natural history of HCV infection; the impact of age on clinical outcomes in HCV-infected persons; and current knowledge regarding safety and efficacy of HCV treatment regimens in the older patient.

Norovirus is the leading cause of acute gastroenteritis. In older adults, it is responsible for an estimated 3.7 million illnesses, 320,000 outpatient visits, 69,000 emergency department visits, 39,000 hospitalizations, and 960 deaths annually in the United States. Older adults are particularly at risk for severe outcomes, including prolonged symptoms and death. Long-term care facilities and hospitals are the most common settings for norovirus outbreaks in developed countries. Diagnostic platforms are expanding. Several norovirus vaccines in clinical trials have the potential to reap benefits. This article summarizes current knowledge on norovirus infection in older adults.

INFECTIOUS DISEASE CLINICS OF NORTH AMERICA

RELATED INTEREST

Medical Clinics of North America, March 2015 (Vol. 99, Issue 2)
Geriatric Medicine
Susan E. Merel and Jeffrey Wallace, *Editors*

THE CLINICS ARE AVAILABLE ONLINE!
Access your subscription at:
www.theclinics.com

Preface

Aging Has Unique Effects on the Risks, Presentation, Diagnosis, Treatment, and Prognosis of Infectious Diseases

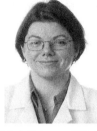 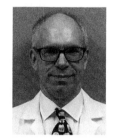

Robin L.P. Jump, MD, PhD   David H. Canaday, MD
Editors

By the year 2040, 1 out of every 5 Americans will be over the age of 65, with greater proportions of them living into their 80s than ever before.[1] According to the US Congressional Budget Office, the outlay by Medicare is overwhelmingly for care of citizens age 65 and older. These currently account for 3.7% (710 billion USD) of the US Gross Domestic Product, with an estimated rise to 7.0% (4.3 trillion USD) in the next 30 years.[2] From a purely economic perspective, the incentive to provide optimal and appropriate medical care in this older population is enormous.

With aging comes increased risk of infection. This is in part due to aging of the immune system, termed immunosenescence, and, in part to the short- and long-lasting effects of other medical illnesses. Of the top 10 leading causes of death in older adults, 2 (influenza and pneumonia, and septicemia) are directly related to infection. Furthermore, infections likely play an important role in several of the other leading causes of death, including chronic low respiratory disease, Alzheimer disease, diabetes, and potentially even myocardial infarction and cerebrovascular deaths due to the infection-induced prothrombotic state.[3]

Geriatrics emerged as a unique discipline in the 1940s, expanding from Britain to the United States, with the first certifying examination in geriatric medicine in the United States finally offered in 1988.[4] The medical field was slow to recognize the unique and important role of medical providers specializing in older adults, relegating

Infect Dis Clin N Am 31 (2017) xiii–xv
http://dx.doi.org/10.1016/j.idc.2017.08.001
0891-5520/17/© 2017 Published by Elsevier Inc.

geriatricians to primary care or nursing homes. As our population ages, however, their medical and concomitant social, psychological, and rehabilitation needs become increasing complex. Involving clinicians with geriatrics training, even when the problem seems straightforward and the acuity is low, can improve the quality and safety of the care provided to older adults.[5]

To that end, this issue of *Infections Disease Clinics of North America* seeks to bring a geriatric perspective to the diagnosis and treatment of infections in older adults. In general, treating infections in people greater than 65 years of age follows the same general principles as it does in all age groups, namely, source control and pathogen-directed therapy. Other important considerations, however, influence the recognition and response to infections in this population. While never asymptomatic, older adults manifest presenting signs and symptoms differently from younger adults. In addition, goals of therapy must consider not only effective treatment but also preventing loss of function, avoidance of adverse drug events, minimizing the risk of acquiring drug-resistant pathogens, and fending off other unintended consquences of antibiotic exposure, namely *Clostridium difficile* infection. Finally, sometimes attempting to diagnose and respond to concerns for infection may cause discomfort for older adults. Active monitoring or, in select cases, permitting an infection to be an end-of-life event, may constitute good medical care.

Our hope is that the content in this issue will inspire further work in this understudied yet ever-more important area. We offer our sinere thanks to the authors for their dedication to improving the care of older adults with infections.

Robin L.P. Jump, MD, PhD
Division of Infectious Diseases and HIV Medicine
Department of Medicine
Case Western Reserve University
Geriatric Research Education and Clinical Center (GRECC)
Specialty Care Center of Innovation
Louis Stokes Cleveland Veterans Affairs Medical Center
10701 East Boulevard
Cleveland, OH 44106, USA

David H. Canaday, MD
Division of Infectious Diseases and HIV Medicine
Department of Medicine
Case Western Reserve University
Geriatric Research Education and Clinical Center (GRECC)
Louis Stokes Cleveland Veterans Affairs Medical Center
10701 East Boulevard
Cleveland, OH 44106, USA

E-mail addresses:
robin.jump@va.gov (R.L.P. Jump)
David.Canaday@case.edu (D.H. Canaday)

REFERENCES

1. Aging Statistics. Available at: http://www.aoa.acl.gov/Aging_Statistics/index.aspx. Accessed August 8, 2016.

2. Congressional Budget Office. The 2017 long-term budget outlook. 2017. Available at: https://www.cbo.gov/publication/52480. Accessed June 6, 2017.

3. Xu J, Murphy SL, Kochanek KD, et al. Deaths: final data for 2013. Natl Vital Stat Rep 2016;64:1–119.
4. Morley JE. A brief history of geriatrics. J Gerontol A Biol Sci Med Sci 2004;59: 1132–52.
5. Deschodt M, Flamaing J, Haentjens P, et al. Impact of geriatric consultation teams on clinical outcome in acute hospitals: a systematic review and meta-analysis. BMC Med 2013;11:48.

Influence of Aging and Environment on Presentation of Infection in Older Adults

Nadim G. El Chakhtoura, MD, MPH[a,b], Robert A. Bonomo, MD[a,b,c,d,e,f,g,h], Robin L.P. Jump, MD, PhD[a,b,c,d,*]

KEYWORDS

- Older adults • Immunosenescence • Frailty • Thermoregulation • Malnutrition

KEY POINTS

- Age-related physiologic changes affect several organ systems and contribute to increased vulnerability to infections.
- With aging comes immunosenescence, affecting both the adaptive and innate immune systems, and contributing to an increased risk of infection.
- Older adults experience a reduced febrile response caused by altered thermoregulation and a decrease in mean body temperature.
- Addressing malnutrition and dehydration among older adults may reduce their risk of infection.
- Knowledge of debilitated older adults' functional and cognitive baseline may support early recognition of infection and discernment of conditions not related to infection.

Disclosure: See at the last page.
[a] Geriatric Research Education and Clinical Center (GRECC), Louis Stokes Cleveland Department of Veterans Affairs Medical Center (LSCVAMC), 10701 East Boulevard, Cleveland, OH 44106, USA; [b] Division of Infectious Diseases and HIV Medicine, Department of Medicine, Case Western Reserve University, 11100 Euclid Avenue, Cleveland, OH 44195-5029, USA; [c] Specialty Care Center of Innovation, LSCVAMC, 10701 East Boulevard, Cleveland, OH 44106, USA; [d] Research Services, LSCVAMC, 10701 East Boulevard, Cleveland, OH 44106, USA; [e] Department of Pathology, Case Western Reserve University School of Medicine, 11100 Euclid Avenue, Cleveland, OH 44195-5029, USA; [f] Department of Pharmacology, Case Western Reserve University School of Medicine, 11100 Euclid Avenue, Cleveland, OH 44195-5029, USA; [g] Department of Molecular Biology and Microbiology, Case Western Reserve University School of Medicine, 11100 Euclid Avenue, Cleveland, OH 44195-5029, USA; [h] Department of Biochemistry, Case Western Reserve University School of Medicine, 11100 Euclid Avenue, Cleveland, OH 44195-5029, USA
* Corresponding author. GRECC 111C(W), Louis Stokes Cleveland VA Medical Center, 10701 East Boulevard, Cleveland, OH 44106.
E-mail address: robinjump@gmail.com

Infect Dis Clin N Am 31 (2017) 593–608
http://dx.doi.org/10.1016/j.idc.2017.07.017
0891-5520/17/Published by Elsevier Inc.

INTRODUCTION

The topic of human longevity has invited extensive scientific and philosophic debate. Haller, a prominent Swiss physiologist of the 18th century, thought that people ought to live to 200 years. Buffon, an 18th century French naturalist, was of the opinion that when someone did not die from some accident or disease they would reach 90 or 100 years.[1] Nobel laureate Élie Metchnikoff, arguably the father of modern immunology and gerontology, found it "impossible to accept the view that the high mortality between the ages of 70 and 75 indicates a natural limit of human life." In his 1907 book, *The Prolongation of Life*, he equated aging with a disease process that can be studied and possibly cured until death inevitably settles in from "natural causes." He suggested that, similar to the instinct of sleep, there could be an instinct of death that is neither due to diseases nor accidents, but rather the result of age-related physiologic changes. He thought these changes were the result of self-digesting macrophages and poisoning by intestinal microbiota.[1] Although this theory has been disproved, his contributions to immunology and gerontology were groundbreaking and continue to shape our understanding of infectious processes in older adults.

A testament to the contributions by these pioneers in the field of gerontology, people are living longer such that the number of older adults is rapidly increasing, both in the United States and globally. In 2015, approximately 617 million people were 65 years or older, representing 8.5% of the 7.3 billion people worldwide.[2] Projections estimate that by 2050, approximately 1.6 billion people will be 65 years or older, with the proportion nearly doubling to 16.6% of the total world population. In the United States, the proportion of people projected to be 65 years or older by 2050 will constitute more than 20% of our total population.[2] Bartels and Naslund[3] famously described this demographic trend as the "silver tsunami." Understanding the process of aging and how it influences the clinical presentation of diseases in general, and infectious diseases in particular, is a necessity for modern practitioners.

Aging changes the risk of and the clinical presentation of infection. This is due to factors intrinsic to individuals fortunate enough to age and to the environment in which they reside. Intrinsic factors include age-related physiologic changes, which can sometimes result in frailty, a pathologic state. Some age-related changes also influence the clinical manifestation of infection, presenting as alterations in temperature regulation, cognitive decline, and malnutrition.[4] Environmental factors also play a role, particularly those related to the living situation (eg, nursing home), and the health care setting to which older adults present. In combination, these factors make it difficult for health care workers to determine whether changes in clinical status are due to infection. This may contribute to a low threshold for prescribing systemic antimicrobials, which in turn increases older adults' risk for acquiring multidrug-resistant organisms (MDRO) and *Clostridium difficile*.

Herein we review the age-related physiologic changes that may progress to frailty; these include both immune and organ-specific changes. We also address clinical factors that influence the manifestation of infections in older adults. Finally, we consider the influence of the external environment on the presentation and evaluation of infections in older adults, with consideration of the subjective roles and perspectives of caregivers within different settings.

PATHOPHYSIOLOGIC FACTORS INFLUENCING INFECTION RISK AND PRESENTATION IN OLDER ADULTS

With aging, physiologic changes occur that affect the immune system as well as various organ systems. Aging itself is not a disease, yet as time passes, the accumulation of such changes can sometimes lead to a clinical condition in older adults known as frailty. In this section, we discuss these changes and introduce the concept of frailty.

Age-related Immune Changes

Gavazzi and Krause[5] describe immunosenescence as "an age-related dysfunction of the immune system which leads to enhanced risk of infection." This phenomenon is an area of active research and encompasses a large body of evidence. Globally, the total number of immune cells does not decrease with aging, but studies demonstrate a functional decline in both innate immunity and adaptive immunity that encompasses cell mediated and humoral immunity.

Changes in innate immunity include reduced phagocytic activity of neutrophils, macrophages, and natural killer cells.[5–7] This is accompanied by upregulation of a number of proinflammatory cytokines, including interleukin (IL)-6, C-reactive protein, tumor-necrosis factor-α, and CXC chemokine ligand-10.[6,8–10] This increase in cytokine and chemokine production results in a heightened chronic proinflammatory state in older adults that may contribute to the development of infection and other diseases (eg, atherosclerosis, arthritis, diabetes mellitus).[11,12] Franceschi and Campisi[13] referred to this chronic proinflammatory state as "inflammaging," which can result in anorexia, nutritional compromise, muscle weakness, and weight loss, all of which could be presentations of infection in older adults, but also represent characteristics of frailty, as discussed elsewhere in this article.[5,6] As such, the distinction between the clinical condition of frailty and presentation of infection becomes challenging, particularly for health care workers who encounter an individual patient for the first time in an acute care setting. Knowledge of older adults' clinical baseline is, therefore, of great benefit when evaluating a suspected infectious process in this population.

One of the changes in cell-mediated immunity is the decline in the proportion of naïve T cells with aging. This occurs as a consequence of thymus involution and an increase in the proportion of circulating memory T cells in the setting of continued antigenic stimulation. This increase in the number of memory T cells is offset by their restricted clonal diversity (**Fig. 1**).[12,14–16] These changes in turn limit the antibody response to foreign antigens due to reduced regulatory control of T cells on B cells. Interestingly, Van Epps and colleagues[17] recently demonstrated in vitro that although naïve T cells are reduced in number in older adults, they had enhanced functional ability, mainly the CD8[+] T cells. The clinical relevance of these findings is unclear at this time, but this increased functionality may also contribute, along with cytokine upregulation, to "inflammaging." Some chronic infections also contribute to generalized chronic inflammation and through accumulation of damage to host cells, hasten the aging process.[5] The best investigated example is human immunodeficiency virus (HIV), which results in accelerated aging. Gross and colleagues[18] have demonstrated that HIV-infected individuals on sustained antiretroviral therapy have an epigenetic age about 5 years older than healthy controls. Smith and colleagues[19] proposed that in addition to inflammation caused by HIV, adverse effects of antiretroviral drugs, specifically those that affect the mitochondria, also contribute to the accelerated aging of treated HIV-infected patients. Viruses other than HIV, namely cytomegalovirus and herpes simplex virus, also seem to correlate with premature immune aging.[5] Given that most individuals do not receive antiviral therapy for these viruses, the implication is that these viral infections directly contribute to this phenomenon.[5]

As a result of the changes to adaptive and innate immune responses, although the incidence of severe infections is higher in older adults, the protective effect elicited by vaccines is lower.[12] This is the case for influenza,[20,21] hepatitis B,[22] and

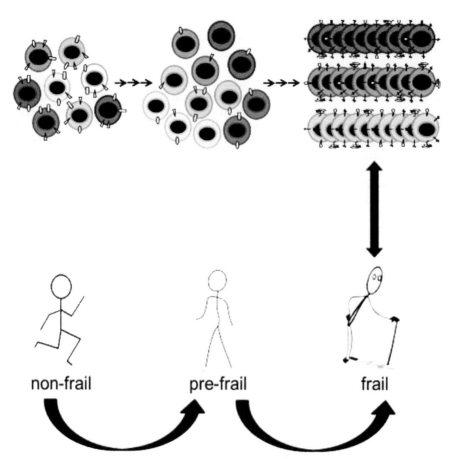

Fig. 1. Antigen-specific clonal expansion of T cells in older adults leads to an increased proportion of replicative senescent cell populations, filling the immunologic space and resulting in decreased repertoire diversity.

pneumococcal vaccines,[23] supporting the idea that vaccination in older adults is associated with modest clinical effectiveness.

Finally, it is important to appreciate that immunosenescence and chronic inflammation are gradual, relentless processes. Their clinical impact may not be fully apparent until progression to frailty. Coupled with other factors, such as comorbidities and declining functional status, frailty results in increased morbidity and mortality, including from infection.

Age-related Organ-specific Physiologic Changes

In addition to immunosenescence, aging also causes physiologic changes that affect nearly every organ system, independent of existing comorbidities and disease. This process is the result of a lifelong accumulation of molecular and cellular damage caused by a number of mechanisms regulated by a complex maintenance and repair network.[6,24] Described in **Table 1**, these changes include structural transformations, altered anatomy, and decreased function in multiple physiologic systems, as well as loss of feedforward and feedback mechanisms between interacting systems.[11,25]

Table 1
Age-related organ-specific physiologic changes that increase the risk of infection and affect the clinical presentation of infectious syndromes

Organ System	Physiologic Changes
Urinary	Mechanical changes: reduction in bladder capacity, uninhibited contractions, decreased urinary flow rate and postvoid residual volume Urothelial change: enhanced bacterial adherence Bladder prolapse in women and prostatic disease in men increase urinary stasis Diminished estrogen in postmenopausal women
Pulmonary	Blunting of cough and other reflexes that protect the airway Decreased mucociliary clearance, lung elasticity, chest compliance, and respiratory muscle strength Decreased immunoglobulin in respiratory secretion
Skin and soft tissue	Loss of subcutaneous tissue Loss of collagen from the dermis and slower wound healing Reduction in the size of blood vessels in the dermis impairs delivery of immune cells Dry skin resulting from diminished water-binding capacity of the stratum corneum Flattened dermal–epidermal junctions and reduced dermal–epidermal adhesion
Gastrointestinal	Decreased saliva production and alterations in antimicrobial proteins in the saliva Decreased tongue strength and slower swallowing Decreased gastric acidity (mucosal gastric atrophy, proton pump inhibitors, surgery) Decreased intestinal motility Modifications of resident intestinal flora (protective Bifidobacteria and anaerobes decrease, *Enterobacteriaceae* increase) Slow recovery of the gut microbiome following antimicrobial use in older adults
CNS	Structural and functional changes to microglial cells (resident immune cell population of the CNS and CNS equivalents of macrophages)
Endocrine system	Gradual increase in cortisol release with age and increased catabolism with resultant anorexia, weight loss, reduced energy expenditure, and decreased muscle mass (all components of frailty)
Musculoskeletal system	Sarcopenia (loss of skeletal muscle mass, often catabolism induced, after acute disease events) leads to decreased strength and functionality

Abbreviation: CNS, central nervous system.
Data from Refs.[5,6,29,34,64,78]

The resulting constellation of physiologic changes results in progressive homeostatic dysregulation and may contribute to vulnerability to infections.[6,25]

An example is the increased risk of pneumonia in older adults. The strength of respiratory muscles, compliance of the chest wall, and static elastic recoil all progressively decrease with aging, making the lungs less resistant to environmental insults, such as infectious agents and pollutants.[26,27] Older adults are also at an increased risk of aspiration pneumonia. Aging is associated with a higher incidence of dysphagia, which can lead to aspiration as a result of misdirection of oropharyngeal secretions with a high bacterial load or gastric material into the lower respiratory tract.[11] Decreased respiratory muscle strength and cough reflexes increase the risk of aspiration.

Skin and skin structure infections offer a second example of organ-specific changes contributing to an increase risk of infection. By age 70, about 70% of people have at least 1 underlying skin problem, such as keratoses, dermatitides, or pressure sores. Physiologic changes that occur with age contribute to skin fragility. Reduction in the size of blood vessels in the dermis impairs delivery of immune cells, and loss of collagen from the dermis results in thinner skin. Beyond these physiologic changes, older adults may also have pathologic conditions such as edema or trauma that further impair the integrity of the skin. All of these changes place older adults at a higher risk for skin and skin structure infections.[28]

In summary, consideration of how age-related, organ-specific physiologic changes may alter the clinical presentation of infections may not only improve early recognition of infection in older adults, but may also help to discriminate conditions and changes not related to infection.[11,29]

Frailty

Frailty affects 13% to 28% of older adults and up to one-third of those 80 years and older.[30,31] Fried and colleagues[32] defined a frequently adopted phenotypic definition of frailty as the presence of 3 or more of the following readily identifiable characteristics: unintended weight loss, exhaustion, weakness, slow gait speed, and low physical activity.[29] Other clinical features include falls, delirium, and fluctuating disability, all of which may overlap with presentation of infections in the older adults. Although several definitions of frailty exist, the criteria proposed by Fried and colleagues,[32] which are based on phenotypic features, are the most feasible to assess clinically. That said, frailty extends beyond an apparent physical phenotype to include functional and cognitive statuses of the individual, as well as the setting in which they evolve or present. Additionally, continuous low-intensity inflammatory processes, detectable by moderately elevated levels of inflammatory cytokines, may also contribute to frailty.[10,11,30]

Differentiation of the physiologic changes that accompany aging, the clinical entity of frailty, and the baseline clinical features of individual subjects may help to improve recognition of manifestations of infection in older adults. Notwithstanding the aging process and the resulting decline in various organ systems, these systems are resilient and do not immediately fail, owing to the gradual nature of that decline and to redundancy that provides for significant physiologic reserve.[6] This reserve is unfortunately not inexhaustible, and a threshold is eventually reached beyond which vulnerability for subsequent morbidity and mortality becomes significant, triggered even by minor stressors.[6,29] Fried and colleagues[25] showed that the likelihood of frailty increases nonlinearly in relationship to the number of abnormal physiologic systems, and that the number of abnormal systems is more predictive of frailty than any of the individual affected systems. This aggregate loss results in frailty, which in turn is associated with increased morbidity and mortality.

CLINICAL FACTORS INFLUENCING INFECTION RISK AND PRESENTATION IN OLDER ADULTS
Temperature Regulation

The evidence suggesting a lower baseline temperature and fever suppression in older adults, albeit mitigated by concerns over measurement difficulties, is unanimous in showing that mean body temperature decreases with age.[33–36] A recent analysis of cross-sectional data from more than 18,000 adults shows a difference of 0.3°F between the oldest and youngest groups after controlling for sex, body mass index, and white blood cell count.[37] This is commensurate with the adage, "the older, the colder."[38]

Fever, or at least an increase in temperature over baseline, occurs in most cases of infection in older adults.[33] In a landmark study of mostly male veteran nursing home residents, Castle and colleagues[39] showed that a single temperature reading of 101°F (38.3°C) had a sensitivity of 40% for predicting infection, compared with 70% when lowered to 100°F (37.8°C), while maintaining a specificity of 90%. Studies of specific syndromes confirm this observation and show a blunted fever response in older compared with younger adults in the contexts of bloodstream infections, endocarditis, meningitis, intraabdominal infection, nosocomial infections, and tuberculosis.[34] It is important to recognize that a robust fever of 38.3°C or higher in a geriatric patient is indicative of a serious infection and needs to be promptly addressed.[40]

The definition of fever is relative and depends in part on the population for which it is intended (**Box 1**), making its recognition challenging for caregivers.[41,42] One of the criteria offered by the Infectious Disease Society of America is an increase in temperature of greater than 2°F (1.1°C) over the baseline temperature.[4] The relative temperature change indicative of infection varies among individuals. Accordingly, knowledge of an older adult's baseline temperature, such as might be available in electronic health records, may help caregivers to ascertain if a change in temperature truly indicates a fever.

Reasons for decreased body temperature in older adults reflect thermoregulatory changes in cutaneous vasomotor and sudomotor responses. Other physiologic mechanisms responsible for temperature variations in older adults remain unclear.[33,36] Previous studies indicate that they experience alterations in the circadian temperature rhythms, with flatter and earlier phased rhythms.[43,44] In the context of infection, animal data show that quantitative and qualitative abnormalities occur in the production and response to peripheral endogenous mediators, such as IL-1, IL-6 and tumor necrosis

---

Box 1
Fever definitions by the Infectious Diseases Society of America

Fever in patients with neutropenia (one of the following):

- Oral temperature measurement of greater than 101°F (38.3°C).

- Temperature of greater than 100.4°F (38.0°C) sustained over a 1-hour period.

Fever in older adult residents of long-term care facilities (one of the following):

- Single oral temperature greater than 100°F (>37.8°C)

- Repeated oral temperatures greater than 99°F (>37.2°C) or rectal temperatures greater than 99.5°F (>37.5°C), or

- An increase in temperature of greater than 2°F (1.1°C) over the baseline temperature.

Data from High KP, Bradley SF, Gravenstein S, et al. Clinical practice guideline for the evaluation of fever and infection in older adult residents of long-term care facilities: 2008 update by the Infectious Diseases Society of America. J Am Geriatr Soc 2009;57(3):375–94; and Freifeld AG, Bow EJ, Sepkowitz KA, et al. Clinical practice guideline for the use of antimicrobial agents in neutropenic patients with cancer: 2010 Update by the Infectious Diseases Society of America. Clin Infect Dis 2011;52(4):427–31.

factor-α, induced by bacterial products, such as lipopolysaccharide.[33,45–47] Furthermore, peripheral endogenous mediators are unable to cross the blood–brain barrier to exert their effect on the central nervous system,[33,46] resulting in a blunted fever response in older adults.

Finally, some evidence suggests that lower body temperature might confer a survival advantage in humans. Analysis from the Baltimore Longitudinal Study of Aging over 25 years of follow-up showed that men with body temperatures below the median had significantly higher survival rates than those with body temperatures above the median temperature.[37,48] Nonetheless, mounting a fever in the context of infection is part of overall health defense and the absence of fever in response to a serious infection is a poor prognostic sign.[34,49,50]

Cognitive Decline

Cognitive decline in older adults encompasses a clinical spectrum ranging from mild cognitive impairment to overt dementia. Memory deficits but intact activities of daily living and preserved general cognitive function characterize mild cognitive impairment. Overt dementia is manifested by progressive deterioration in cognitive ability and in capacity for independent living.[51,52] Here we focus on overt dementia, because infections are often exceptionally difficult to ascertain in this population.

The global burden of dementia in adults 60 years of age or older is estimated at 5% to 7% in most world regions and at 6.8% in the United States.[52] In 2010, the United States had the second largest estimated number of people living with dementia (3.9 million), surpassed only by China (5.4 million). Nursing home residents with advanced dementia have significant functional impairment and may be effectively mute. In a retrospective study of 148 hospitalized older adults with pneumonia, Johnson and colleagues[53] compared nonspecific presenting symptoms, with the exception of delirium, between older (>65 years) and younger adults (<65 years). When subjects with dementia were excluded, nonspecific symptoms (eg, generalized weakness, decreased appetite, falls, and delirium) were similar in both groups. They found that the presence of dementia, not age, explained the difference in the clinical presentation of pneumonia in their cohort.

Estimating the exact contribution of dementia to the clinical presentation of infection in older adults is difficult. Misdiagnosis of infection, and frequent and inappropriate antimicrobial use are common in older adults, particularly nursing home residents, contributing to increasing antimicrobial resistance in this setting.[54,55] In a prospective cohort of 362 nursing home residents with advanced dementia, Mitchell and colleagues[55] showed that 66% of residents experienced at least 1 suspected infection over 12 months. They defined advanced dementia in this study as a nurse-measured Global Deterioration Scale score of 7 of 7 (manifested as profound memory deficits, severely curtailed verbal ability with command of <5 words, incontinence, and inability to walk). The most commonly observed infections in these residents were respiratory tract infections, followed by urinary tract and skin infections. More than 90% of skin infections met treatment criteria, compared with only 19% of urinary tract infections.[55] The authors attributed this discrepancy to the fact that objective changes support the diagnosis of skin infections, whereas subjective symptoms obtained from nursing homes residents or observed from health care workers may trigger a concern for a urinary tract infection.

Just as cognitive decline may influence presentation of infection, chronic infection and inflammation are linked with cognitive decline.[56–60] As discussed, chronic infections such as HIV contribute to the aging process through chronic inflammation. Infection causes immune activation in the form of cytokines, chemokines, adhesion molecules, and matrix metalloproteinases that in turn activate microvascular endothelial cells, facilitating vascular leukocyte adhesion and dissolving the basement membrane. Vessel leakage, microbleeds, and inflammatory progression of cerebrovascular lesions ensue, precipitating cognitive decline.[56] Support for this theory comes from the Honolulu Aging Study, which linked elevated C-reactive protein to all cause dementia.[59] A subset of the Northern Manhattan Study also suggests that the accumulation of infectious burden (measured as an index based on serum titers of antibodies against 5 common viruses and bacteria) correlates with cognitive decline.[56,60] Other clinical data suggest an association between hospitalization with pneumonia and increased risk of dementia,[57] as well as an association between *Helicobacter pylori* infection and dementia.[58]

Malnutrition

After retiring to his country estate in 44 BC, the Roman philosopher and politician Marcus Cicero wrote a short treatise on the subject of old age, *De Senectute*, which offers the earliest known account of malnutrition of aging.[61] Malnutrition affects 20% to 30% of older adults and is more prevalent in institutionalized and hospitalized individuals.[5,62,63] It is the result of the interplay of multiple factors: socioeconomic, psychological (eg, depression, stress), and biological (eg, decreased senses of smell and taste, dental problems, increased proinflammatory cytokines associated with excess catabolism, and alterations in the production of appetite-regulating peptides and hormones).[62–64] Dehydration is also a common problem in older adults, specifically during a febrile illness. Reasons include poor oral intake and impaired vasopressin responses in older adults, manifested as decreased thirst.[4] Polypharmacy may also be a factor leading to malnutrition and dehydration in older adults.

Malnutrition contributes to immune dysregulation in older adults and results in increased susceptibility to infections. It is also a significant predictor of mortality in this group.[65,66] For example, in a study of 188 nursing home residents with physical and cognitive impairment, urinary tract infection during the preceding year was independently associated with poor nutritional status.[67] Similar to the association between frailty and infection, there is a 2-way association between malnutrition and infection, as well as between dehydration and infection. In contrast with frailty, however, age-related immune and organ-specific changes that occur in older adults, malnutrition and dehydration both respond to intervention.[5] For example, Langkamp-Henken and colleagues[66] studied EXP, an experimental nutritional formula, and found that it enhanced immune function in nursing home residents older than 65 years of age, indicated by increased influenza vaccine response and lymphocyte activation, less fever, and fewer newly prescribed antimicrobials compared with those consuming a standard ready-to-drink nutritional supplement.

On the other end of the spectrum, obesity is also problematic in older adults. Along with diabetes, it is a recognized cause of accelerated aging triggered by increased inflammation resulting from macrophage infiltration of the adipose tissue, which in turn increases cytokine levels (eg, tumor necrosis factor-α and IL-6). That said, obesity in older adults is a controversial topic. Some data suggest that it correlates with an increased risk of morbidity in older adults, whereas other studies found that it may confer a protective effect in older adults.[68]

In summary, recognizing and addressing nutritional concerns may help to mitigate some complications in older adults, while recognizing that only some aspects of poor oral intake may be remediable.

THE INFLUENCE OF THE LIVING ENVIRONMENT ON INFECTION RISK AND PRESENTATION IN OLDER ADULTS

Older adults reside in a variety of settings (eg, home, nursing homes, assisted living facilities) and may also come to medical attention in a number of different settings (eg, physician's office, nursing homes, emergency departments [ED] or hospitals). Currently in the United States, approximately 1.4 million people reside in 15,600 nursing homes.[69] Despite ongoing efforts to help people "age in place,"[70] as our population ages, the need for postacute and long-term care will continue to increase.

Nursing home residents share dining, recreation and therapeutic facilities. They are also highly dependent upon health care workers for assistance with activities of daily living, namely bathing, toileting, dressing, eating, and mobility.[69] Hospitals are closely linked to nursing homes with frequent patient transfers between the 2 types of facilities and as many opportunities for the spread of MDROs and C difficile from one setting to the other. During hospitalization, older adults may acquire drug-resistant pathogens and, upon transfer to a nursing home, become a reservoir and source of transmission to others.

In addition, inappropriate antimicrobial use has been shown to be a significant problem in nursing homes, with as many as 25% to 75% of antimicrobial prescriptions in nursing homes being inappropriate.[71] The magnitude of the antimicrobial resistance problem in nursing homes is potentially substantial knowing that by 2030, 70 million US residents will be aged 65 years or older and that 3.5% are nursing home residents.[71] Fear of infection in long-term care residents with cognitive decline may promote injudicious antimicrobial use, MDRO selection, and C difficile infection. In the study by Mitchell and colleagues,[55] most nursing home residents with suspected infections received antimicrobials (72%) and the cumulative incidence of MDRO acquisition was 48%; acquisition was independently associated with exposure to antimicrobials. Other contributing factors include lack of time and reimbursement, and the fact that nursing home practitioners are often family or internal medicine physicians without specialty training in geriatrics or infectious diseases. As such, their expertise in addressing complicated infections in the absence of further support might be limited.[4,71,72] Antimicrobial stewardship programs in nursing homes, made mandatory by the Centers for Medicare and Medicaid Services starting 2017, might aid practitioners and help reduce antimicrobial misuse and the prevalence of MDROs.[73]

In an attempt to assist in the diagnosis of infection and the initiation of antimicrobials in residents of long-term care facility, the Society for Healthcare Epidemiology of America convened a consensus conference that established minimum criteria for initiating antimicrobials in this population. The conference elaborated criteria for the most common infectious syndromes in residents of long-term care facility, namely respiratory tract infections, urinary tract infections, skin and soft tissue infections, and fever where the focus of infection is unknown.[54] These criteria, commonly referred to as the Loeb minimum criteria and detailed in **Table 2**, can facilitate the diagnosis of infection in long-term care facility residents as well as in older adults with advanced dementia.

Caregivers are important in establishing a baseline description of the clinical status of long-term care residents under their care. It is therefore important, during history taking, to obtain a detailed account of baseline clinical features from caregivers, including patients' relatives and friends. This includes knowledge of residents' baseline frailty, temperature as well as their cognitive, functional, and psychological status. A good understanding of these baseline parameters will significantly aid in discerning clinical changes that might be related to infection or other new stressors. This

Table 2
Loeb minimum criteria for initiating antibiotics in residents of long-term care facilities for selected infectious syndromes

Infection/Site	Criteria	Notes
Urine tract infection in resident without catheter	Acute dysuria alone or Fever (>37.9°C [100°F] or 1.5°C [2.4°F] increase above baseline temperature) and at least one of the following: suprapubic pain, gross hematuria, costovertebral angle tenderness, or new or worsening urgency, frequency or urinary incontinence	Foul smelling or cloudy urine is not a valid indication for initiating antibiotics Asymptomatic bacteriuria should not be treated with antibiotics
Urine tract infection in resident with catheter	Presence of at least one of the following: Fever (>37.9°C [100°F] or 1.5°C [2.4°F] increase above baseline temperature) New costovertebral tenderness Rigors (shaking chills) with or without identified cause New onset of delirium	
Respiratory Infections in the febrile patients	If temperature >38.9°C [102°F]: Respiratory rate >25 breaths per minute or productive cough If temperature >37.9°C [100°F] (or a 1.5°C [2.4°F] increase above baseline temperature) but <38.9°C [102°F]: Presence of a cough and at least one of the following: (1) pulse >100; (2) delirium; (3) rigors (shaking chills); or (4) respiratory rate >25	Epidemiologic setting (eg, influenza outbreak) in interpreting clinical features is essential Fever and the sudden onset of new pleuritic chest pain are an indication for transfer to hospital for diagnostic testing to rule out a pulmonary embolus. Congestive heart failure must be considered within the differential diagnosis of residents with acute respiratory symptoms and signs
Respiratory infections in the afebrile patients	Afebrile residents with COPD New or increased cough with purulent sputum production. Afebrile residents with no COPD New cough with purulent sputum production and at least one of the following: respiratory rate >25 breaths per minute or delirium	
Skin and soft-tissue infections	New or increasing purulent drainage at a wound, skin, or soft-tissue site or At least two of the following: Fever (temperature >37.9°C [100°F] or an increase of 1.5°C [2.4°F] above baseline temperatures taken at any site) Redness Tenderness Warmth Swelling that was new or increasing at the affected site	Erythema alone is not adequate as a minimum criterion for initiating antibiotics Deeper infections, such as olecranon bursitis, may present with similar symptoms Thromboembolic disease should be considered with an erythematous or swollen leg Gout can be mistaken for cellulitis

Abbreviation: COPD, chronic obstructive pulmonary disease.

Data from Loeb M, Bentley DW, Bradley S, et al. Development of minimum criteria for the initiation of antibiotics in residents of long-term-care facilities: results of a consensus conference. Infect Control Hosp Epidemiol 2001;22(2):120–4.

contributes, in turn, to improving diagnostic accuracy, which supports reducing inappropriate and unnecessary antimicrobial use.

Although it is possible for caregivers in nursing homes to observe and understand the baseline clinical features of their residents, this is not usually possible for caregivers in other settings. Older adults account for 12% to 24% of all ED visits with pneumonia (25%), urinary tract infection (22%), and sepsis and bacteremia (18%) representing the most frequently cited infections.[74] They also visit the ED more frequently than younger adults, arrive more often by ambulance, have a higher level of medical acuity, higher rates of test use, longer durations of ED stays, higher rates of hospital admission, and more serious medical illnesses.[74] Absent detailed communication with nursing home staff or other caregivers accompanying older adults, ED personnel have no reference while evaluating geriatric patients. As a result, these patients are more likely to be misdiagnosed, and more frequently discharged with unrecognized health problems.[74,75] A common scenario is an older adult with a change in mental status who receives treatment for a urinary tract infection based on the results of a urinalysis. This may not only expose them to unnecessary antimicrobials, but also overlook more common and treatable causes for a mental status change, such as dehydration, pain, recent change in medications, or sleep deprivation.

Although several risk assessment and screening tools are available for use by ED personnel in caring for older adults, there is a need for more guidance in optimizing the evaluation of older adults in the ED setting. Comprehensive geriatric evaluation of older adults in the ED by trained specialized nurses or interdisciplinary teams is effective. Coupled with risk assessment and screening tools, it helps in detecting geriatric syndromes and other missed diagnoses, increasing community referrals, and avoiding hospital admission on the ED index visit.[74,75]

SUMMARY

We have summarized the pathophysiologic, clinical, and environmental influences on the presentation of infections in older adults. Health care professionals should understand those changes and the specific features that affect presentation of illness in older adults, especially at a time when the increasing geriatric population is referred to as the "geriatric demographic imperative"[76] or the "silver tsunami."[3] Pope John XXIII once joked that, "Men are like wine - some turn to vinegar, but the best improve with age."[77] Recognition of age-related changes as well as their treatable effects will aid in the prevention, early diagnosis, and treatment of infections and other illnesses, ultimately improving clinical outcomes in this population.

DISCLOSURE

N.G. El Chakhtoura has no conflicts of interest. AstraZeneca, grant investigator/recipient; Merck, grant investigator/recipient (R.A. Bonomo). Pfizer (ID 13162823), grant investigator/recipient; Steris, grant investigator/recipient (R.L.P. Jump).

Research reported in this publication was supported in part by the National Institute of Allergy and Infectious Diseases of the National Institutes of Health under Award Numbers R01AI100560, R01AI063517, R21AI114508, and R01AI072219 to R. A. Bonomo. This study was also supported in part by funds and/or facilities provided by the Cleveland Department of Veterans Affairs, the Geriatric Research Education and Clinical Center and the VA Office of Research and Development under Award Numbers 1I01BX001974 to R.A. Bonomo, and PPO 16-118-1 to R.L.P. Jump. The content is solely the responsibility of the authors and does not necessarily represent the official views of the U.S. Department of Veterans Affairs, the National Institutes of Health or the United States Government.

ACKNOWLEDGMENTS

The authors gratefully acknowledge Puja Van Epps for providing the figure for this article.

REFERENCES

1. Metchnikoff E, Mitchell PC. The prolongation of life; optimistic studies. London, New York: W. Heinemann; G.P. Putnam's Sons; 1907.
2. He W, Goodkind D, Kowal P. An aging world: 2015. Washington, DC: U.S. Census Bureau; 2016. Available at: https://www.census.gov/content/dam/Census/library/publications/2016/demo/p95-16-1.pdf. Accessed February 6, 2017.
3. Bartels SJ, Naslund JA. The underside of the silver tsunami–older adults and mental health care. N Engl J Med 2013;368(6):493–6.
4. High KP, Bradley SF, Gravenstein S, et al. Clinical practice guideline for the evaluation of fever and infection in older adult residents of long-term care facilities: 2008 update by the Infectious Diseases Society of America. J Am Geriatr Soc 2009;57(3):375–94.
5. Gavazzi G, Krause K-H. Ageing and infection. Lancet Infect Dis 2002;2(11): 659–66.
6. Clegg A, Young J, Iliffe S, et al. Frailty in elderly people. Lancet 2013;381(9868): 752–62.
7. Aspinall R, Del Giudice G, Effros RB, et al. Challenges for vaccination in the elderly. Immun Ageing 2007;4:9.
8. Qu T, Walston JD, Yang H, et al. Upregulated ex vivo expression of stress-responsive inflammatory pathway genes by LPS-challenged CD14(+) monocytes in frail older adults. Mech Ageing Dev 2009;130(3):161–6.
9. Qu T, Yang H, Walston JD, et al. Upregulated monocytic expression of CXC chemokine ligand 10 (CXCL-10) and its relationship with serum interleukin-6 levels in the syndrome of frailty. Cytokine 2009;46(3):319–24.
10. Collerton J, Martin-Ruiz C, Davies K, et al. Frailty and the role of inflammation, immunosenescence and cellular ageing in the very old: cross-sectional findings from the Newcastle 85+ Study. Mech Ageing Dev 2012;133(6):456–66.
11. Heppner HJ, Sieber C, Walger P, et al. Infections in the elderly. Crit Care Clin 2013;29(3):757–74.
12. Grubeck-Loebenstein B, Wick G. The aging of the immune system. Adv Immunol 2002;80:243–84.
13. Franceschi C, Campisi J. Chronic inflammation (inflammaging) and its potential contribution to age-associated diseases. J Gerontol A Biol Sci Med Sci 2014; 69(Suppl 1):S4–9.
14. Sahin E, Depinho RA. Linking functional decline of telomeres, mitochondria and stem cells during ageing. Nature 2010;464(7288):520–8.
15. Miller RA. The aging immune system: primer and prospectus. Science 1996; 273(5271):70–4.
16. Herndler-Brandstetter D, Landgraf K, Tzankov A, et al. The impact of aging on memory T cell phenotype and function in the human bone marrow. J Leukoc Biol 2012;91(2):197–205.
17. Van Epps P, Banks R, Aung H, et al. Age-related differences in polyfunctional T cell responses. Immun Ageing 2014;11:14.

18. Gross AM, Jaeger PA, Kreisberg JF, et al. Methylome-wide analysis of chronic HIV infection reveals five-year increase in biological age and epigenetic targeting of HLA. Mol Cell 2016;62(2):157–68.

19. Smith RL, de Boer R, Brul S, et al. Premature and accelerated aging: HIV or HAART? Front Genet 2012;3:328.

20. Shahid Z, Kleppinger A, Gentleman B, et al. Clinical and immunologic predictors of influenza illness among vaccinated older adults. Vaccine 2010;28(38): 6145–51.

21. Deng Y, Jing Y, Campbell AE, et al. Age-related impaired type 1 T cell responses to influenza: reduced activation ex vivo, decreased expansion in CTL culture in vitro, and blunted response to influenza vaccination in vivo in the elderly. J Immunol 2004;172(6):3437–46.

22. Rosenberg C, Bovin NV, Bram LV, et al. Age is an important determinant in humoral and T cell responses to immunization with hepatitis B surface antigen. Hum Vaccin Immunother 2013;9(7):1466–76.

23. Ridda I, Macintyre CR, Lindley R, et al. Immunological responses to pneumococcal vaccine in frail older people. Vaccine 2009;27(10):1628–36.

24. Kirkwood TB. Understanding the odd science of aging. Cell 2005;120(4):437–47.

25. Fried LP, Xue QL, Cappola AR, et al. Nonlinear multisystem physiological dysregulation associated with frailty in older women: implications for etiology and treatment. J Gerontol A Biol Sci Med Sci 2009;64(10):1049–57.

26. Angulo J, El Assar M, Rodriguez-Manas L. Frailty and sarcopenia as the basis for the phenotypic manifestation of chronic diseases in older adults. Mol Aspects Med 2016;50:1–32.

27. Janssens J-P, Krause K-H. Pneumonia in the very old. Lancet Infect Dis 2004; 4(2):112–24.

28. Anderson DJ, Kaye KS. Skin and soft tissue infections in older adults. Clin Geriatr Med 2007;23(3):595–613, vii.

29. Cruz-Jentoft AJ, Baeyens JP, Bauer JM, et al. Sarcopenia: European consensus on definition and diagnosis: report of the European Working Group on Sarcopenia in Older People. Age Ageing 2010;39(4):412–23.

30. Yao X, Li H, Leng SX. Inflammation and immune system alterations in frailty. Clin Geriatr Med 2011;27(1):79–87.

31. Theou O, Cann L, Blodgett J, et al. Modifications to the frailty phenotype criteria: systematic review of the current literature and investigation of 262 frailty phenotypes in the Survey of Health, Ageing, and Retirement in Europe. Ageing Res Rev 2015;21:78–94.

32. Fried LP, Tangen CM, Walston J, et al. Frailty in older adults: evidence for a phenotype. J Gerontol A Biol Sci Med Sci 2001;56(3):M146–56.

33. Norman DC. Fever in the elderly. Clin Infect Dis 2000;31(1):148–51.

34. Yoshikawa T, Norman D. Infectious disease in the aging: a clinical handbook. Springer Science & Business Media; 2009.

35. Kenney WL, Munce TA. Invited review: aging and human temperature regulation. J Appl Physiol (1985) 2003;95(6):2598–603.

36. Blatteis CM. Age-dependent changes in temperature regulation - a mini review. Gerontology 2012;58(4):289–95.

37. Waalen J, Buxbaum JN. Is older colder or colder older? The association of age with body temperature in 18,630 individuals. J Gerontol A Biol Sci Med Sci 2011;66(5):487–92.

38. Castle SC, Norman DC, Yeh M, et al. Fever response in elderly nursing home residents: are the older truly colder? J Am Geriatr Soc 1991;39(9):853–7.

39. Castle SC, Yeh M, Toledo S, et al. Lowering the temperature criterion improves detection of infections in nursing home residents. Aging Immunol Infect Dis 1993;4:67–76.
40. Keating HJ 3rd, Klimek JJ, Levine DS, et al. Effect of aging on the clinical significance of fever in ambulatory adult patients. J Am Geriatr Soc 1984;32(4):282–7.
41. O'Grady NP, Barie PS, Bartlett JG, et al. Guidelines for evaluation of new fever in critically ill adult patients: 2008 update from the American College of Critical Care Medicine and the Infectious Diseases Society of America. Crit Care Med 2008; 36(4):1330–49.
42. Freifeld AG, Bow EJ, Sepkowitz KA, et al. Clinical practice guideline for the use of antimicrobial agents in neutropenic patients with cancer: 2010 Update by the Infectious Diseases Society of America. Clin Infect Dis 2011;52(4):427–31.
43. Vitiello MV, Smallwood RG, Avery DH, et al. Circadian temperature rhythms in young adult and aged men. Neurobiol Aging 1986;7(2):97–100.
44. Weitzman ED, Moline ML, Czeisler CA, et al. Chronobiology of aging: temperature, sleep-wake rhythms and entrainment. Neurobiol Aging 1982;3(4):299–309.
45. Blatteis CM. A personal recollection: 60 years in thermoregulation. Temperature (Austin) 2016;3(1):1–7.
46. Plata-Salaman CR, Peloso E, Satinoff E. Interleukin-1beta-induced fever in young and old Long-Evans rats. Am J Physiol 1998;275(5 Pt 2):R1633–8.
47. Scarpace PJ, Borst SE, Bender BS. The association of E. coli peritonitis with an impaired and delayed fever response in senescent rats. J Gerontol 1992;47(4): B142–5.
48. Roth GS, Lane MA, Ingram DK, et al. Biomarkers of caloric restriction may predict longevity in humans. Science 2002;297(5582):811.
49. Weinstein MP, Murphy JR, Reller LB, et al. The clinical significance of positive blood cultures: a comprehensive analysis of 500 episodes of bacteremia and fungemia in adults. II. Clinical observations, with special reference to factors influencing prognosis. Rev Infect Dis 1983;5(1):54–70.
50. Kluger MJ, Kozak W, Conn CA, et al. The adaptive value of fever. Infect Dis Clin North Am 1996;10(1):1–20.
51. Burns A, Zaudig M. Mild cognitive impairment in older people. Lancet 2002; 360(9349):1963–5.
52. Prince M, Bryce R, Albanese E, et al. The global prevalence of dementia: a systematic review and metaanalysis. Alzheimers Dement 2013;9(1):63–75.e62.
53. Johnson JC, Jayadevappa R, Baccash PD, et al. Nonspecific presentation of pneumonia in hospitalized older people: age effect or dementia? J Am Geriatr Soc 2000;48(10):1316–20.
54. Loeb M, Bentley DW, Bradley S, et al. Development of minimum criteria for the initiation of antibiotics in residents of long-term-care facilities: results of a consensus conference. Infect Control Hosp Epidemiol 2001;22(2):120–4.
55. Mitchell SL, Shaffer ML, Loeb MB, et al. Infection management and multidrug-resistant organisms in nursing home residents with advanced dementia. JAMA Intern Med 2014;174(10):1660–7.
56. Swardfager W, Black SE. Dementia: a link between microbial infection and cognition? Nat Rev Neurol 2013;9(6):301–2.
57. Tate JA, Snitz BE, Alvarez KA, et al. Infection hospitalization increases risk of dementia in the elderly. Crit Care Med 2014;42(5):1037–46.
58. Huang WS, Yang TY, Shen WC, et al. Association between Helicobacter pylori infection and dementia. J Clin Neurosci 2014;21(8):1355–8.

59. Schmidt R, Schmidt H, Curb JD, et al. Early inflammation and dementia: a 25-year follow-up of the Honolulu-Asia Aging Study. Ann Neurol 2002;52(2):168–74.
60. Katan M, Moon YP, Paik MC, et al. Infectious burden and cognitive function: the Northern Manhattan Study. Neurology 2013;80(13):1209–15.
61. Cicero MT, Freeman P, Cicero MT, et al. How to grow old: ancient wisdom for the second half of life. Princeton (NJ): Princeton University Press; 2016.
62. Sanford AM. Anorexia of aging and its role for frailty. Curr Opin Clin Nutr Metab Care 2017;20(1):54–60.
63. Donini LM, Poggiogalle E, Piredda M, et al. Anorexia and eating patterns in the elderly. PLoS One 2013;8(5):e63539.
64. Htwe TH, Mushtaq A, Robinson SB, et al. Infection in the elderly. Infect Dis Clin North Am 2007;21(3):711–43, ix.
65. Lilamand M, Kelaiditi E, Demougeot L, et al. The Mini Nutritional Assessment-Short Form and mortality in nursing home residents–results from the INCUR study. J Nutr Health Aging 2015;19(4):383–8.
66. Langkamp-Henken B, Wood SM, Herlinger-Garcia KA, et al. Nutritional formula improved immune profiles of seniors living in nursing homes. J Am Geriatr Soc 2006;54(12):1861–70.
67. Carlsson M, Haglin L, Rosendahl E, et al. Poor nutritional status is associated with urinary tract infection among older people living in residential care facilities. J Nutr Health Aging 2013;17(2):186–91.
68. Vaughan KL, Mattison JA. Obesity and aging in humans and nonhuman primates: a mini-review. Gerontology 2016;62(6):611–7.
69. Harris-Kojetin L, Sengupta M, Park-Lee E, et al. Long-Term Care Providers and services users in the United States: data from the National Study of Long-Term Care Providers, 2013-2014. Vital Health Stat 3 2016;(38):x–xii, 1–105.
70. United States Congress. Older Americans Act Amendments of 2006. 2006. Available at: https://www.congress.gov/bill/109th-congress/house-bill/6197. Accessed February 6, 2017.
71. Jump RL, Olds DM, Jury LA, et al. Specialty care delivery: bringing infectious disease expertise to the residents of a Veterans Affairs long-term care facility. J Am Geriatr Soc 2013;61(5):782–7.
72. Caprio TV, Karuza J, Katz PR. Profile of physicians in the nursing home: time perception and barriers to optimal medical practice. J Am Med Dir Assoc 2009;10(2):93–7.
73. United States Department of Health and Human Services. Centers for Medicare and Medicaid Services Survey and Certification Group 2016/2017 Nursing Home Action Plan. 2016. Available at: https://www.cms.gov/Medicare/Provider-Enrollment-andCertification/CertificationandComplianc/Downloads/2016-2017-Nursing-Home-Action-Plan.pdf. Accessed February 6, 2017.
74. Samaras N, Chevalley T, Samaras D, et al. Older patients in the emergency department: a review. Ann Emerg Med 2010;56(3):261–9.
75. Aminzadeh F, Dalziel WB. Older adults in the emergency department: a systematic review of patterns of use, adverse outcomes, and effectiveness of interventions. Ann Emerg Med 2002;39(3):238–47.
76. Crossley KB, Peterson PK. Infections in the elderly. Clin Infect Dis 1996;22(2):209–15.
77. Bingham J. Pope Francis: 'like good wine we get better with age'. 2013. Available at: http://www.telegraph.co.uk/news/worldnews/the-pope/9932391/Pope-Francis-like-good-wine-we-get-better-with-age.html. Accessed February 6, 2017.
78. Amelia EJ. Presentation of illness in older adults. AORN J 2006;83(2):372–89.

Antimicrobial Pharmacokinetics and Pharmacodynamics in Older Adults

John M. Benson, PharmD[a,b],*

KEYWORDS

- Elderly • Antimicrobial therapy • Pharmacokinetics • Pharmacodynamics

KEY POINTS

- Although the adage "start low, go slow" is applicable for most medications in elderly patients, it is inappropriate for most antimicrobials.
- In the elderly, the therapeutic indices of drugs that require serum concentration monitoring (eg, vancomycin, aminoglycosides) may be narrower because of increased sensitivity to adverse effects.
- For time-dependent antibiotics (eg, β-lactams), decreasing the dose and continuing the same dosing interval maximizes efficacy while reducing the risk of toxicity in elderly patients with reduced clearance.
- For concentration-dependent antibiotics (eg, aminoglycosides), using the same dose and increasing the dosing interval maximizes efficacy while reducing the risk of toxicity in elderly patients with reduced clearance.
- Because of their central nervous system side effect profile, clinicians should only select fluoroquinolones for older patients when other options are unavailable due to bacterial resistance, allergy, or other compelling reasons.

INTRODUCTION

Although it is now the eighth decade of the antibiotic era, with the commensurate wealth of data, there are still areas that require greater exploration. The pharmacokinetic (PK), and especially the pharmacodynamic (PD), behavior of systemic antimicrobial agents in elderly patients (>65 years) is a topic that has been inadequately studied.[1,2] Notably, the efforts of a growing number of intrepid investigators are

The author has no conflicts of interest to disclose.
[a] Promise Hospital of Salt Lake, 8th Avenue and C Street, Salt Lake City, UT 84143, USA;
[b] College of Pharmacy, University of Utah, 30 South 2000 East, Salt Lake City, UT 84112, USA
* Promise Hospital of Salt Lake, 8th Avenue and C Street, Salt Lake City, UT 84143.
E-mail address: john.benson@promisehealthcare.com

Infect Dis Clin N Am 31 (2017) 609–617
http://dx.doi.org/10.1016/j.idc.2017.07.011
0891-5520/17/© 2017 Elsevier Inc. All rights reserved.

id.theclinics.com

gratefully received. There are valid reasons for this. Studies undertaken by manufacturers intended to secure US Food and Drug Administration, European Medicines Evaluation Agency, and other governmental agency approvals frequently exclude elderly patients because of their altered clearance, increased risk for adverse events, and more frequent use of concomitant medications that could interact with the investigational drugs, all of which would confound the results of such research.[3]

Pharmacokinetics is the study of the movement of drugs from the moment of administration through elimination from the body and has been described as "what the body does to the drug." Each of the four phases (absorption, distribution, metabolism, and excretion) has age-related alterations, which are discussed in the next section.

Pharmacodynamics describes the relationship between drug concentration in the body and patient response, or "what the drug does to the body." For most nonantimicrobial drugs PD behavior is directly related to the pharmacologic effect as they interact at the molecular level with host receptors in target (efficacy) and nontarget (toxicity) organs. For antimicrobial agents, however, the target receptors are found in invading pathogens, rather than host organs' receptors. The desired effect of these target receptor-ligand interactions is fatal interference with normal cellular function. Indeed, any interplay of antimicrobial agents with host receptors usually produces only adverse effects, although some antibiotics may have pleiotropic effects, such as modest immunomodulation or other favorable actions.[4–6] Thus, the impact of age on PD results either from alterations in PK, which may affect efficacy and toxicity, or possibly from changes in host receptors responsible only for adverse effects.[7]

Within the elderly population, the frail elderly are especially susceptible to the toxic effects of drugs, including antimicrobials, because of their diminished physiologic reserve. This diminished reserve is attributed to a lower baseline function of one or more organs because of extreme age, a higher incidence of concomitant chronic diseases, and frequent polypharmacy with its attendant increases in adverse effect- and drug interaction-related stressors to physiologic systems.[2,8] Although the adage "start low, go slow" is often applied to drug use in such patients, this is inappropriate for most antimicrobials. Ample evidence shows delayed and inadequate dosing of antimicrobials correlates with increased adverse outcomes, including development of resistance and mortality.[1]

PHARMACOKINETIC CHANGES IN THE ELDERLY

Several PK changes are known to correlate with age.[9–12] For some drugs, however, they are minor changes that do not reach clinical significance or are absent.[13–15] Moreover, there is significant interpatient heterogeneity in the effects of age on PK, resulting in greater variability in these parameters than in younger patient groups. Current data are inadequate to enable identification of which elderly patients will exhibit clinically significant changes and which will not.[2,8] Nevertheless, some general statements can be made.

Absorption

Several alterations in the gastrointestinal tract occur with increasing age and may affect drug absorption. Increased gastric pH, either caused by an age-related reduction in acid production, or the frequent use of acid-reducing medications in older patients, may alter the absorption of low pH-dependent (decreased absorption, seen with ampicillin, ketoconazole, and itraconazole) or acid-labile (increased absorption, seen with penicillin and erythromycin lactobionate) antibiotics. Although acid lability and pH-dependent absorption of antibiotics may be of historical interest, they bear little clinical relevance in the modern era because of innovations in drug delivery, such as enteric coatings and delayed-release formulations, which bypass the low pH environment of the stomach. Older patients often have decreased intestinal surface area and splanchnic blood flow, which may reduce the absorption of most antimicrobials, and decreased gastric emptying and peristaltic activity, which may decrease and/or delay absorption. In general, these changes may slow the rate (lower peak concentration and longer time to peak), but do not significantly decrease the extent (area under the curve [AUC]) of absorption, and are of minor clinical consequence.[1–3,7,8,16] The effects of age on absorption seem to be most pronounced when active transport mechanisms are involved.[16] Several antimicrobials now available have good to excellent oral bioavailability (eg, fluoroquinolones, triazoles, and oxazolidinones), but it is currently unknown whether advanced age correlates with any changes in the absorption of these agents. Age-related changes also affect other routes of absorption, such as dermal, buccal, and conjunctival, but because these routes lack the capacity for systemic delivery of antibiotics, they are not discussed here.

Distribution

The apparent volume of distribution (volume) is a mathematical contrivance that allows the effective concentration of a drug to be derived from its dose. It does not represent actual anatomic or physiologic compartments, and is affected by a variety of factors including plasma protein binding, lipophilicity, tissue binding, and membrane transporters.[2] With age, adipose tissue increases and muscle mass decreases, both of which decrease the elimination of highly lipophilic antimicrobial agents, such as rifampin, fluoroquinolones, macrolides, oxazolidinones, tetracyclines, amphotericin B, and most of the imidazole antifungals. Age-related decreases in total body water contract the volume of hydrophilic drugs (aminoglycosides, β-lactams, and glycopeptides). Hydrophilic drugs that are also weak acids (eg, penicillin, ceftriaxone, and clindamycin) are further affected by the decrease in circulating albumin that also accompanies aging, the net result being increased concentrations of unbound drug.[1,3,7,12,16,17] Plasma α_1-acid glycoprotein, another drug-binding protein, increases with age, which may reduce the free concentration of alkaline antibiotics like the macrolides. Volume is the PK value that determines initial loading doses, and for hydrophilic drugs it correlates closely with body weight. Importantly, for elderly patients with severe infections, treatment with hydrophilic drugs, such as aminoglycosides and glycopeptides, must always be initiated with full loading doses, when such are recommended. Adjustments for renal function are only applied to the ensuing maintenance regimens.[10]

Metabolism

Splanchnic blood flow decreases with age, which also reduces first-pass metabolism and thus increases the serum concentrations of metabolized drugs, such as macrolides, fluoroquinolones (except levofloxacin), clindamycin, tetracyclines, imidazole antifungals (except fluconazole), sulfamethoxazole/trimethoprim, and rifampin.[1,3,12,16,17] Alterations in first-pass metabolism affect only orally administered antimicrobials. Phase I hepatic metabolism (oxidation, reduction, hydrolysis) declines with age, the cytochrome P-450 enzyme systems being the primary pathways. Phase II pathways (methylation, sulfation, acetylation, glucuronidation, and so forth) are largely unaffected by age.[2,7,10,17,18] Some medications are metabolized by phase I pathways, followed by phase II metabolism, but many others are metabolized only by one or the other. Because of the increased number of medications typically prescribed for elderly patients, many of which may interact with antimicrobials via cytochrome P-450 interference or other mechanisms, and the paucity of data in this area, there currently is no clear delineation regarding which of these metabolic changes will predominate in any given patient. Moreover, evidence suggests that the magnitude of interpatient genetic variability overshadows the effects of age on drug metabolism.[16]

Elimination

With age, renal blood flow and glomerular filtration rate decrease, both of which decrease the clearance of renally eliminated drugs.[17,19] Patients greater than 80 years of age have a 40% decline in renal function compared with adults of middle age.[20] Decreased renal clearance of antimicrobials is directly proportional to increases in half-life. Importantly, increased half-life not only necessitates a decrease in daily dose to avoid toxicity, but also prolongs the time necessary to achieve steady-state serum concentrations, which is of particular importance for drugs with narrow therapeutic indices (the ratio of effective to toxic serum concentrations) that require serum concentration monitoring (eg, vancomycin, aminoglycosides). In the elderly, the therapeutic indices of such drugs may be narrower still.[2]

Some published research has challenged the common notion that renal function declines as a function of age per se, independent of other factors.[16,17] The association of aging with decreased renal function is confounded by the high incidence of hypertension, heart disease, and other chronic conditions that also strongly correlate with age. Approximately one-third of elderly patients have a normal glomerular filtration rate.[3,8]

Irrespective of the cause, most elderly patients have decreased renal function and appropriate adjustments must be made for renally cleared antimicrobial agents.[1,3,11,21] Accurate estimates of renal function in older patients are achieved with standard equations,[22] and the equation developed by Cockcroft and Gault[23] is the most commonly used in published guidelines.[2] However, because of the strong correlation of aging with chronic conditions that reduce renal function, this equation may underestimate renal function for the healthiest segment of elderly patients. Age, independent of renal function, has been shown to correlate with several PK changes, which are shown in **Table 1**.

PHARMACODYNAMIC MODELS

With age-related changes in PK as a background, we now review the impact of aging on PD models and discuss what adjustments may be needed when using these models in older patients. For nonantibiotic medications, in addition to altered PK, there may be age-related changes at the receptor level, including differences in receptor density, affinity, or action, which would alter drug PD. In the special case of antimicrobial agents, however, microbial target receptors are "external" to the host and,

Table 1 Drug measures that correlate with age, independent of renal function		
Measure	**Direction of Change**	**References**
Vd (hydrophilic drugs)	Decreased	[24]
Cl	Decreased	[25–27]
Serum concentrations	Increased	[28–31]
AUC	Increased	[32,33]
Toxicity	Increased	[34]

Abbreviations: Cl, clearance; Vd, volume of distribution.

therefore, drug effects at those receptors (once the drug is delivered to the site) are unaffected by patient age.

As with most drugs, delivery of antimicrobial molecules to their site of action depends largely on chemical properties, including lipophilicity, molecular weight, and protein binding, whereas the action of the antimicrobial at the target receptor depends almost entirely on its molecular structure, shape, and charge. In the elderly, fluoroquinolones in particular have a higher incidence of central nervous system toxicities (anxiety, restlessness, insomnia, confusion, hallucinations, psychosis, and seizures), which, in addition to reduced renal function, may be attributable to a more permeable blood-brain barrier, concomitant medications that lower seizure threshold (eg, nonsteroidal anti-inflammatory drugs), or possibly central nervous system receptor changes.[12,20,35,36] For this patient group, clinicians should select fluoroquinolones only when other options are unavailable because of bacterial resistance, drug allergy, or other compelling reasons.

PD models have been developed for antibiotics that take many of these factors into account and accurately describe the relationships between certain PK parameters and the desired clinical outcome (microbial inhibition or eradication). By understanding such models, optimal use of these drugs in the aged is more likely.

Time-Dependent Bacterial Killing

For some antibiotics, bacterial killing best correlates with the amount of time serum concentrations exceed a certain threshold, usually the organism's minimum inhibitory concentration (MIC), a PD model known as time-dependent bacterial killing (T > MIC). Time dependence implies concentration independence. For these drugs, once an optimal concentration is reached, further increasing the concentration does not increase the rate of bacterial killing, possibly because of available binding sites approaching saturation. All of the β-lactam antibiotics (penicillins, cephalosporins, carbapenems, and monobactams) exhibit this behavior.[37] β-Lactams are small molecules that inhibit cell wall synthesis, the target binding sites being located external to the cell membrane. Reducing doses of these drugs to avoid toxicity caused by decreased renal clearance in elderly patients is best done by decreasing the dose and continuing the same dosing interval. This approach optimizes time greater than MIC.[10]

Concentration-Dependent Bacterial Killing

The rate of bacterial killing of antibiotics whose sites of action lie intracellularly (inhibition of protein synthesis via ribosome binding, interference with DNA supercoiling and transcription, and so forth) is usually concentration-dependent, with the strongest correlation being either peak concentration to MIC ratio, or AUC greater than the MIC. Drugs that fit these concentration-dependent PD models include aminoglycosides, macrolides, clindamycin, metronidazole, fluoroquinolones, daptomycin, and tetracyclines.[37] Despite their action on the cell wall similar to the β-lactams, glycopeptides exhibit concentration-dependent bacterial killing with AUC greater than MIC being the strongest correlate. For older patients with decreased renal function being treated with such drugs, reducing dosage regimens is best done by increasing the dosing interval (eg, changing from 6 to 8 hours, 12 to 24 hours) and maintaining the same dose, thus maximizing peak serum concentrations.[10]

MODIFICATIONS IN DRUG DELIVERY BASED ON PHARMACODYNAMIC MODELS

During the past few decades, the body of published medical literature has significantly increased the understanding of how antibiotics work, the PD models that best describe their actions, and how to maximize efficacy and/or minimize toxicity. We next examine these approaches and the potential age-related changes in each.

Once-Daily Aminoglycoside Therapy

It has been well documented that total daily doses of aminoglycosides given as a single infusion are at least as effective as divided daily doses,[38,39] and this has been validated in elderly patients.[40] This method exploits several PD principles that have been observed with aminoglycosides. The higher dose achieves high serum concentrations, maximizing the peak to MIC ratio. The longer interval between doses is possible because of the postantibiotic effect (continued bacterial killing or inhibition when serum concentrations have declined less than the MIC) seen with drugs of this class. The higher serum concentrations seem to increase bacterial killing without increasing toxic effects. In fact, there is substantial evidence that adverse effects decrease with this method.[39]

The introduction of newer antibiotics with similar spectra and lower toxicities has resulted in the aminoglycosides being seldom used, especially in patients older than 65 years of age who are at higher risk of toxicity. Nevertheless, for an elderly patient with normal renal function, and for whom other options have less favorable risk/benefit ratios, once-daily aminoglycosides may be used with published dosing recommendations.[39] In such cases, the prudent clinician chooses the lower end of the range for loading doses (to correct for reduced total body water), and stops aminoglycoside therapy at the shortest recommended duration once appropriate outcomes are reached.

Prolonged Infusions

In the United States, there was a period when nearly all of the most active antibiotics available (eg, extended-spectrum carbapenems, penicillins, and cephalosporins) were under patent protection, and thus expensive. This prompted investigation into whether the time-dependent bacterial killing of these agents could be used to achieve similar outcomes while reducing total antibiotic use. Prolonging the infusion for normal or reduced doses of carbapenems (imipenem, meropenem, and doripenem), and extended-spectrum penicillins (piperacillin, ticarcillin) and cephalosporins (ceftazidime, cefepime) blunts the peak concentration and prolongs the T > MIC. Continuous infusions of β-lactams have similar effects.[41,42] Clinical outcomes, including mortality, have been found to be superior with extended infusions[42] and it is reasonable to expect no difference in older patients. In the current era of increasing bacterial resistance, prolonged infusions of normal or high doses may increase the activity of these drugs against pathogens with intermediate susceptibility or low-level resistance, although this has yet to be studied.

Lower, More Frequent Doses

Another approach that maximizes the time-dependent nature of bacterial killing with β-lactams is to give smaller doses at more frequent intervals. For example, meropenem, 500 mg every 6 hours, has been compared with 1000 mg given every 8 hours, both by 30-minute infusions. For most susceptible organisms, the T > MIC for these two regimens has been shown to be equivalent.[43,44] As with prolonged infusions, this approach is expected to yield similar efficacy in elderly patients, and potentially decrease adverse events and resistance because of the lower total daily exposure to drug.

SUMMARY

The expectations of antimicrobial agents are starkly dichotomous in that one intends for them to be harmless to host cells, and yet be lethal to the cell (the pathogen) against which they are deployed. (Alas, the search for medications that bind the intended receptor and no other, colloquially the "magic bullet," continues.) This, at least in part, may explain the difficulties faced by those pharmaceutical manufacturers who endeavor to produce novel antimicrobial agents. Nearly all studies that have examined the effects of age on the PK and PD of drugs used cross-sectional study designs that compared young patients with old, rather than the more ideal but also more difficult longitudinal study of patients as they age. That these patients use more medications than any other group, and are a growing segment of the population, heightens the need for more research. Further investigation into the PK and PD of antimicrobial agents in the elderly, with its resultant innovation into better regimen design, will increase the ability of clinicians to use these agents with optimal efficacy and safety in this expanding population.

REFERENCES

1. Bellmann-Weiler R, Weiss G. Pitfalls in the diagnosis and therapy of infections in elderly patients: a mini-review. Gerontology 2009;55:241–9.
2. Hilmer SM. ADME-tox issues for the elderly. Expert Opin Drug Metab Toxicol 2008;4:1321–31.
3. Corsonello A, Pedone C, Antonelli Incalzi R. Age-related pharmacokinetic and pharmacodynamic changes and related risk of adverse drug reactions. Curr Med Chem 2010;17:571–84.
4. Zarogoulidis P, Papanas N, Kioumis I, et al. Macrolides: from in vitro anti-inflammatory and immunomodulatory properties to clinical practice in respiratory diseases. Eur J Clin Pharmacol 2012;68:479–503.
5. Parnham MJ, Erakovic Haber V, Giamarellows-Bouboulis EJ, et al. Azithromycin: mechanisms of action and their relevance for clinical applications. Pharmacol Ther 2014;143:225–45.
6. Pradhan S, Madke B, Kabra P, et al. Anti-inflammatory and immunomodulator effects of antibiotics and their use in dermatology. Indian J Dermatol 2016;61: 469–81.
7. Colloca G, Santoro M, Gambassi G. Age-related physiologic changes and perioperative management of elderly patients. Surg Oncol 2010;19(3):124–30.
8. Hubbard RE, O'Mahony MS, Woohouse KW. Medication prescribing in trial older people. Eur J Clin Pharmacol 2013;69:319–26.
9. Riccobene T, Jakate A, Rank D. A series of pharmacokinetic studies of ceftaroline fossil in select populations: normal subjects, healthy elderly subjects, and subjects with renal impairment or end-stage renal disease requiring hemodialysis. J Clin Pharmacol 2014;54:742–52.
10. Petrosillo N, Cataldo MA, Pea F. Treatment options for community-acquired pneumonia in the elderly people. Expert Rev Anti Infect Ther 2015;13:473–85.
11. Chien SC, Chow AT, Nathan J, et al. Absence of age and gender effects on the pharmacokinetics of a single 500-milligram oral dose of levofloxacin in health subjects. Antimicrob Agents Chemother 1997;41:1562–5.
12. Cefalu CA. Theories and mechanisms of aging. Clin Geriatr Med 2011;27: 491–506.

13. Chandrokar G, Xiao A, Moukasassi MS, et al. Population pharmacokinetic of ceftolozane/tazobactam in healthy volunteers, subjects with varying degrees of renal function and patients with bacterial infections. J Clin Pharmacol 2015;55:230–9.

14. Meagher AK, Forrest A, Rayner CR, et al. Population pharmacokinetics of linezolid in patients treated in a compassionate-use program. Antimicrob Agents Chemother 2003;47:548–53.

15. Goldberg MR, Wong SL, Shaw JP, et al. Single-dose pharmacokinetics and tolerability of telavancin in elderly men and women. Pharmacotherapy 2010;30: 806–11.

16. Shi S, Klotz U. Age-related changes in pharmacokinetics. Curr Drug Metab 2011; 12:601–10.

17. Thompson CM, Johns DO, Sonawane B, et al. Database for physiologically based pharmacokinetic (PBPK) modeling: physiological data for healthy and health-impaired elderly. J Toxicol Environ Health B Crit Rev 2009;12:1–24.

18. Coates P, Daniel R, Houston AC, et al. An open study to compare the pharmacokinetics, safety and tolerability of a multiple-dose regimen of azithromycin in young and elderly volunteers. Eur J Clin Microbiol Infect Dis 1991;10:850–2.

19. Triggs EFJ, Johnson JM, Learoyd B. Absorption and disposition of ampicillin in the elderly. Eur J Clin Pharmacol 1980;18:195–8.

20. Stahlmann R, Lode H. Safety considerations of fluoroquinolone in the elderly: and update. Drugs Aging 2010;27:193–209.

21. Dvorchik B, Damhousse D. Single-dose pharmacokinetics of daptomycin in young and geriatric volunteers. J Clin Pharmacol 2004;44:612–20.

22. Drenth-van Maanen AC, Jansen PAF, Proost JH, et al. Renal function assessment in older adults. Br J Clin Pharmacol 2013;76:616–23.

23. Cockcroft DW, Gault MH. Prediction of creating clearance from serum creatinine. Nephron 1976;16:31–41.

24. Rubino CM, Bhvnani SM, Moeck G, et al. Population pharmacokinetic analysis for a single 1,200-milligram dose of oritavancin using data from two pivotal phase 3 clinical trials. Antimicrob Agents Chemother 2015;59:3365–72.

25. Li C, Kuti JL, Nightingale CH, et al. Population pharmacokinetic analysis and dosing regimen optimization of meropenem in adult patients. J Clin Pharmacol 2006;46:1171–8.

26. Rubino CM, Van Wart SA, Bhavnani SM, et al. Oritavancin population pharmacokinetics in healthy subjects and patients with complicated skin and skin structure infections or bacteremia. Antimicrob Agents Chemother 2009;53:4422–8.

27. Sjovall J, Alvan G, Huitfeldt B. Intra- and inaner-individual variation in pharmacokinetics of intravenously infused amoxycillin and ampicillin to elderly volunteers. Br J Clin Pharmacol 1986;21:171–81.

28. Paladino JA, Forrest A, Wilton JH. Predictors of trough concentrations for oral ciprofloxacin. Pharmacotherapy 1993;13:504–7.

29. Reesor Nimmo C, Mamdani F, Baker A, et al. Development and implementation of simplified amino glycoside empiric dosing guidelines. Pharmacotherapy 1993;13:408–14.

30. Conil JM, Georges B, Ravat F, et al. Ceftazidime dosage recommendations in burn patients: from a population pharmacokinetic approach to clinical practice via Monte Carlo simulations. Clin Ther 2013;35:1603–12.

31. Sullivan JT, Letter JT, Liu P, et al. The influence of age and gender on the pharmacokinetics of moxifloxacin. Clin Pharmacokinet 2001;40(Suppl 1):11–8.

32. Samara E, Shaw JP, Barriere SL, et al. Population pharmacokinetics of telavancin in healthy subjects and patients with infections. Antimicrob Agents Chemother 2012;56:2067–73.
33. Tarral A, Merdjan H. Effect of age and sex on the pharmacokinetics and safety of avibactam on healthy volunteers. Clin Ther 2015;37:877–86.
34. Cosgrove SE, Vigliani GA, Camion M, et al. Initial low-dose gentamicin for staph-ylococcus aureus bacteremia and endocarditis is nephrotoxic. Clin Infect Dis 2009;48:713–21.
35. Wallace J, Paauw DS. Appropriate prescribing and important drug interactions in older adults. Med Clin North Am 2015;99:295–310.
36. Asín-Prieto E, Rodríguez-Gascón A, Isla A. Applications of the pharmacokinetic/pharmacodynamic (PK/PD) analysis of antimicrobial agents. J Infect Chemother 2015;21(5):319–29.
37. Ambrose PG, Bhavanni SM, Rubino CM, et al. Pharmacokinetics-pharmacody-namics of antimicrobial therapy: it's not just for mice anymore. Clin Infect Dis 2007;44:79–86.
38. Prins JM, Buller HR, Kuijper EJ, et al. Once versus thrice daily gentamicin in pa-tients with serious infections. Lancet 1993;341:335–9.
39. Bauer LA. Clinical pharmacokinetics and pharmacodynamics. In: DiPiro JT, Talbert RL, Yee GC, et al, editors. Pharmacotherapy: a pathophysiologic approach. 10th edition. New York: McGraw-Hill; 2017. Chapter e4.
40. Koo J, Tight R, Rajkumar V, et al. Comparison of once-daily versus pharmacoki-netic dosing of aminoglycosides in elderly patients. Am J Med 1996;101:177–83.
41. Lal A, Jaoude P, El-Solh AA. Prolonged versus intermittent infusion of beta-lactams for the treatment of nosocomial pneumonia: a meta-analysis. Infect Chemother 2016;48:81–90.
42. Yost RJ, Cappelletty DM. The retrospective cohort of extended-infusion piperacil-lin-tazobactam (RECEIPT) study: a multicenter study. Pharmacotherapy 2011;31:767–75.
43. Kotapati S, Nicolau DP, Nightingale CH, et al. Clinical and economic benefits of a meropenem dosage strategy based on pharmacodynamic concepts. Am J Health Syst Pharm 2004;61:1264–70.
44. Kuti JL, Maglio D, Nightingale CH, et al. Economic benefit of a meropenem dosage strategy based on pharmacodynamic concepts. Am J Health Syst Pharm 2003;60:565–8.

Antibiotic Stewardship in Nursing Facilities

Miranda McElligott, RN, MS[a], Grace Welham, PharmD, PhD[a], Aurora Pop-Vicas, MD[a,b], Lyndsay Taylor, MD[b], Christopher J. Crnich, MD, PhD[a,b,c,*]

KEYWORDS

- Long-term care • Antimicrobial stewardship • Antimicrobial resistance • Elderly

KEY POINTS

- Overuse and misuse of antibiotics is a major cause of adverse drug events, antibiotic resistance, and *Clostridium difficile* in nursing facilities.
- Antibiotic prescribing decisions in nursing facilities are complex and influenced by several factors.
- Antibiotic stewardship structure and process in many nursing facilities remains rudimentary.
- Focus on several key tasks and improvement strategies can have a meaningful impact on antibiotic prescribing in nursing facilities.

INTRODUCTION

The 15,600 nursing facilities (NFs) in the United States provide medical and residential care for 1.4 million persons on a daily basis. Each year, 3.2 million persons will reside in one of these facilities.[1] No longer exclusively tasked with providing long-term custodial care, NFs provide care for an increasingly complex patient population that requires a wide array of skilled care services, including intensive rehabilitation, wound care, and parenterally administered medications. Infections are a common problem in NFs; residents experiencing an infection are at significant risk of hospitalization and death, which promotes the overuse of antibiotics in this setting. Approximately 75% of residents who stay in an NF for 6 months or longer will receive at least one course of antibiotics.[2] More than half of the antibiotic courses initiated in NFs are

Disclosure statement: All the authors have no conflicts of interest. Dr C.J. Crnich is supported by research grants from the Agency for Healthcare Research and Quality (R18HS022465, R18 HS022465-01 A1) and the Veterans Health Services Research & Development (RFA# HX-16-006, CRE-12-291, and PPO 16-118-1).

[a] University of Wisconsin, School of Medicine and Public Health, Madison, WI, USA; [b] University of Wisconsin Hospital and Clinics, Madison, WI, USA; [c] William S. Middleton Veterans Affairs Hospital, Madison, WI, USA
* Corresponding author. 2500 Overlook Terrace, B5112E, Madison, WI 53705.
E-mail address: cjc@medicine.wisc.edu

Infect Dis Clin N Am 31 (2017) 619–638
http://dx.doi.org/10.1016/j.idc.2017.07.008
0891-5520/17/Published by Elsevier Inc.

id.theclinics.com

unnecessary[3–9]; even when necessary, the antibiotics prescribed are often excessively broad spectrum[5,7] or administered for a duration longer than necessary for treatment of the underlying infection.[10] The overuse and misuse of antibiotics in NFs are major causes of adverse drug events and future infections such as those caused by *Clostridium difficile* and antibiotic-resistant bacteria. Once acquired by a resident, *C difficile* and/or antibiotic-resistant bacteria may then be spread to other residents and to patients in hospitals when resident illness requires a higher level of care.[11]

An antibiotic stewardship program (ASP) is a coordinated effort that monitors patterns of antibiotic use and antibiotic-related outcomes as well as oversees identification and implementation of strategies to improve these measures.[12] Until recently, ASPs existed almost exclusively in the hospital setting. However, human consumption of antibiotics in nonhospital settings greatly exceeds that in hospitals, which has led to calls for implementation of ASPs across the health care continuum.[13] Recent revisions to regulations governing NFs will require facilities to have an ASP in place by November of 2017 in order to participate in the Medicare and Medicaid programs.[14] Although hospitals and NFs share common antibiotic stewardship goals, the structure and process of ASPs in these two settings differ considerably. In this review, the authors (1) describe the factors that influence antibiotic prescribing decisions in NFs; (2) review the evidence supporting strategies to improve antibiotic prescribing in these facilities; (3) describe the current state of ASPs in NFs; and (4) provide suggestions for how antibiotic stewardship activity can be further expanded in NFs.

FACTORS DRIVING ANTIBIOTIC USE IN NURSING FACILITIES

Antibiotic prescribing is a multistep, often iterative process that involves consideration of the potential diagnoses, a decision to initiate antibiotic therapy, consideration of the different therapeutic options, and, ideally, reevaluation of patients and available diagnostic information to determine if treatment modification is indicated (**Fig. 1**). These decisions are complex and often involve high levels of uncertainty as well as risk. Most NF residents are frail and may not always exhibit classic signs and symptoms of infection. Fever, the cardinal symptomatic response to serious bacterial or viral systemic infections, may be blunted 20% to 30% of the time in older patients.[15] Difficulty in distinguishing between asymptomatic colonization and infection is further complicated by resident inability to communicate symptoms due to advanced dementia or other medical conditions associated with impairments in verbal capacity. Many facilities lack on-site laboratory or radiologic diagnostics, necessitating transfer of the resident or their specimens to an outside facility. These transfers impose additional burdens on residents and their health care givers and may result in either decreased use of diagnostic investigations or delays in obtaining test results.[16]

Although social and contextual influences play a role in antibiotic prescribing in all health care settings,[17–19] they seem particularly strong in the NF setting.[20] In other clinical settings, the prescribing provider assesses patients before engaging in the

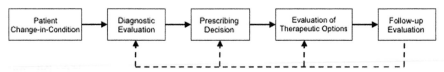

Fig. 1. The antibiotic decision-making process.

decisions detailed in **Fig. 1**. In NFs, however, clinicians may not always be available to physically evaluate the residents before prescribing an antibiotic[21] or, if they operate primarily in a cross-cover capacity, may be unfamiliar with the resident.[22] Consequently, most antibiotic decisions in NFs rely heavily on the content of information communicated by nurses, nursing assistants, or other on-site health care personnel, with medical decision-making largely influenced by the quality of these communications.[23,24] Physicians practicing in general clinics outside of the NF setting may be difficult to reach directly during working hours, increasing the chance of losing important clinical information during repeated attempts at communication.[25] Biases related to staff knowledge, attitudes, and beliefs regarding the appropriate course of action or existent prescriber-nursing relationships are, therefore, easily introduced.[26] In addition to nursing staff's points of view,[27,28] pressures from patients and their families may also contribute to prescribing decisions, as physicians may feel inclined to comply with family wishes, especially for uncertain clinical situations or during end-of-life care.[22,24,29] This circumstance seems to be particularly true for the NF environment in the United States, Canada, and Australia,[29,30] though less so for the Netherlands.[31] Hospitals have significantly invested in the development of information technology infrastructure that can provide clinicians with access to updated information on local antimicrobial resistance patterns and institution-specific antibiotic prescribing guidelines. The same is not necessarily true in the NF setting,[9] which further complicates medical decision-making.

Rather than a relatively straight forward dyadic interaction between patient and provider, what emerges from this literature is a complex interaction between multiple factors and individuals that may enhance, but more commonly degrade, the quality of antibiotic decision-making in NFs (**Fig. 2**). Efforts to improve antibiotic stewardship in NFs will likely need to target several of these factors in order to be successful.

EFFECTS OF ANTIBIOTIC STEWARDSHIP INTERVENTIONS IN NURSING FACILITIES

Antibiotic stewardship is accomplished through centralized (programmatic) and/or decentralized (nonprogrammatic) approaches. Centralized approaches include formulary restriction, preauthorization, as well as prospective audit and feedback. With notable exceptions, these approaches have been primarily used in hospitals and typically rely on individuals with specific training and expertise in the diagnosis and management of infectious diseases (IDs).[32] Noncentralized antibiotic stewardship interventions seek to positively impact antibiotic prescribing quality through education as well as introduction of guidelines and decision-support tools. These interventions have been the predominant strategies used in NFs and generally do not rely on individuals with ID and/or antibiotic stewardship expertise.[33,34]

Centralized Antibiotic Stewardship Interventions

There have been 3 studies that have examined the impact of a centralized antibiotic stewardship approach in NFs. Implementation of an ID consultative service in a Veterans Affairs (VA) Community Living Center, the VA equivalent of an NF, was associated with significant improvements in antibiotic utilization.[35] The ID service performed in-person consultation on residents once weekly and was available for remote consultations the remainder of the week. They completed 291 consults on 250 study facility residents during the 18-month intervention period (~7 patient visits and 5–10 calls per week). Ninety-five percent of the consultative team

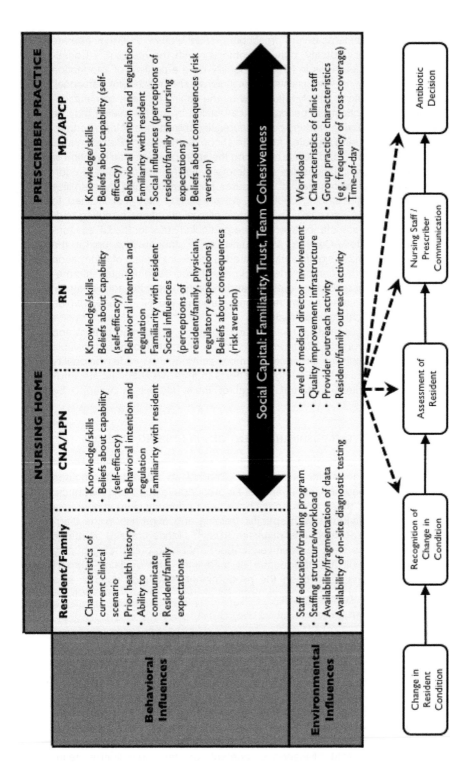

Fig. 2. Framework of the factors influencing antibiotic decision-making in NFs. Antibiotic decisions in NFs often occur off-site during communication events with nursing staff who have performed the primary resident evaluation on behalf of the prescriber. Characteristics of the individuals involved in this process as well as the nursing facility and prescriber practice environment likely play an important role in the quality of the decision-making that emerges from this process. APCP, advanced practice care provider; CNA, certified nursing assistant; LPN, licensed practical nurse; MD, doctor of med-

recommendations were accepted. Compared with a 3-year baseline period, total antibiotic use in the study facility decreased by 30% (175–122 days of therapy [DOT] per 1000 resident-days, $P<.01$) with statistically significant reductions in the use of fluoroquinolones, sulfamethoxazole/trimethoprim, β-lactam/β-lactamase inhibitors, clindamycin, and tetracycline antibiotics. Rates of hospitalization during the intervention period did not change; however, rates of positive C difficile tests declined significantly relative to the baseline period.

Although current levels of pharmacist involvement in stewardship activities in most NFs are limited,[36] pharmacist-driven interventions have been shown to positively impact the quality of antibiotic prescribing in this setting.[9,37] A pharmacist-led prospective audit and feedback intervention focused on antibiotics initiated for treatment of culture-positive infections was associated with a 50% reduction in inappropriate antibiotic therapy in a single hospital-affiliated NF.[37] More recently, prospective audit and feedback intervention of antibiotics initiated for treatment of urinary tract infections (UTIs) in 3 California NFs was associated with a significant reduction in UTI-specific and all-cause antibiotic starts.[9] The intervention in this study involved once-weekly site visits by an ID-trained pharmacist who performed chart reviews, discussed the cases with an off-site ID physician, and communicated recommendations to facility prescribers. The ID pharmacist reviewed 57% (104 of 183) of UTI treatment events during the intervention phase and left specific modification recommendations for 40 of these cases, 10 of which were accepted by providers (25%). The investigators hypothesized that notifying providers of the intent of the study, to improve the quality of antibiotic prescribing, created an unexpected normative influence that may have led to reductions in antibiotic utilization independent of those driven by pharmacist recommendations.

Decentralized Antibiotic Stewardship Interventions

Given existing limitations in access to clinicians with ID expertise, current efforts to influence antibiotic prescribing behaviors in NFs have predominantly focused on noncentralized interventions based on education, practice guidelines, and decision-support tools.[11,38–40] Several of the interventions described in published studies have targeted the decision to initiate antibiotic therapy in NF residents with a suspected UTI. A cluster randomized controlled trial in 24 US and Canadian NFs found that implementation of UTI testing and treatment pathways was associated with a short-term reduction in antibiotic treatment of UTIs.[41] Treatment effects waned over the study period; the intervention did not have a significant impact on urine culture utilization, suggesting some issues with intervention sustainability and fidelity.[42] In contrast, a subsequent study in a single VA long-term care facility using the same testing and treatment pathways demonstrated a 59% reduction in urine culture utilization (incidence rate ratio [IRR] = 0.41; 95% confidence interval [CI] 0.27–0.64), a 63% reduction in treatment of asymptomatic bacteriuria (IRR = 0.37; 95% CI 0.19–0.72), and 30% reduction in overall days of antibiotic therapy per 1000 patient-days when comparing the 3-month preintervention phase, the 6-month postintervention phase, and the subsequent 2 years.[43] Although these two studies addressed both testing and treatment decision-making, other studies have shown that interventions focusing on testing decision-making can positively impact antibiotic prescribing in NFs. Implementation of a testing decision-support pathway in 10 acute and long-term care units at a VA medical center was associated with a significant reduction in urine culture utilization and overtreatment of asymptomatic bacteriuria.[44] Similarly, there was a significant decrease in utilization of urine cultures and antibiotic therapy for UTIs following introduction of a UTI diagnostic pathway in 17 Massachusetts NFs.[45]

There is substantial evidence that suboptimal assessment of NF residents experiencing a change in condition coupled with poor interdisciplinary communication has an untoward influence on antibiotic decision-making by off-site providers.[3,4,27] Not surprisingly, interventions focused on improving nursing assessments of residents and standardizing the content of communication with prescribers have been associated with reductions in antibiotic use in NFs.[46,47] A quality-improvement intervention focused on education of NF staff and families and implementation of tools to improve nurse-provider communication led to a 14% reduction in antibiotic utilization in 6 North Carolina NFs relative to control NFs in the same region that did not participate in the quality-improvement intervention.[47] Similarly, antibiotic prescribing in Texas NFs was 33% lower in facilities that implemented a standardized communication and UTI decision-support form with high fidelity compared with control facilities that implemented the form with low fidelity.[46]

Efforts to improve the spectrum and duration of antibiotic therapy through educational interventions have had modest success in NFs. Case-based educational sessions on intervention units in a Chicago long-term care facility were associated with a 28% improvement in the frequency of guideline-concordant treatment courses and a 30% reduction in the days of antibiotic therapy. No changes were noted on care units that did not receive the educational intervention.[48] The impact of education-based interventions on a larger scale has been less impressive. A cluster randomized controlled study was performed in 8 Canadian NFs in which providers in intervention NFs were mailed an antibiotic guide describing treatment of common infections (UTI, lower respiratory tract infection, skin and soft tissue infection) as well as a report of their personal prescribing patterns over the previous 3 months.[49] Although initial guideline-adherent prescribing improved in intervention NFs, adherence rates were no better when compared with control NFs at the conclusion of the study.[49] Similarly, a cluster randomized controlled study in Swedish NFs in which printed educational materials and in-person small group educational sessions were delivered to staff and providers in intervention facilities did not demonstrate a significant impact on the targeted prescribing behavior (reduction in use of fluoroquinolone antibiotics) but was associated with a modest reduction in the numbers of residents treated with antibiotics (difference in difference: −0.12; 95% CI −0.23 to −0.02).[50] Interestingly, the effectiveness of educational interventions may rely on the simultaneous delivery of content to facility nursing staff and prescribing providers. A cluster randomized controlled trial of an educational intervention to improve antibiotic prescribing for pneumonia in New York NFs demonstrated significant improvement in adherence to prescribing guidelines (from 50% to 82%) in facilities where education targeted both types of clinical staff.[51] In contrast, guideline adherence remained essentially unchanged in NFs where education was targeted solely at prescribing providers (from 65% to 69%).[51]

Although most of the stewardship interventions studied in NFs have focused on reducing unnecessary antibiotic use, there is ample evidence that the quality of antibiotic prescribing in NFs could be improved through efforts to reduce length of treatment courses[10,52] and decreasing use of broad-spectrum agents.[7] These two goals have been successfully achieved through a centralized prospective audit and feedback approach as detailed earlier but the scalability of this approach in NFs remains uncertain. Self-directed postprescriptive review, which has been shown to be modestly effective in the hospital setting,[33,34] has been studied on a limited basis in NFs. A cluster randomized controlled study of a multicomponent intervention that included protocol-guided postprescription review of antibiotic courses initiated in 30 NFs in London demonstrated a 5% reduction in antibiotic consumption in intervention facilities compared with control facilities despite only a 26% adherence to the postprescription review protocol.[53]

CURRENT STATE OF ANTIBIOTIC STEWARDSHIP PROGRAMS IN NURSING FACILITIES

Although many NFs may be capable of implementing the stewardship interventions described earlier, adoption and sustainment of these practice changes are likely to be more successful in facilities with infrastructure and procedures dedicated to the improvement of antibiotic use (ie, an ASP). Although there is significant variability, ASPs in hospitals are typically built around a team with broad expertise in IDs, pharmacodynamics/pharmacokinetics, and informatics.[54] Although ASPs in hospitals engage in several activities to promote more judicious use of antibiotics, the most effective strategies are built around prior authorization, postprescribing review and feedback interventions.[55,56] Although the data are limited, there are several studies that have begun to characterize the status of ASPs in US NFs.[36,57–61] Perhaps, not surprisingly, these studies show that most NFs lack the resources to achieve models of ASP like those observed in the hospital setting.

Although most NFs report having written policies and procedures that address antibiotic prescribing in some form, less than half of the facilities queried in published survey studies had a formally recognized ASP.[36,57–61] Unlike the situation in hospitals, ASP programs in NFs are largely overseen by facility nursing staff and infection preventionists.[36,57–60] The medical director and pharmacist are actively engaged in NF ASPs in less than 50% of facilities,[36,57–60] and involvement of individuals with formal ID training is seen in less than 15% of facilities.[60]

From 52% to 92% of NFs report tracking antibiotic use,[36,57–61] although a minority employ standardized utilization metrics or trend data longitudinally.[36] Most NFs track antibiotic-related outcomes like *C difficile* and methicillin-resistant *Staphylococcus aureus* (MRSA) infections and several NFs (9%–89%) report availability of an antibiogram.[36,57–60] However, on closer inspection less than 10% of NFs employ a facility-specific antibiogram[59] and most repurpose microbiological data generated in their referring hospitals.

Education on the appropriate use of antibiotics is provided to nursing staff is common in NFs, but the providers ultimately responsible for antibiotic orders are rarely targeted by these efforts.[57,59–61] Antibiotic prescribing guidelines, although often present, predominantly focus on nursing practices; a limited number of NFs report having infection-specific (eg, UTI) treatment guidelines or protocols.[36] A minority of NFs use antibiotic formularies, and less than 25% report use of preauthorization as a strategy to improve the quality of antibiotic prescribing.[57,59,61] Finally, although most NFs report tracking appropriateness of antibiotic prescribing,[57–59] these data are rarely fed back to providers; less than 15% of facilities use postprescribing review and feedback as a means of improving prescribing practices.[36]

EXPANDING ANTIBIOTIC STEWARDSHIP PROGRAMS IN NURSING FACILITIES

The findings of the survey studies described in the preceding section speak to a critical need to enhance the spread and scope of ASPs in NFs. The Centers for Disease Control and Prevention (CDC) has identified the core elements of ASPs in NFs.[62] It is expected that facilities will tailor implementation of the core elements based on existing organizational structure and resource availability (**Table 1**). Importantly, NFs are encouraged to develop their ASP in a stepwise fashion, starting with

Table 1
Core elements of antibiotic stewardship in nursing facilities

Component	Description	Comments
1. Leadership commitment	Dedicate support and commitment to safe and appropriate antibiotic use in the facility.	• Medical director, chief nursing official, and director of pharmacy should be visible and vocal champions for the facility ASP. • Structure, roles, and responsibilities of facility ASP should be detailed in a policy that is reviewed and approved by the facility leadership (the QAPI committee). • Other policies and guidelines developed by the facility ASP should be reviewed and approved through these same committees. • The facility ASP program should periodically report to the QAPI committee.
2. Accountability	Identify which members of the facility will be part of the stewardship team and clearly delineate their roles and responsibilities. Assign administrative leadership of the stewardship team to a single individual.	• Antibiotic stewardship is a team-based process that requires involvement and collaboration between leadership, providers, nursing staff, and pharmacy. • Although responsibility for completing the various stewardship-related tasks (eg, policy/guideline development, staff education/training, process/outcome tracking and reporting, stewardship intervention development and implementation) may be delegated to different members of the team, administrative oversight should be assigned to a single individual. • The stewardship team leader should have a clinical background plus a demonstrated capacity to work and communicate well with stakeholders in other disciplines who operate in the facility. The director of nursing, infection preventionist, nurse educator, or facility pharmacist are appropriate for this position.

3. Drug expertise	Ensure access to individuals with experience and/or training in antibiotic stewardship.	• Ideally, the individual selected to lead the facility stewardship team will have prior training/expertise in ID and/or antibiotic stewardship; but this will be unusual in most NFs.
		• In the absence of local expertise, the facility should
		  ○ Provide support for the stewardship team to attend stewardship training opportunities and pursue formal certification, if available.
		  ○ Identify and collaborate with experts in the region (eg, referring acute care hospital) who can help develop facility policies/guidelines and provide input on selection and implementation of different stewardship interventions.

(continued on next page)

Table 1 (continued)		
Component	Description	Comments
4. Action	Implement at least one policy or practice to improve antibiotic use in the facility.	• Specific strategies should be chosen based on facility resources and needs identified through tracking measures. • Strategies that focus on reducing unnecessary testing of urine samples and treatment of asymptomatic bacteriuria seem to have the greatest potential for immediate impact (see text).
5. Tracking	Monitor at least one *antibiotic utilization outcome* and one *clinical outcome* measure of antibiotic use in the facility.	• At a minimum, track facility-initiated antibiotic starts on a monthly basis (ideally, denominate by resident-days). Other measures to consider include proportion of antibiotic starts prescribed for >7 d[75] and proportion of antibiotic starts that meet appropriateness criteria.[74] • Clinical outcomes that should be considered include the monthly number of residents colonized or infected with different multidrug-resistant organisms (eg, MRSA), *C difficile*, and the facility antibiogram.[85]
6. Reporting	Provide regular feedback of antibiotic use and antibiotic resistance to staff and providers in the facility.	• Antibiotic utilization and clinical outcomes data should be presented at least quarterly at the facility QAPI meeting. • Providing individual feedback to providers on their prescribing patterns relative to their peers may have a beneficial normative influence on outliers.[77,89]
7. Education	Provide resources to staff, providers, and patients/residents about the risks of antibiotics and opportunities for improving antibiotic use.	• Education on the importance of antibiotic stewardship and the strategies the facility is using to promote better antibiotic stewardship should be delivered at hire and periodically thereafter. • Education should target both nursing staff and prescribers.[90,91]

Abbreviation: QAPI, quality assurance/performance improvement.

From Centers for Disease Control and Prevention. The core elements of antibiotic stewardship for nursing homes. Atlanta (GA): US Department of Health and Human Services, CDC; 2015; with permission.

one or 2 activities and gradually adding new strategies over time. Assessment checklists such as those developed by the CDC[63] are an excellent starting point for facilities and can help leadership identify and prioritize resource needs and also develop a road map for implementation of the various policies and procedures that can be used to improve antibiotic prescribing practices.

Leadership Commitment

There is little doubt that NFs will face increasing external pressures to demonstrate action focused around judicious use of antibiotics. Revised Centers for Medicare and Medicaid Services' (CMS) regulatory requirements[14] will require all NFs to have an ASP in place by November of 2017; facilities that fail to meet this standard are at risk of receiving a state survey deficiency citation (F-tag), which can incur significant financial penalties. Although external pressures such as those from CMS provide a needed initial impetus for change, it is critical that commitment for developing ASPs be internally motivated. Failure to proactively identify local needs, opportunities, and resources for improvement will likely result in a stewardship program that reacts only in response to regulatory actions and is unlikely to improve the outcomes of patients and residents. Consequently, it is critical that facility leadership, including the chief executive officer, medical director, and director of nursing (DON), provide visible support for facility ASPs and their attendant activities. Several arguments can be used to secure the support of leadership, including (1) a need to satisfy regulatory requirements focused on appropriate use of medications; (2) federal mandates to demonstrate meaningful organizational quality assurance and performance improvement[64]; (3) emerging federal policies to promote and ultimately require antibiotic stewardship activities across all health care settings[65]; (4) organizational costs of treating antibiotic-resistant and C difficile infections[66,67]; (5) avoidance of financial penalties arising from survey deficiencies for inappropriate medication use; and (6) how antibiotic stewardship interventions, particularly those focused around enhancing interdisciplinary communication, can generate corollary benefits in other processes and outcomes (eg, enhanced management of resident change in condition). Although the day-to-day involvement of these individuals in running the ASP may be minimal, leadership is responsible for making stewardship an organizational priority and communicating this to providers and staff, identifying the key stakeholders responsible for implementing the facility ASP, and providing the necessary resources and support needed for these stakeholders to be successful.

Programmatic Structure (Accountability and Expertise)

Guidelines recommend that the individual or individuals responsible for developing the facility ASP will possess ID expertise and/or specific training in antibiotic stewardship operations.[54,62] It is unrealistic to assume that NFs will be able to employ or even contract with individuals who have specific antibiotic stewardship expertise, although this may change in the future. Nevertheless, it is important that NFs, at a minimum, identify a local champion to develop and implement the facility's ASP. Ideally, the local champion will possess operational skills and expertise, including (1) long-term care clinical expertise; (2) an ability to meaningfully engage nursing staff and providers; (3) an understanding of facility pharmacy operations and how medication administration data are structured and stored; (4) an understanding of facility laboratory services and how results are structured and stored; and (5) an ability to interact with other key operational staff (eg, the infection preventionist as well as pharmacy, laboratory, and information technology staff) to identify opportunities to standardize and automate methods for tracking and reporting important process and outcome measures (see later discussion). Although a pharmacist may be the individual best positioned to fill this role, most NFs do not use pharmacists directly. Most pharmacists who work in NFs are contracted by the facilities to provide core services (eg, monthly medication reconciliation), and these individuals often play a limited role in the facility's day-to-day operations.[36] The infection preventionist or DON, who often performs double duty as the facility infection preventionist, may be the individuals best positioned to assume leadership responsibilities for the facility's ASP.

When available, the NF should attempt to cultivate collaborative or even formal consultative relationships with ID and antibiotic stewardship experts in referring hospitals. These individuals can be particularly helpful in the development and delivery of educational content for nursing staff and providers, development of guidelines for the treatment of commonly encountered infections, and development of effective antibiotic utilization tracking and reporting systems. The medical director and DON, even if they are not the designated ASP leaders, can play a critical role in growing the facility ASP by publicly affirming its importance and supporting improvement efforts. For example, NFs often have limited organizational influence over providers and the medical director can exert important social influence on his or her peers to adhere to ASP policies and practices. A recent case report of a Wisconsin NF identified medical director support and involvement as a key facilitator in the implementation of a facility ASP.[68] High levels of frontline staff turnover is a continuing problem in many NFs[69]; the DON plays an important role in bringing on new staff, continuing education of existing staff, as well as reinforcing expectations of staff responsible for assessment and communication of resident change in condition, both of which factor into provider decisions regarding initiation of antibiotics.[3,4,27]

Tracking and Reporting Antibiotic Utilization and Related Outcomes

A capability to track and report process and outcomes is a fundamental characteristic of successful quality improvement.[70] The infection preventionists in NFs are already engaged in tracking infections[71,72] and adapting this process to track antibiotic utilization and related outcomes (C difficile and multidrug-resistant organisms) should be feasible in most NFs. The penetration of electronic medical records in NFs remains limited; however, tracking methods to identify residents experiencing a change in condition, including those residents who are currently receiving antibiotics, is a common practice in these facilities.[73] Consequently, information on antibiotic starts is readily available and can be tracked at predefined time periods by the individual responsible for infection surveillance in the facility. At a minimum, facilities should periodically assess antibiotic utilization in the facility using a cross-sectional approach (eg, the number of residents on antibiotics during a given day, week, or month). However, cross-sectional assessments are not as sensitive to change as measures that are tracked more regularly. In order to monitor the effects of improvement interventions and detect aberrant prescribing patterns, post–acute care facilities should ideally track antibiotic starts and/or antibiotic DOT prospectively. Although tracking counts may be reasonable in settings where monthly census patterns are stable, tracking antibiotic utilization using incidence density measures (eg, antibiotic starts or DOT per 1000 resident-days) is more appropriate in settings where there is variation in monthly census data. Stratifying tracking measures by indication (eg, UTI) and antibiotic class (eg, fluoroquinolones) can help facilities better ascertain conditions in need of focused attention and follow the effects of condition-specific interventions. Supplementing utilization measures with assessments of appropriateness (eg, proportion of monthly antibiotic courses meeting explicit criteria[72,74] or proportion of monthly antibiotic courses exceeding 7 days[75]) can provide additional insights into opportunities for improvement.

Staff and Provider Education

Education is a foundational activity of the ASP. Educational content should cover the importance of antibiotic stewardship, plans for implementation of specific ASP activities, and the responsibilities of clinical staff in achieving ASP goals. Education should be targeted and tailored to nursing assistants, nursing staff, providers, residents, and families. Resident and family education, when combined with staff and provider education as well as interventions to enhance interdisciplinary communication, has also been shown to be associated with reductions in antibiotic use in NFs.[47] Studies such as these demonstrate that educational interventions can be powerful tools for changing behaviors but likely need to target multiple individuals[51] and be delivered via several modalities, including in-service training sessions, newsletters, pocket guides, posters, and brochures, in order to be maximally effective.

Giving providers feedback on their antibiotic prescribing patterns and engaging in interactive academic detailing are strategies that have been used to improve antibiotic prescribing in hospitals and outpatient settings[76,77] but has not been well studied in NFs. An educational intervention in which the aggregate prescribing practices of providers in a Chicago NF were compared with existing guideline recommendations was associated with a significant reduction in antibiotic utilization and improvement in adherence to prescribing guidelines.[48] However, giving providers a summary of the quality of their antibiotic prescribing did not have a sustained impact on antibiotic utilization in a cluster randomized controlled trial in French NFs.[49]

Antibiotic Stewardship Program Improvement Activities

There are several ASP activities from which post–acute care facilities can choose to implement. In general, these strategies map to one of 4 categories: (1) antibiotic prescribing policies/guidelines; (2) broad interventions; (3) pharmacy-driven interventions; and (4) syndrome-specific interventions. NFs should not attempt to implement all of these strategies simultaneously but rather should start with a single intervention, particularly one that is feasible based on available resources within a given setting.

Antibiotic prescribing policies

NFs should have policies stipulating that antibiotic orders include clear documentation of the drug, dose, duration and indication for treatment (eg, UTI).[62] Many hospitals use standardized antibiotic order forms to ensure that this information is captured reliably.[78] Use of standardized order forms can help the local ASP leader track antibiotic use more effectively and, when adapted to include decision-support content (eg, preferred agents, dosage adjustments for renal function and appropriateness criteria[74]), these tools can be a mechanism for educating facility providers. Unnecessary laboratory testing is a driver of antibiotic overuse.[79] There is considerable evidence that positive urine culture results exert an undue influence on prescriber decisions to initiate antibiotics, particularly in the post–acute care setting.[80–82] Accordingly, policies focused on reducing utilization of urine cultures should be assigned a high priority. Policies should specifically address testing urine samples with reagent strips (ie, the dipstick)[83,84] and performing urine cultures to confirm test of cure both of which are unnecessary and likely promote antibiotic overuse in NFs.[81] Other policy topics that facilities should consider include (1) appropriate testing for C difficile; (2) prohibitions against the routine use of broad-spectrum antibiotics (eg, fluoroquinolones)[85,86]; and (3) guidelines on how to treat commonly encountered infections. However, drafting effective treatment guidelines may require input from individuals with ID expertise who may not be easily available.[48]

Broad interventions

Two resource-intensive ASP interventions commonly used in hospitals include (1) formulary restrictions with prior authorization and (2) expert-led prospective audit and feedback to frontline providers.[55] It is unlikely that most NFs will have the resources to implement either of these intensive ASP activities successfully. Strategies focused on promotion of self-directed stewardship, in which prescribers are trained and/or prompted to engage in review of empirically initiated antibiotics and modify the therapeutic dose, spectrum, and/or duration when appropriate (antibiotic time-out), have been implemented successfully in a hospital setting with limited access to individuals with stewardship expertise.[33] Implementation of a checklist tool to foster self-directed

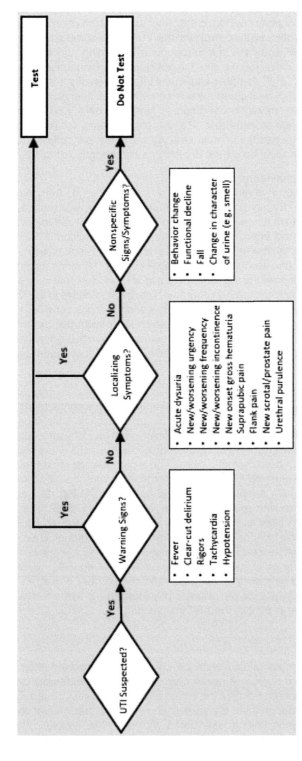

Fig. 3. Decision pathway to reduce unnecessary diagnostic testing of urine samples in long-term care facilities. (*Adapted from* Crnich CJ, Drinka P. Improving the management of urinary tract infections in nursing homes: it's time to stop the tail from wagging the dog. Ann Long Term Care 2014;43–7.)

stewardship activities in a cluster randomized controlled trial in 30 UK NFs was associated with a 5% reduction in systemic antibiotic use in intervention facilities versus a 5% increase in antibiotic use in control facilities.[53] Another broad strategy that should be feasible in the NF setting is the introduction of training and tools focused on improving resident assessments and interdisciplinary communication of resident change in condition.[44,87,88] As noted earlier, the introduction of standardized communication forms as part of multicomponent interventions has been associated with significant reductions in antibiotic utilization in North Carolina and Texas NFs.[46,47] Although the CDC recommends that NFs use antibiograms, facility-specific instruments are not widely available in most settings and there is insufficient evidence of their impact on prescribing behaviors to justify routine adoption at this time.[85]

Pharmacy-driven interventions

Examples of pharmacy interventions include automatic changes from intravenous to oral antibiotic therapy for highly bioavailable antibiotics (ie, ciprofloxacin, levofloxacin, trimethoprim-sulfamethoxazole, linezolid, and so forth), which reduces the need for intravenous access and improves patient safety and satisfaction. Pharmacists can perform automatic renal dose adjustments and dose optimization based on therapeutic drug monitoring (ie, vancomycin, aminoglycosides). Although postprescription review and feedback seem to be most effective with models that pair pharmacists with ID specialists, pharmacist-only programs have been effective in the NF setting.[37] Pharmacists engaged in postprescription review and feedback activities in this study possessed antibiotic stewardship expertise, which likely limits the implementation of this approach in most NFs. Unfortunately, pharmacists with this advanced antibiotic stewardship training are not typically available in most post–acute care facilities currently.[36]

Syndrome-specific interventions

Several practices that promote the overuse of antibiotics are common in many post–acute care facilities, specifically NFs. Prescribing prophylactic antibiotics to prevent recurrent UTIs, sending urine cultures to confirm test of cure and culturing open wounds are just some examples of questionable practices still encountered in NFs. However, treatment of asymptomatic bacteriuria is probably the most prevalent problem encountered in most NFs.[81,82] Implementation of protocols that restrict urine testing to residents with a high probability of having a UTI (**Fig. 3**)[45] and similarly designed protocols to limit antibiotic therapy in residents without clear signs and symptoms of UTI[41,43] have been associated with significant reductions in antibiotic utilization in NFs. These protocols should be operationalized through education of providers[27,28] and procedures that empower nursing staff to discourage providers from ordering diagnostic tests of the urine in the absence of specific, evidence-based criteria. Tracking the frequency of urine cultures and number of treated UTI events that do not satisfy surveillance definitions[72] provides targets that a facility can follow in order to assess the impact of the ASP intervention.

FUTURE DIRECTIONS

The emerging crisis in antibiotic resistance will require a concerted effort to improve antibiotic stewardship across all health care settings.[65] Considerable progress has been made in our understanding of the extent and determinants of inappropriate antibiotic use in NFs. Although there is accumulating evidence that interventions focused on processes (eg, urine testing) associated with the initial antibiotic decision can reduce unnecessary antibiotic use, there remains a critical need to identify the effectiveness of interventions that target postprescribing decision-making (eg, review and de-escalation) and how these interventions can be delivered in a cost-effective manner. There is also a need for more research on how to implement stewardship interventions with fidelity and sustain them over time, particularly in NFs with limited quality-improvement resources. Finally, there is a need for studies that evaluate the effects of stewardship interventions on facility and resident outcomes, including health care costs and rates of infections caused by C difficile and multidrug-resistant bacteria.

REFERENCES

1. Harris-Kojetin LD, Sengupta M, Park-Lee E, et al. Long-term care services in the United States: 2013 overview. National health care statistics report; no. 1. Hyattsville (MD): National Center for Health Statistics; 2013.
2. van Buul LW, van der Steen JT, Veenhuizen RB, et al. Antibiotic use and resistance in long term care facilities. J Am Med Dir Assoc 2012;13(6):568.e1-13.
3. Zimmer JG, Bentley DW, Valenti WM, et al. Systemic antibiotic use in nursing homes. A quality assessment. J Am Geriatr Soc 1986;34(10):703–10.
4. Warren JW, Palumbo FB, Fitterman L, et al. Incidence and characteristics of antibiotic use in aged nursing home patients. J Am Geriatr Soc 1991;39(10):963–72.
5. Pickering T, Gurwitz J, Zaleznik D, et al. The appropriateness of oral fluoroquinolone-prescribing in the long-term care setting. J Am Geriatr Soc 1994;42(1):28–32.
6. Loeb M, Simor AE, Landry L, et al. Antibiotic use in Ontario facilities that provide chronic care. J Gen Intern Med 2001;16(6):376–83.
7. Rotjanapan P, Dosa D, Thomas KS. Potentially inappropriate treatment of urinary tract infections in two Rhode Island nursing homes. Arch Intern Med 2011;171(5): 438–43.
8. Vergidis P, Hamer DH, Meydani SN, et al. Patterns of antimicrobial use for respiratory tract infections in older residents of long-term care facilities. J Am Geriatr Soc 2011;59(6):1093–8.
9. Doernberg SB, Dudas V, Trivedi KK. Implementation of an antimicrobial stewardship program targeting residents with urinary tract infections in three community long-term care facilities: a quasi-experimental study using time-series analysis. Antimicrob Resist Infect Control 2015;4(1):54.
10. Daneman N, Gruneir A, Newman A, et al. Antibiotic use in long-term care facilities. J Antimicrob Chemother 2011;66(12):2856–63.
11. Crnich CJ, Jump R, Trautner B, et al. Optimizing antibiotic stewardship in nursing homes: a narrative review and recommendations for improvement. Drugs Aging 2015;32(9):699–716.
12. Dellit TH, Owens RC, McGowan JE, et al. Infectious Diseases Society of America and the Society for Healthcare Epidemiology of America guidelines for developing an institutional program to enhance antimicrobial stewardship. Clin Infect Dis 2007;44(2):159–77.
13. Society for Healthcare Epidemiology of America, Infectious Diseases Society of America, Pediatric Infectious Diseases Society. Policy statement on antimicrobial stewardship by the Society for Healthcare Epidemiology of America (SHEA), the Infectious Diseases Society of America (IDSA), and the Pediatric Infectious Diseases Society (PIDS). Infect Control Hosp Epidemiol 2012;33(4):322–7.
14. Centers for Medicare & Medicaid Services (CMS). HHS reform of requirements for long-term care facilities. Final rule. Fed Regist 2016;81(192):68688–872.

15. Norman D, Grahn D. Yoshikawa T fever and aging. J Am Geriatr Soc 1985;33(12): 859–63.

16. Nicolle L, Bentley D, Garibaldi R, et al. Antimicrobial use in long-term-care facilities. Infect Control Hosp Epidemiol 2000;21(8):537–45.

17. Borg MA. National cultural dimensions as drivers of inappropriate ambulatory care consumption of antibiotics in Europe and their relevance to awareness campaigns. J Antimicrob Chemother 2012;67(3):763–7.

18. Charani E, Castro-Sanchez E, Sevdalis N, et al. Understanding the determinants of antimicrobial prescribing within hospitals: the role of "prescribing etiquette". Clin Infect Dis 2013;57(2):188–96.

19. Livorsi D, Comer A, Matthias MS, et al. Factors influencing antibiotic-prescribing decisions among inpatient physicians: a qualitative investigation. Infect Control Hosp Epidemiol 2015;36(9):1065–72.

20. Tjia J, Gurwitz JH, Briesacher BA. Challenge of changing nursing home prescribing culture. Am J Geriatr Pharmacother 2012;10(1):37–46.

21. Richards CL, Darradji M, Weinberg A, et al. Antimicrobial use in post-acute care: a retrospective descriptive analysis in seven long-term care facilities in Georgia. J Am Med Dir Assoc 2005;6(2):109–12.

22. Kistler CE, Sloane PD, Platts-Mills TF, et al. Challenges of antibiotic prescribing for assisted living residents: perspectives of providers, staff, residents, and family members. J Am Geriatr Soc 2013;61(4):565–70.

23. Whitson HE, Hastings SN, Lekan DA, et al. A quality improvement program to enhance after-hours telephone communication between nurses and physicians in a long-term care facility. J Am Geriatr Soc 2008;56(6):1080–6.

24. van Buul LW, van der Steen JT, Doncker SMMM, et al. Factors influencing antibiotic prescribing in long-term care facilities: a qualitative in-depth study. BMC Geriatr 2014;14:136.

25. Perkins A, Gagnon R, deGruy FA. Comparison of after-hours telephone calls concerning ambulatory and nursing home patients. J Fam Pract 1993;37(3): 247–50.

26. Tjia J, Mazor KM, Field T, et al. Nurse-physician communication in the long-term care setting: perceived barriers and impact on patient safety. J Patient Saf 2009; 5(3):145–52.

27. Walker S, McGeer A, Simor AE, et al. Why are antibiotics prescribed for asymptomatic bacteriuria in institutionalized elderly people? A qualitative study of physicians "and nurses" perceptions. CMAJ 2000;163(3):273–7.

28. Schweizer AK, Hughes CM, Macauley DC, et al. Managing urinary tract infections in nursing homes: a qualitative assessment. Pharm World Sci 2005;27(3):159–65.

29. Lim CJ, Kwong MWL, Stuart RL, et al. Antibiotic prescribing practice in residential aged care facilities–health care providers' perspectives. Med J Aust 2014;201(2): 98–102.

30. Stuart RL, Marshall C, Orr E, et al. Survey of infection control and antimicrobial stewardship practices in Australian residential aged-care facilities. Intern Med J 2015;45(5):576–80.

31. van der Steen JT, Ooms ME, Ribbe MW, et al. Decisions to treat or not to treat pneumonia in demented psychogeriatric nursing home patients: evaluation of a guideline. Alzheimer Dis Assoc Disord 2001;15(3):119–28.

32. Gross R, Morgan AS, Kinky DE, et al. Impact of a hospital-based antimicrobial management program on clinical and economic outcomes. Clin Infect Dis 2001;33(3):289–95.

33. Lee TC, Frenette C, Jayaraman D, et al. Antibiotic self-stewardship: trainee-led structured antibiotic time-outs to improve antimicrobial use. Ann Intern Med 2014;161(10 Suppl):S53–8.
34. Hamilton KW, Gerber JS, Moehring R, et al. Point-of-prescription interventions to improve antimicrobial stewardship. Clin Infect Dis 2015;60(8):1252–8.
35. Jump RLP, Olds DM, Seifi N, et al. Effective antimicrobial stewardship in a long-term care facility through an infectious disease consultation service: keeping a LID on antibiotic use. Infect Control Hosp Epidemiol 2012;33(12):1185–92.
36. Taylor L, Adibhatla S, Nace DA, et al. Antibiotic stewardship structure and process in Wisconsin nursing homes: a follow-up telephone survey. IDWeek a Joint Scientific Meeting of the Infectious Disease Society of America, Society for Healthcare Epidemiology of America, HIV Medical Association, and Pediatric Infectious Disease Society, New Orleans, LA. 2016.
37. Gugkaeva Z, Franson M. Pharmacist-led model of antibiotic stewardship in a long-term care facility. Ann Long Term Care 2012;20(10):22–6.
38. Nicolle LE. Antimicrobial stewardship in long term care facilities: what is effective? Antimicrob Resist Infect Control 2014;3(1):6.
39. Rhee SM, Stone ND. Antimicrobial stewardship in long-term care facilities. Infect Dis Clin North Am 2014;28(2):237–46.
40. Dyar OJ, Pagani L, Pulcini C. Strategies and challenges of antimicrobial stewardship in long-term care facilities. Clin Microbiol Infect 2015;21(1):10–9.
41. Loeb M, Brazil K, Lohfeld L, et al. Effect of a multifaceted intervention on number of antimicrobial prescriptions for suspected urinary tract infections in residents of nursing homes: cluster randomised controlled trial. BMJ 2005;331(7518):669.
42. Lohfeld L, Loeb M, Brazil K. Evidence-based clinical pathways to manage urinary tract infections in long-term care facilities: a qualitative case study describing administrator and nursing staff views. J Am Med Dir Assoc 2007;8(7):477–84.
43. Zabarsky TF, Sethi AK, Donskey CJ. Sustained reduction in inappropriate treatment of asymptomatic bacteriuria in a long-term care facility through an educational intervention. Am J Infect Control 2008;36(7):476–80.
44. Trautner BW, Grigoryan L, Petersen NJ, et al. Effectiveness of an antimicrobial stewardship approach for urinary catheter-associated asymptomatic bacteriuria. JAMA Intern Med 2015;175(7):1120–7.
45. Doron S, McElroy N, Salem-Schatz S, et al. Improved practice and decreased antibiotic utilization for urinary indications in long term care facilities after an educational intervention. Poster Presentation at: IDWeek a Joint Scientific Meeting of the Infectious Disease Society of America, Society for Healthcare Epidemiology of America, HIV Medical Association, and Pediatric Infectious Disease Society, Philadelphia, PA.
46. Frentzel E, Moudouni DKM, Garfinkel S, et al. Standardizing antibiotic use in long-term care settings (SAUL Study): final report. Agency for Healthcare Research and Quality accelerating (AHRQ) ACTION Contract No. 290-2006-000-191, Task Order No. 8. Washington, DC: American Institutes for Research; 2013.
47. Zimmerman S, Sloane PD, Bertrand R, et al. Successfully reducing antibiotic prescribing in nursing homes. J Am Geriatr Soc 2014;62(5):907–12.
48. Schwartz DN, Abiad H, DeMarais PL, et al. An educational intervention to improve antimicrobial use in a hospital-based long-term care facility. J Am Geriatr Soc 2007;55(8):1236–42.
49. Monette J, Miller M, Monette M, et al. Effect of an educational intervention on optimizing antibiotic prescribing in long-term care facilities. J Am Geriatr Soc 2007;55(8):1231–5.

50. Pettersson E, Vernby A, Mölstad S, et al. Can a multifaceted educational intervention targeting both nurses and physicians change the prescribing of antibiotics to nursing home residents? A cluster randomized controlled trial. J Antimicrob Chemother 2011;66(11):2659–66.

51. Naughton BJ, Mylotte JM, Ramadan F, et al. Antibiotic use, hospital admissions, and mortality before and after implementing guidelines for nursing home-acquired pneumonia. J Am Geriatr Soc 2001;49(8):1020–4.

52. Daneman N, Gruneir A, Bronskill SE, et al. Prolonged antibiotic treatment in long-term care: role of the prescriber. JAMA Intern Med 2013;173(8):673–82.

53. Fleet E, Gopal Rao G, Patel B, et al. Impact of implementation of a novel antimicrobial stewardship tool on antibiotic use in nursing homes: a prospective cluster randomized control pilot study. J Antimicrob Chemother 2014;69(8):2265–73.

54. Barlam TF, Cosgrove SE, Abbo LM, et al. Implementing an antibiotic stewardship program: guidelines by the Infectious Diseases Society of America and the Society for Healthcare Epidemiology of America. Clin Infect Dis 2016;62(10):e51–77.

55. Mehta JM, Haynes K, Wileyto EP, et al. Comparison of prior authorization and prospective audit with feedback for antimicrobial stewardship. Infect Control Hosp Epidemiol 2014;35(9):1092–9.

56. Bushen JL, Mehta JM, Hamilton KW, et al. Impact of two different antimicrobial stewardship methods on frequency of streamlining antimicrobial agents in patients with bacteremia. Infect Control Hosp Epidemiol 2017;38(1):89–95.

57. Van Schooneveld T, Miller H, Sayles H, et al. Survey of antimicrobial stewardship practices in Nebraska long-term care facilities. Infect Control Hosp Epidemiol 2011;32(7):732–4.

58. Malani AN, Brennan BM, Collins CD, et al. Antimicrobial stewardship practices in Michigan long-term care facilities. Infect Control Hosp Epidemiol 2016;37(2):236–7.

59. Crnich CJ, Adibhatla S, Van Schooneveld T, et al. A survey of antibiotic stewardship structure and process in Wisconsin nursing homes. IDWeek a Joint Scientific Meeting of the Infectious Disease Society of America, Society for Healthcare Epidemiology of America, HIV Medical Association, and Pediatric Infectious Disease Society, San Diego, CA.

60. Morrill HJ, Mermel LA, Baier RR, et al. Antimicrobial stewardship in Rhode Island long-term care facilities: current standings and future opportunities. Infect Control Hosp Epidemiol 2016;37(8):979–82.

61. Yang M, Vleck K, Bellantoni M, et al. Telephone survey of infection-control and antibiotic stewardship practices in long-term care facilities in Maryland. J Am Med Dir Assoc 2016;17(6):491–4.

62. Centers for Disease Control and Prevention. The core elements of antibiotic stewardship for nursing homes. Atlanta (GA): US Department of Health and Human Services, CDC; 2015.

63. Centers for Disease Control and Prevention checklist: the core elements of antibiotic stewardship for nursing homes. Available at: http://www.cdc.gov/longtermcare/pdfs/core-elements-antibiotic-stewardship-checklist.pdf. Accessed April 12, 2016.

64. Dellefield ME, Kelly A, Schnelle JF. Quality assurance and performance improvement in nursing homes: using evidence-based protocols to observe nursing care processes in real time. J Nurs Care Qual 2013;28(1):43–51.

65. The White House. National action plan for combating antibiotic-resistant bacteria. 2015. Available at: https://www.whitehouse.gov/sites/default/files/docs/national_action_plan_for_combating_antibotic-resistant_bacteria.pdf.

66. Capitano B, Leshem O, Nightingale C, et al. Cost effect of managing methicillin-resistant Staphylococcus aureus in a long-term care facility. J Am Geriatr Soc 2003;51(1):10–6.

67. Dubberke ER, Olsen MA. Burden of Clostridium difficile on the healthcare system. Clin Infect Dis 2012;55(Suppl 2):S88–92.

68. The Pew Charitable Trusts. A path to better antibiotic stewardship in inpatient settings. Available at: http://www.pewtrusts.org ~/media/assets/2016/04/apathto betterantibioticstewardshipininpatientsettings.pdf.

69. Castle N. Measuring staff turnover in nursing homes. Gerontologist 2006;46(2):210–9.

70. Pronovost PJ, Berenholtz SM. Needham DM translating evidence into practice: a model for large scale knowledge translation. BMJ 2008;337:a1714.

71. Smith P, Bennett G, Bradley S, et al. SHEA/APIC guideline: infection prevention and control in the long-term care facility. Infect Control Hosp Epidemiol 2008;29(9):785–814.

72. Stone ND, Ashraf MS, Calder J, et al. Surveillance definitions of infections in long-term care facilities: revisiting the McGeer criteria. Infect Control Hosp Epidemiol 2012;33(10):965–77.

73. Fisch J, McNamara SE, Lansing BJ, et al. The 24-hour report as an effective monitoring and communication tool in infection prevention and control in nursing homes. Am J Infect Control 2014;42(10):1112–4.

74. Loeb M, Bentley DW, Bradley S, et al. Development of minimum criteria for the initiation of antibiotics in residents of long-term-care facilities: results of a consensus conference. Infect Control Hosp Epidemiol 2001;22(2):120–4.

75. Mylotte JM. Antimicrobial stewardship in long-term care: metrics and risk adjustment. J Am Med Dir Assoc 2016;17(7):672.e13-8.

76. Davey P, Brown E, Fenelon L, et al. Interventions to improve antibiotic prescribing practices for hospital inpatients. Cochrane Database Syst Rev 2005;(4):CD003543.

77. Gerber JS, Prasad PA, Fiks AG, et al. Effect of an outpatient antimicrobial stewardship intervention on broad-spectrum antibiotic prescribing by primary care pediatricians: a randomized trial. JAMA 2013;309(22):2345–52.

78. Gyssens IC, Blok WL, van den Broek PJ, et al. Implementation of an educational program and an antibiotic order form to optimize quality of antimicrobial drug use in a department of internal medicine. Eur J Clin Microbiol Infect Dis 1997;16(12):904–12.

79. Morgan DJ, Croft LD, Deloney V, et al. Choosing wisely in healthcare epidemiology and antimicrobial stewardship. Infect Control Hosp Epidemiol 2016;37(7):755–60.

80. Phillips CD, Adepoju O, Stone N, et al. Asymptomatic bacteriuria, antibiotic use, and suspected urinary tract infections in four nursing homes. BMC Geriatr 2012;12:73.

81. Crnich CJ, Drinka P. Improving the management of urinary tract infections in nursing homes: it's time to stop the tail from wagging the dog. Ann Long Term Care 2014;43–7.

82. Nace DA, Drinka PJ, Crnich CJ. Clinical uncertainties in the approach to long term care residents with possible urinary tract infection. J Am Med Dir Assoc 2014;15(2):133–9.

83. Ducharme J, Neilson S, Ginn JL. Can urine cultures and reagent test strips be used to diagnose urinary tract infection in elderly emergency department patients without focal urinary symptoms? CJEM 2007;9(2):87–92.

84. Arinzon Z, Peisakh A, Shuval I, et al. Detection of urinary tract infection (UTI) in long-term care setting: is the multireagent strip an adequate diagnostic tool? Arch Gerontol Geriatr 2009;48(2):227–31.

85. Furuno JP, Comer AC, Johnson JK, et al. Using antibiograms to improve antibiotic prescribing in skilled nursing facilities. Infect Control Hosp Epidemiol 2014; 35(Suppl 3):S56–61.

86. Wenisch JM, Equiluz-Bruck S, Fudel M, et al. Decreasing Clostridium difficile infections by an antimicrobial stewardship program that reduces moxifloxacin use. Antimicrob Agents Chemother 2014;58(9):5079–83.

87. Ouslander JG, Lamb G, Tappen R, et al. Interventions to reduce hospitalizations from nursing homes: evaluation of the INTERACT II collaborative quality improvement project. J Am Geriatr Soc 2011;59(4):745–53.

88. Linnebur SA, Fish DN, Ruscin JM, et al. Impact of a multidisciplinary intervention on antibiotic use for nursing home-acquired pneumonia. Am J Geriatr Pharmacother 2011;9(6):442–50.e1.

89. Meeker D, Linder JA, Fox CR, et al. Effect of behavioral interventions on inappropriate antibiotic prescribing among primary care practices: a randomized clinical trial. JAMA 2016;315(6):562–70.

90. Jump RLP, Heath B, Crnich CJ, et al. Knowledge, beliefs, and confidence regarding infections and antimicrobial stewardship: a survey of Veterans Affairs providers who care for older adults. Am J Infect Control 2015;43(3):298–300.

91. Heath B, Bernhardt J, Michalski TJ, et al. Results of a Veterans Affairs employee education program on antimicrobial stewardship for older adults. Am J Infect Control 2016;44(3):349–51.

Antimicrobial Use at the End of Life

Adam Baghban, MD, Manisha Juthani-Mehta, MD*

KEYWORDS

- Antimicrobials • Antibiotics • End of life • Palliative care

KEY POINTS

- Antimicrobials are overused in the final weeks of life.
- Common goals of antimicrobial use at the end of life are prolongation of survival and relief of symptoms.
- End-of-life patients are a heterogeneous population. Antimicrobials are more likely to achieve specific goals within some subgroups than others.
- Decisions regarding antimicrobial use at the end of life should incorporate the patients' goals and the likelihood of achieving those goals.

INTRODUCTION

Health care providers of patients at the end of life (EOL) have the responsibility of reevaluating an evolving balance between potential benefits and harms of a variety of otherwise common medical interventions. Medicine is failing at this task across many medical specialties. Recent data suggest that 33% to 38% of patients at the EOL receive interventions that they are unlikely to benefit from, and 22.4% to 42% of patients die in the intensive care unit (ICU).[1,2] These statistics include antimicrobial use, which tends to be one of the last interventions withdrawn or withheld, with 27% to 88% of patients receiving antimicrobials during the final weeks of life.[3–7] In EOL patients with documentation of a suspected infection, antimicrobials are withheld in a small number of cases.[8] For example, as many as 92% to 100% of patients with cancer receiving hospice and palliative care are treated with antimicrobials in this setting.[8] This high rate of antimicrobial use may be because providers view antimicrobials differently from invasive interventions, such as mechanical ventilation and cardiopulmonary resuscitation. Many providers may believe that antimicrobials carry a lower potential for harm.

Disclosure Statement: Both authors have no commercial or financial conflicts of interest.
Section of Infectious Diseases, Department of Internal Medicine, Yale School of Medicine, PO Box 208022, New Haven, CT 06520, USA
* Corresponding author.
E-mail address: manisha.juthani@yale.edu

Infect Dis Clin N Am 31 (2017) 639–647
http://dx.doi.org/10.1016/j.idc.2017.07.009
0891-5520/17/© 2017 Elsevier Inc. All rights reserved.

Although there is a high utilization of antimicrobials at the EOL, data suggest that much of this use is in the absence of a documented infection. One study found that 15.6% of patients who transitioned to a comfort care protocol remained on antimicrobials, and 31% of those on antimicrobials did not have a documented infectious diagnosis.[9] Another study found that among hospice patients who received antibiotics in the last 7 days of life, only 15% had a documented infectious diagnosis.[3] These high rates of antimicrobial use delineate the importance of clearly defining the goals of these therapies in patients at the EOL. To date, most available data on antimicrobial use at the EOL are retrospective.[10] Not only are prospective studies uncommon but ethical considerations also limit the feasibility of randomized controlled trials.[11,12] Consensus guidelines were previously unavailable. However, newly published antimicrobial stewardship guidelines by the Infectious Diseases Society of America have broached the subject of antimicrobials at the EOL by suggesting that antimicrobial stewardship programs should provide support to clinicians in decisions related to antibiotic use.[13]

PATIENT POPULATIONS AND POPULATION-SPECIFIC CONSIDERATIONS

For this review, EOL is defined as the final weeks before death. The most commonly studied patient populations are those with advanced dementia, those with advanced malignancies, and those enrolled in hospice programs. Studies in palliative care units and hospice programs often include mixed populations. Because data on antimicrobial use at the EOL are limited, studies from one patient population may guide others. However, it is important to keep patient-specific nuances in mind.

A study by Ahronheim and colleagues[6] compared management of patients with metastatic solid tumors to those with advanced dementia before their deaths at a tertiary care hospital. These 2 groups of patients had similar rates of nonpalliative invasive treatments (eg, hemodialysis, enteral tube feeding) and cardiopulmonary resuscitation attempts. Patients with cancer were more likely to receive invasive (eg, lumbar puncture, bronchoscopy) and noninvasive (eg, blood work, radiographs) diagnostic testing, much of which was for suspected infection. The overall rate of antibiotic administration in the 2 groups was high at 88%, most of which was empiric, particularly for patients with cancer.

Patients with cancer at the EOL have been found to receive antibiotics more often than advanced dementia patients, frequently in the absence of a documented infection.[3,14] These results highlight not only overall similarities but also subtle differences in health care providers' approaches to these 2 EOL populations. Some of these differences may reflect the tempo of the underlying disease process. In advanced dementia patients in whom deterioration typically occurs over a longer period of time, patients, families, and providers may alter their approach to medical management decisions by favoring less aggressive measures with each stepwise decline in overall health. In advanced cancer where a more acute deterioration can occur, patients, families, and providers may be attached to the goal for cure or prolongation of life, thereby favoring more aggressive diagnostic and treatment strategies.

Noninfectious fever is an important reason for overuse of antimicrobials and may occur at different rates in patients with malignancies and dementia. When fever occurs without other localizing signs of infection, alternative causes of an elevated temperature such as drug-induced, venous thromboembolism and neoplastic fever should be considered. Although patients both with dementia and with cancer can develop noninfectious fever, this diagnosis is particularly relevant to patients with advanced malignancies. The finding that antimicrobials are used empirically more often in patients with cancer may be related to the fact that malignancies can be the direct cause of fever, with cancer identified as the underlying cause of fever of unknown origin in 7% to 19% of cases.[15–18] The incidence of neoplastic fever is increased in patients with hematologic malignancies and metastatic tumors, although it has been described with a wide variety of cancers. Fevers caused by malignancy are associated with fewer symptoms than those resulting from infection,[19] a greater antipyretic response to nonsteroidal anti-inflammatory drugs than acetaminophen,[19–21] and a low procalcitonin.[22–24] Typically, neoplastic fever is a diagnosis of exclusion, and empiric antimicrobials are administered while undertaking further evaluation. However, this approach may not be universally appropriate for patients with advanced cancer at the EOL, for whom the primary goal is palliation, particularly if fever is the only sign of potential infection and symptoms are minimal.

For patients with advanced dementia, nursing homes are the most common site of death.[25] Consequentially, care of nursing home residents is complicated by close living quarters and the risk of nosocomial infectious outbreaks. Given the progressive cognitive decline present in these patients, many EOL decisions must be made by health care proxies. Decreased verbalization of symptoms presents a barrier to accurate diagnosis of infections in this patient population. For example, using bacteriuria and pyuria as the sole criteria for diagnosis of urinary tract infection in patients who cannot express symptoms leads to overtreatment of asymptomatic bacteriuria.[26,27]

GOALS OF ANTIMICROBIAL THERAPY

Increased patient survival is a common goal of antimicrobial use. In patients near the EOL, a determination as to whether the goal of prolonged survival is congruent with the overall goals of care should be made. Antimicrobials are unable to alter the natural history of the underlying disease in most patients at the EOL, and hence, this goal of prolonging life should be weighed against the risk of prolonging suffering.[28] Furthermore, data regarding prolongation of life with antimicrobial use in the final weeks of life are mixed. One study evaluated survival in patients who chose either "full use" of antimicrobials, to avoid antimicrobials entirely, or to accept antimicrobials only when there were symptoms attributed to an infection. They did not find a survival difference between these groups.[29] Another survey of inpatients in a palliative care unit did not find a statistically significant difference in survival for patients with an identified bacterial infection.[30] In contrast, prospective data suggest that survival may be increased in EOL patients with pneumonia who receive antimicrobials.[12]

Rather than focusing on extending survival in EOL patients, a goal of palliation is often deemed appropriate by patients and health care providers. An important aspect of this paradigm shift toward symptom relief and minimization of suffering is individualization of care. Antimicrobials likely increase comfort in specific patient populations and infections (eg, urinary tract infections). In one study, antimicrobials administered to patients with advanced cancer with identified infections in the last several weeks of life led to symptomatic relief in only 33% of patients. This benefit was seen in an even smaller minority of those patients (9.2%) in their last week of life.[31] The same study also reported that patients receiving potentially painful invasive measures, such as indwelling catheters and surgical procedures, were less likely to have a perceived symptomatic benefit from antimicrobial therapy in the setting of a suspected infection. These findings suggest that the palliative benefit from anti-infective therapy is not universal, but may have a role for some patients with certain infections.

The Choices, Attitudes, and Strategies for Care of Advanced Dementia at the End-of-Life study conducted by Givens and colleagues[12] is one of the few prospective studies of antimicrobial therapy at the EOL. In this study, the efficacy of antimicrobial therapy on the outcomes of both survival and palliation in nursing home residents with advanced dementia and pneumonia was evaluated. A survival benefit was seen in patients who received antimicrobials for suspected pneumonia. This benefit was present regardless of the route of drug administration. In contrast, lower comfort levels were observed in patients who received antimicrobials. These findings suggest a tradeoff between the goals of prolonging survival and reducing symptoms. They are also in contrast with previously published reports of a possible role for antimicrobials in palliation of EOL patients with pneumonia.[32,33] These discrepancies may reflect the challenges of symptom assessment in patients with advanced dementia.

Despite evidence of significant antimicrobial use described thus far, most patients may have preferences in stark contrast with these practices. A survey of patients with advanced cancer in community-based hospice programs found that 79.2% preferred to either avoid antimicrobials altogether or to use antimicrobials with the goal of symptomatic relief only.[29] Patients and health care proxies may not have the opportunity to address these wishes with health care providers. In a cohort of patients with advanced dementia, despite 94.8% of health care proxies stating that comfort was their primary objective, 72.4% of suspected infections were treated with antimicrobials. Only 45.3% of patients or health care proxies were asked about their preferences for antimicrobial use, and fewer received counseling on this issue.[34] Similarly, another study found that the health care proxies of patients with advanced dementia were aware of suspected infections in 39% of cases, and only 57% of those who were aware of a suspected infection participated in the decision-making process.[35]

POTENTIAL BENEFITS OF ANTIMICROBIAL THERAPY

Although antimicrobial use in EOL patients does not universally result in positive survival and symptomatic outcomes, these patient populations are heterogeneous. There may be subgroups of patients with greater potential for benefit. As outlined above, antimicrobial use for pneumonia at the EOL does not consistently demonstrate an improvement in survival or symptomatic relief in patients with advanced dementia. Beyond these findings, some studies have suggested that antimicrobial therapy for urinary tract infections in EOL patients is more likely to result in resolution of symptoms than therapy for other sites of infection, with the least symptomatic benefit seen in bloodstream infections.[29,36,37] In addition, treatment of symptomatic infections may contribute to improvement in psychological distress.[30] Intuitively, individual patients with painful symptoms directly attributable to particular infections, such as herpes simplex virus, varicella zoster virus, or oral candidiasis, should be treated with antimicrobials with a goal of palliation. Treatment of these infections should not impact mortality, but may provide symptom relief, which is the primary goal of palliative care.

POTENTIAL HARMS OF ANTIMICROBIAL THERAPY

One potential for harm secondary to antimicrobial use relates to the route of drug administration. The use of intravenous devices for parenteral antibiotics carries the risk of phlebitis, local skin and soft tissue infections, and secondary bacteremia. Furthermore, insertion of either central or peripheral venous access catheters is painful and may necessitate mechanical restraints in delirious or demented patients, which are outcomes in direct opposition to a goal of palliation. Despite these risks, as many as 82% of patients with terminal cancer receive parenteral antibiotics.[31] Patients in hospice units are more likely to receive oral antimicrobials, accounting for up to 83% of antimicrobial use in this setting, compared with patients in acute care settings or tertiary palliative care units. In these inpatient settings, intravenous therapy is more frequent, and alternative invasive routes such as intramuscular administration are also reported.[38] A potential explanation for the increased use of parenteral antimicrobials in a tertiary palliative care setting is that many patients in such units have pain that requires intravenous opiates. In addition, some patients may have difficulty with oral medications because of odynophagia related to thrush, mucositis, or their underlying condition, making parenteral therapy the less painful route.

Health care providers should weigh the risk of adverse drug side effects and immunologically mediated allergic reactions against the drug's potential benefit to patients when they prescribe antimicrobials. Undesirable drug reactions may be more clinically significant in EOL patients because of underlying frailty and polypharmacy. Antibiotic-associated diarrhea is one such example. A large prospective study compared rates of antibiotic-associated diarrhea across multiple medical settings and found the highest rate (7.1%) in the geriatrics unit. Half of the patients tested were positive for *Clostridium difficile*.[39] As another example, an association between beta-lactam antibiotics and seizures has been described. The risk of seizure with beta-lactam use is likely higher in patients with underlying central nervous system structural abnormalities and encephalopathy and hence may disproportionately affect patients in their final weeks of life.[40] It is important to consider these adverse effects when using antimicrobials in EOL patients, because antibiotics administered in nonbeneficial scenarios can have devastating consequences for patients and their families.

In addition to adverse patient outcomes, societal costs of nonbeneficial treatments are significant. As mentioned previously, one-fifth to almost one-half of patients die during a hospitalization with an ICU admission. The average cost of a terminal ICU admission is between $24,541 and $39,315, with drugs accounting for 4.1% of these costs.[2,41] Terminal non-ICU admissions cost an average of $8548.[2] A recent comparison between EOL expenditures in 7 countries found that although a lower percentage of patients in the United States die in the hospital compared with several western European countries and Canada, the United States had the highest percentage of ICU admissions in the final 180 days of life.[42] Avoidance of interventions that are not beneficial to patients at the EOL, including antimicrobials in many instances, is a crucial step in reducing these costs.

The increasing prevalence of multidrug-resistant organisms (MDROs) is an additional adverse societal outcome associated with antimicrobial overuse. MDROs are especially significant in nursing homes, where many patients with advanced dementia die. Colonization with any MDRO in a 12-month period can be as high as 66.9% of nursing home residents, and the 12-month incidence of acquisition of an MDRO is 47.9%.[34] A study of ICU patients identified EOL antimicrobial use as a risk factor for colonization with drug-resistant organisms and hypothesized that this patient population is a reservoir for MDROs in the ICU.[43] Antimicrobial stewardship programs limiting the inappropriate use of antimicrobials decrease the prevalence of MDROs in health care settings.[13,44] Reducing the use of nonbeneficial antimicrobials in EOL patients may aid in combating this epidemic.

PROPOSED ALGORITHM FOR MANAGEMENT

The authors propose the following guidelines for management of patients at the EOL with suspected infections (**Fig. 1**). First, the use of antimicrobial agents should be included in a comprehensive goals-of-care discussion, ideally during routine care. This conversation should include the education of patients and health care proxies regarding the harms and benefits of diagnostic testing and antimicrobial therapy.

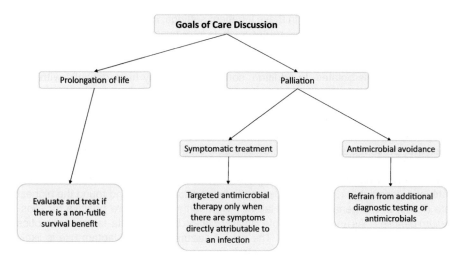

Fig. 1. A proposed algorithm for use of antimicrobial agents at the EOL that begins with discussing antimicrobial use during a comprehensive goals-of-care discussion.

Options, including the limitation of antimicrobials to palliative use and complete abstinence from antimicrobials, should be broached. Future decisions regarding antimicrobial use should take into account the educated wishes of the patient and their health care proxies. Second, when considering antimicrobial therapy for a suspected infection, the patient's life expectancy, symptoms, and the possibility of noninfectious fever should be considered. As discussed thus far, antimicrobials are unable to alter the progression of advanced dementia or cancer, may or may not affect survival time in some patient populations, and conversely may prolong suffering. If the patient has symptoms attributable to an infection (eg, dysuria, odynophagia), it is reasonable to consider treating a suspected infection, with urinary tract infections being the most likely to result in symptomatic improvement. Finally, nonparenteral routes of administration should be used, unless intravenous access is otherwise necessary for therapies such as pain medication or there is severe odynophagia related to their underlying condition.

SUMMARY

Health care providers across medical specialties continue to use societal resources for nonbeneficial treatments at the EOL, which at best will not help and at worst can harm their patients. Antimicrobials are not exempt from this problem. The authors have proposed an approach to management of suspected infections in patients at the EOL. Providers should carefully consider the appropriate goals of such therapy for individual patients and the likelihood of achieving such goals.

REFERENCES

1. Cardona-Morrell M, Kim J, Turner RM, et al. Non-beneficial treatments in hospital at the end of life: a systematic review on extent of the problem. Int J Qual Health Care 2016;28(4):456–69.

2. Angus DC, Barnato AE, Linde-Zwirble WT, et al. Use of intensive care at the end of life in the United States: an epidemiologic study. Crit Care Med 2004;32(3): 638–43.

3. Albrecht JS, McGregor JC, Fromme EK, et al. A nationwide analysis of antibiotic use in hospice care in the final week of life. J Pain Symptom Manage 2013;46(4): 483–90.

4. Oh DY, Kim JH, Kim DW, et al. Antibiotic use during the last days of life in cancer patients. Eur J Cancer Care 2006;15(1):74–9.

5. Thompson AJ, Silveira MJ, Vitale CA, et al. Antimicrobial use at the end of life among hospitalized patients with advanced cancer. Am J Hosp Palliat Care 2012;29(8):599–603.

6. Ahronheim JC, Morrison RS, Baskin SA, et al. Treatment of the dying in the acute care hospital. Advanced dementia and metastatic cancer. Arch Intern Med 1996; 156(18):2094–100.

7. D'Agata E, Mitchell SL. Patterns of antimicrobial use among nursing home residents with advanced dementia. Arch Intern Med 2008;168(4):357–62.

8. Rosenberg JH, Albrecht JS, Fromme EK, et al. Antimicrobial use for symptom management in patients receiving hospice and palliative care: a systematic review. J Palliat Med 2013;16(12):1568–74.

9. Merel SE, Meier CA, McKinney CM, et al. Antimicrobial use in patients on a comfort care protocol: a retrospective cohort study. J Palliat Med 2016;19(11):1210–4.

10. Juthani-Mehta M, Malani PN, Mitchell SL. Antimicrobials at the end of life: an opportunity to improve palliative care and infection management. JAMA 2015; 314(19):2017–8.

11. Stiel S, Krumm N, Pestinger M, et al. Antibiotics in palliative medicine–results from a prospective epidemiological investigation from the HOPE survey. Support Care Cancer 2012;20(2):325–33.

12. Givens JL, Jones RN, Shaffer ML, et al. Survival and comfort after treatment of pneumonia in advanced dementia. Arch Intern Med 2010;170(13):1102–7.

13. Barlam TF, Cosgrove SE, Abbo LM, et al. Implementing an antibiotic stewardship program: guidelines by the Infectious Diseases Society of America and the Society for Healthcare Epidemiology of America. Clin Infect Dis 2016;62(10):e51–77.

14. Furuno JP, Noble BN, Horne KN, et al. Frequency of outpatient antibiotic prescription on discharge to hospice care. Antimicrob Agents Chemother 2014;58(9): 5473–7.

15. Nagy-Agren S, Haley H. Management of infections in palliative care patients with advanced cancer. J Pain Symptom Manage 2002;24(1):64–70.

16. Horowitz HW. Fever of unknown origin or fever of too many origins? N Engl J Med 2013;368(3):197–9.

17. Vanderschueren S, Knockaert D, Adriaenssens T, et al. From prolonged febrile illness to fever of unknown origin: the challenge continues. Arch Intern Med 2003;163(9):1033–41.

18. Bleeker-Rovers CP, Vos FJ, de Kleijn EM, et al. A prospective multicenter study on fever of unknown origin: the yield of a structured diagnostic protocol. Medicine (Baltimore) 2007;86(1):26–38.

19. Zell JA, Chang JC. Neoplastic fever: a neglected paraneoplastic syndrome. Support Care Cancer 2005;13(11):870–7.

20. Chang JC, Gross HM. Utility of naproxen in the differential diagnosis of fever of undetermined origin in patients with cancer. Am J Med 1984;76(4):597–603.

21. Chang JC, Gross HM. Neoplastic fever responds to the treatment of an adequate dose of naproxen. J Clin Oncol 1985;3(4):552–8.

22. Vincenzi B, Fioroni I, Pantano F, et al. Procalcitonin as diagnostic marker of infection in solid tumors patients with fever. Sci Rep 2016;6:28090.
23. Shomali W, Hachem R, Chaftari AM, et al. Can procalcitonin distinguish infectious fever from tumor-related fever in non-neutropenic cancer patients? Cancer 2012; 118(23):5823–9.
24. Sakr Y, Sponholz C, Tuche F, et al. The role of procalcitonin in febrile neutropenic patients: review of the literature. Infection 2008;36(5):396–407.
25. Mitchell SL. CLINICAL PRACTICE. Advanced dementia. N Engl J Med 2015; 372(26):2533–40.
26. Mody L, Juthani-Mehta M. Urinary tract infections in older women: a clinical review. JAMA 2014;311(8):844–54.
27. Nicolle LE, Bradley S, Colgan R, et al. Infectious Diseases Society of America guidelines for the diagnosis and treatment of asymptomatic bacteriuria in adults. Clin Infect Dis 2005;40(5):643–54.
28. Decisions near the end of life. Council on Ethical and Judicial Affairs, American Medical Association. JAMA 1992;267(16):2229–33.
29. White PH, Kuhlenschmidt HL, Vancura BG, et al. Antimicrobial use in patients with advanced cancer receiving hospice care. J Pain Symptom Manage 2003;25(5): 438–43.
30. Vitetta L, Kenner D, Sali A. Bacterial infections in terminally ill hospice patients. J Pain Symptom Manage 2000;20(5):326–34.
31. Nakagawa S, Toya Y, Okamoto Y, et al. Can anti-infective drugs improve the infection-related symptoms of patients with cancer during the terminal stages of their lives? J Palliat Med 2010;13(5):535–40.
32. van der Steen JT, Ooms ME, van der Wal G, et al. Pneumonia: the demented patient's best friend? Discomfort after starting or withholding antibiotic treatment. J Am Geriatr Soc 2002;50(10):1681–8.
33. Van Der Steen JT, Pasman HR, Ribbe MW, et al. Discomfort in dementia patients dying from pneumonia and its relief by antibiotics. Scand J Infect Dis 2009;41(2): 143–51.
34. Mitchell SL, Shaffer ML, Loeb MB, et al. Infection management and multidrug-resistant organisms in nursing home residents with advanced dementia. JAMA Intern Med 2014;174(10):1660–7.
35. Givens JL, Spinella S, Ankuda CK, et al. Healthcare proxy awareness of suspected infections in nursing home residents with advanced dementia. J Am Geriatr Soc 2015;63(6):1084–90.
36. Reinbolt RE, Shenk AM, White PH, et al. Symptomatic treatment of infections in patients with advanced cancer receiving hospice care. J Pain Symptom Manage 2005;30(2):175–82.
37. Clayton J, Fardell B, Hutton-Potts J, et al. Parenteral antibiotics in a palliative care unit: prospective analysis of current practice. Palliat Med 2003;17(1):44–8.
38. Oneschuk D, Fainsinger R, Demoissac D. Antibiotic use in the last week of life in three different palliative care settings. J Palliat Care 2002;18(1):25–8.
39. Wistrom J, Norrby SR, Myhre EB, et al. Frequency of antibiotic-associated diarrhoea in 2462 antibiotic-treated hospitalized patients: a prospective study. J Antimicrob Chemother 2001;47(1):43–50.
40. Sutter R, Ruegg S, Tschudin-Sutter S. Seizures as adverse events of antibiotic drugs: a systematic review. Neurology 2015;85(15):1332–41.
41. Khandelwal N, Benkeser D, Coe NB, et al. Patterns of cost for patients dying in the intensive care unit and implications for cost savings of palliative care interventions. J Palliat Med 2016;19(11):1171–8.

42. Bekelman JE, Halpern SD, Blankart CR, et al. Comparison of site of death, health care utilization, and hospital expenditures for patients dying with cancer in 7 developed countries. JAMA 2016;315(3):272–83.

43. Levin PD, Simor AE, Moses AE, et al. End-of-life treatment and bacterial antibiotic resistance: a potential association. Chest 2010;138(3):588–94.

44. Montoya A, Cassone M, Mody L. Infections in nursing homes: epidemiology and prevention programs. Clin Geriatr Med 2016;32(3):585–607.

Breaking the Chain of Infection in Older Adults

A Review of Risk Factors and Strategies for Preventing Device-Related Infections

Gregory Schrank, MD[a], Westyn Branch-Elliman, MD, MMSc[b],*

KEYWORDS

- Infection prevention • Multidrug-resistant organisms • Indwelling devices
- Older adults • Antimicrobial stewardship

KEY POINTS

- Device-related infections are a leading cause of health care–associated infections in older adults.
- Indwelling devices are a risk factor for multidrug-resistant bacterial colonization.
- Host, pathogen, device, and environmental factors all contribute to the development of infection.
- Limiting utilization of these devices and practicing infection prevention techniques can reduce the likelihood of infection and limit transmission of multidrug-resistant pathogens.

INTRODUCTION

Device-related infections (DRIs) in older adults are a substantial cause of morbidity and mortality, and they place a significant economic burden on the health care system of the United States.[1–4] As the number of persons the over the age of 65 increases to 83.7 million by 2050, comprising 20% of the total US population, the incidence of health care–associated infections (HAIs), and DRIs in particular, is expected to increase accordingly.[5]

At the end of 2014, there were 1.4 million persons residing in long-term care facilities (LTCFs) in the Unites States, almost 10% of whom were over the age of 85.[6] Studies

W. Branch-Elliman is supported by a Veterans' Integrated Service Network (VISN-1) Career Development Award.

Conflicts of Interest: None.

[a] Department of Medicine, Division of Infectious Diseases, Beth Israel Deaconess Medical Center, Harvard Medical School, 330 Brookline Avenue, Boston, MA 02215, USA; [b] Medical Service, Section of Infectious Diseases, VA Boston Healthcare System, Harvard Medical School, 1400 VFW Parkway, West Roxbury, MA 02132, USA

* Corresponding author.

E-mail address: wbranche@bidmc.harvard.edu

Infect Dis Clin N Am 31 (2017) 649–671
http://dx.doi.org/10.1016/j.idc.2017.07.004
0891-5520/17/Published by Elsevier Inc.

id.theclinics.com

suggest that 5% to 7% of these residents will develop an HAI during their stay.[7,8] In the United States alone, up to 3.8 million HAIs occur in residents of LTCFs annually.[1,6]

Indwelling devices provide a portal of entry for potential pathogens to enter a susceptible host and set the stage for future infections. The most common indwelling devices are urinary catheters, which predispose patients to catheter-associated urinary tract infections (CAUTIs). Because of a variety of host factors in older adults, including medical illness and incontinence, approximately 13% of new admissions to skilled nursing facilities from acute care facilities have a urinary catheter in place at the time of admission.[9] Up to 22% of LTCF residents have a urinary catheter in place at any given time, indwelling for an average duration of 105 days.[9–12] In addition, an estimated 9% of home care recipients have an indwelling urinary catheter.[12]

The other 2 most commonly used indwelling devices in older adults are percutaneous feeding tubes and central venous catheters (CVCs), which include peripherally inserted central catheters (PICCs), central venous lines, midline catheters, and ports. An estimated 6% to 8% of all residents in LTCFs have a feeding tube, with higher rates in patients with cognitive impairments.[7,13,14] Because intravenous treatments, such as parenteral nutrition and antimicrobials, are increasingly delivered outside of the acute care setting, use of PICC lines in skilled nursing facilities has increased to a prevalence of at least 22%.[15]

Many factors interact to contribute to the frequency and severity of DRIs in older adults. The "Chain of Infection" is a general infection prevention framework that can be used to evaluate the major elements that lead to HAIs and to identify modifiable risk factors that can be targeted to reduce future infections (**Fig. 1**). Host factors, including immune dysfunction and fragile skin, provide an opening for opportunistic pathogens to invade and cause an infection. Bacterial factors, including antimicrobial resistance and biofilms, provide health care–associated organisms with competitive advantages for invasion and pathogenesis. Environmental factors, including contamination, provide a source of exposure for susceptible hosts. Finally, indwelling devices provide a portal of entry for pathogenic organisms to enter a susceptible host and cause infection. Elements of the model can be used to develop a multifaceted approach to treatment and prevention of these DRIs.[16–18]

Here, the authors first review host, pathogen, environmental, and device-related factors that put older adults at increased risk of DRI and then discuss strategies for reducing future infections.

HOST FACTORS

Host susceptibility is a major determinant of infection; age is a nonmodifiable risk factor that impacts immunity and infection risk in the setting of exposure to a potential pathogen. Physical and functional incapacity, combined with the immunologic changes of aging, including those caused by immunosuppressive medications, make older adults more susceptible to DRIs than their younger counterparts.

Aging is associated with a decline of functional innate and adaptive immunity, a process known as immunosenescence.[19] The underlying mechanisms are unclear, but measurable decreases in functional immunity occur. The total number of circulating immune cells does not decline, although remaining immune cells have diminished capabilities: neutrophils lose some of their capacity for phagocytosis; monocytes and macrophages undergo changes in their ability to release cytokines and provide immune regulation; and natural killer cells have reduced potential to respond to cytokine signaling.[19–21]

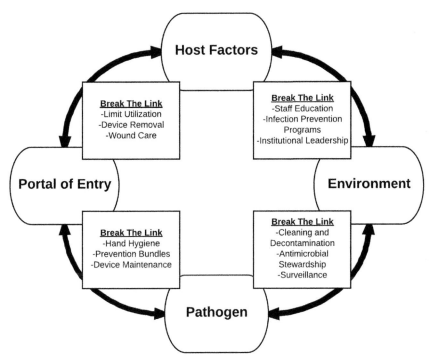

Fig. 1. The "Chain of Infection" is a general infection prevention framework that can be used to evaluate the major elements that lead to HAIs and to identify modifiable risk factors that can be targeted to reduce future infections. Visualized here is the interplay of risk factors contributing to the development of a DRI and potential interventions to "break the link."

Malnutrition can compound the challenges already presented by immunosenescence. Among older adults residing in the community, 2% to 4% are estimated to suffer from protein-energy malnutrition.[22] This most serious form of nutritional deficiency is more common among hospitalized older adults and is associated with increased postdischarge mortality.[22,23] Malnutrition contributes to a vicious cycle, whereby poor nutritional status is a risk factor for infection, and infection can worsen underlying malnutrition, because of the increased metabolic demands of acute and chronic illness.[19,24]

Beyond immune dysfunction, specific organ-system changes contribute to risk of DRIs in older adults. Atrophy of the epidermal and dermal layers of the skin predisposes to breakdown and wound formation. Underscoring the importance of these changes, up to 5% of residents of skilled nursing facilities have pressure ulcers.[6] Skin breakdown is a key element of the link between host and portal of entry; ulcers provide a portal of entry for bacterial pathogens and are often the first step in the pathway to infection. The harms associated with skin breakdown and chronic wounds are compounded because these ulcers are at particularly high risk of colonization with multidrug-resistant organisms (MDROs), such as methicillin-resistant *Staphylococcus aureus* (MRSA) and vancomycin-resistant *Enterococci* (VRE), which can complicate management if the ulcer becomes infected.[6,25]

In the genitourinary system, a reduction in bladder capacity, diminished rate of urine outflow, and increased postvoid residual volume all contribute to bacterial urinary colonization, independent of the risk associated with indwelling urinary catheters.[19,26] In addition, approximately 1 in 3 residents of skilled nursing facilities suffers from bowel or bladder incontinence, which itself influences the risk of infection.[6] First, incontinence leads to increasing use of invasive devices, such as urinary catheters. Indwelling catheters increase infection risk by providing a portal of entry for potentially pathogenic organisms. Second, incontinent patients who do not have urinary catheters placed are at increased risk of skin breakdown, which can provide a separate portal of entry for opportunistic bacterial organisms.

Neurocognitive deficits also play a role. Almost 15% of skilled nursing facility residents have severe cognitive impairment and near-complete dependence for activities of daily living.[6] Within nursing homes, higher levels of nursing needs, often due to chronic wounds or indwelling devices, are independent predictors of early MRSA and VRE acquisition.[27] Use of antipsychotic medications, used in up to 20% of skilled nursing facility residents, is associated with increased risk of pneumonia.[6,28] Delirium in older adults can also hinder proper care of other indwelling devices and cause unplanned removal of indwelling devices, placing patients at even higher risk of infection. Furthermore, obtaining and interpreting microbiologic specimens in the cognitively impaired may be more difficult than in other patient groups.[25]

ENVIRONMENTAL FACTORS

MDRO transmission from health care personnel to patients occurs during patient-provider encounters and is common among older adults with indwelling devices present. The duration and nature of the interaction also play a role. There is a dose-dependent association between nursing dependency, defined by physical and self-maintenance assessments, and MRSA/VRE co-colonization.[29] These data suggest that longer durations of contact with health care personnel lead to increases in MDRO exposure, which in turn lead to more MDRO colonization.[29] Bedbound status and receipt of rehabilitation care are both risk factors for MRSA acquisition, in part due to the high rate of direct contact between these patients and health care personnel.[30] A prospective study of more than 400 residents of residential care and a rehabilitation facilities found that residents receiving rehabilitation services that involve frequent and intense contact with health care personnel are at 4-fold greater risk of new MRSA acquisition compared with their counterparts receiving less direct contact.[30]

Contact with contaminated environmental services also facilitates the transfer of bacterial pathogens to susceptible older adults and sets the stage for future DRIs.[31–34] Rates of environmental contamination in the rooms of patients with VRE colonization or infection can be as high as 70%.[35] Compounding high rates of contamination is the environmental persistence of MDRO organisms. Without appropriate cleaning and decontamination, bacterial organisms can survive on the surfaces of objects for prolonged periods, up to months at a time, and serve as a reservoir for colonization and infections of subsequent patients.[36,37]

Environmental cleaning and contamination are directly related to patient outcomes and prevention of HAIs: In the nursing home setting, higher rates of MRSA environmental contamination are associated with a higher prevalence of MRSA among residents and less frequent room cleaning.[38] These data suggest that cleaning practices may be modified to decrease the bacterial burden of the environment and thereby limit MDRO exposure and reduce HAIs.[38]

PATHOGEN FACTORS

Exposure to, and colonization with, pathogenic bacteria often precede clinical infection; rates of MDRO colonization may exceed 35% in residents of LTCFs.[17] Colonization with MDROs such as MRSA is associated with increased mortality among older adults, although teasing out the independent effect of MDRO colonization from other patient comorbidities is challenging.[39,40]

Those with indwelling devices are at particularly high risk. Device insertion sites are the most common location of new MRSA acquisition in previously uncolonized individuals; molecular-typing demonstrates that the new acquisition is typically due to a health care–associated MRSA strain, and that persistent carriage after initial colonization is the norm.[17,41] A cross-sectional study of 200 residents of 14 community nursing homes in Southeast Michigan found that residents with any type of indwelling device, including urinary catheters, percutaneous feeding tubes, and PICC lines, were more likely to be colonized with MRSA compared with those without devices, after adjusting for functional status, comorbidity, and age (odds ratio 1.97, $P = .04$).[42] Compounding the concern, residents with indwelling devices were also more likely to be colonized with MDROs, such as ceftazidime-resistant gram-negative bacilli, despite no difference in antibiotic exposure history compared with their counterparts without indwelling devices.[42]

THE ROLE OF BIOFILMS

A diverse array of gram-positive and gram-negative pathogens, including *S aureus*, *Enterococcus faecalis*, and *Pseudomonas aeruginosa*, is able to produce biofilms on indwelling devices.[43,44] Organisms that reside within biofilms can originate from multiple different sources, including the host, health care personnel involved in the placement or maintenance of the device, the surrounding environment, and, in the case of CVCs, contaminated infusates.[44] Although the portal of entry is specific to the type of indwelling device, in all circumstances, attachment of bacteria to the device is required before a dynamic biofilm can be established.

Biofilms adhere to device surfaces and protect bacterial populations by encasing organisms in a complex extracellular matrix that is impervious to external protections that would normally help to prevent infection: Biofilms protect bacterial inhabitants from host immune systems and also from antibacterial medications. Because of their dynamic and active nature, biofilms are particularly insidious because they facilitate cellular growth and communication between different bacterial organisms, including transfer of genetic elements that confer antimicrobial resistance.[45] An additional management challenge is that some bacteria contained within the biofilm exist in a nutrient-limited state and have a very slow growth rate. Because many antibacterials work most effectively against actively dividing bacteria, the slow growth rate may further decrease antimicrobial effectiveness.[46] Because of all of these factors, once a biofilm develops on an indwelling device, eradication of these organisms becomes extremely challenging.

IMPACT OF INDWELLING DEVICES ON ANTIMICROBIAL USE

In addition to predisposing patients to infection, indwelling devices place older adults at risk of other adverse events, including overdiagnosis of infections that leads to unnecessary antibiotic use. For example, among nursing homes residents with indwelling urinary catheters, up to 95% have significant bacteriuria with greater than 50,000 colony forming units per milliliter; the high prevalence of bacteriuria diminishes the positive predictive value of culture results.[47] Due in part to difficulties with diagnosis in the catheterized population, up to one-third of antimicrobials prescribed for suspected urinary tract infections (UTIs) in LTCFs are for residents with asymptomatic bacteriuria that does not merit treatment.[48,49]

BREAKING THE LINKS
General Prevention Strategies for Reducing Device-Related Infections

Indwelling devices are risk factors for MDRO colonization and acquisition, particularly in wounds, at the groin, and at device insertion sites.[50,51] Indwelling devices also contribute to colonization with multiple MDROs: After controlling for other host factors, the presence of an indwelling device is associated with a 5.2-fold increase in the incidence of MRSA and VRE co-colonization.[29] Thus, the challenge is 2-fold: Patients with invasive devices are at significantly higher risk for infection, and also at higher risk for antimicrobial-resistant infections. These challenges underscore the need for prevention efforts that focus on reducing the use of indwelling devices and also on stewardship efforts to reduce the development and spread of antibiotic-resistant infections, thereby breaking the link between the portal of entry and the bacterial pathogen.

Device Management

Training in device management and care is a fundamental prevention strategy. Despite the frequency with which older adults have an indwelling device present in skilled nursing facilities, several studies demonstrate that device management training is limited.[52] One survey found that although most nurses in post–acute care facilities received specific training on the management of indwelling urinary catheters, only 40% of other health care personnel providing direct patient care, including nursing assistants, nursing students, and environmental service workers, received similar focused training.[52] These nonnurse health care personnel may be directly involved in activities associated with device management, and potentially contamination.[17,29,52] Thus, formal training and the expectation of all front-line health care personnel to be able to identify and address risk factors for contamination and infection, such as the presence of a urine collection bag on the floor, is important when developing a DRI prevention program.

A critical and often overlooked element of programs to reduce DRI is ongoing health care personnel education. Urinary catheters are most commonly placed by nurses; however, a recent study found that only 64% of nurses underwent training to prevent CAUTIs when starting at their position, and less than half had validated competency.[53] Closed catheter systems and limiting bladder irrigation are 2 interventions that can reduce CAUTI by preventing pathogens from gaining entry. Despite the importance of these simple interventions, a recent survey in Michigan skilled nursing facilities found that more than 50% of health care personnel were unaware of how to maintain a closed catheter drainage system, and a larger number were unaware of recommendations against bladder irrigation.[54] Likely contributing to the lack of appreciation for infection prevention guidelines is the high rate of nursing assistant turnover in the United States, which has been associated with increases in adverse outcomes among older adults, including UTIs.[55]

In addition to specific training about optimal device management to reduce exposure, educational efforts directed toward hand hygiene, proper device insertion with aseptic technique, maintenance, and prompt removal once no longer medically needed are crucial aspects of successful programs for reducing DRIs.[17] These educational efforts should be directed across the spectrum of health care personnel at the facility, because the primary caregiver may vary depending on the setting. Because of the transient nature of the effect that individual educational efforts may have on health care personnel behaviors, these initiatives should be ideally accompanied by intermittent outreach, observation and feedback, and possible recertification at designated intervals to ensure appropriate infection prevention techniques are being applied.[56,57]

Surveillance and Device Removal

Among patients admitted to LTCFs, there is a dose-dependent increase in infection rates when multiple indwelling devices are present.[13] Most DRIs can be prevented by simply removing the indwelling device; this is the single most important DRI prevention intervention.[13] Surveillance of device use and DRIs with direct feedback to providers can be used to reduce device-days and improve practice, thereby reducing patient risk.

A national Centers for Medicare and Medicaid (CMS) mandate requires that nursing homes report appropriateness of urinary catheter use.[6] As nursing homes are now evaluated to "ensure each resident who enters the nursing home without a catheter is not given a catheter, unless medically necessary, and that incontinent patients receive proper services to prevent urinary tract infection and restore normal bladder functions," use of indwelling urinary catheters is decreasing.[6]

The Federal Steering Committee for the Prevention of Health Care–Associated Infections established metrics of reporting from LTCFs, including CAUTI incidence rates and a urinary catheter utilization ratio: catheter-days/resident-days.[16] The goal of urinary catheter utilization ratio reporting is to encourage the implementation of prevention practices that reduce catheter-days, such as avoidance of indwelling urinary catheters whenever possible, performing regular assessments of ongoing need, and early catheter removal. In the acute care setting, stop orders for device removal and catheter assessment protocols increase catheter discontinuation when they are no longer medically indicated.[58,59] Nursing-driven initiatives to evaluate catheter necessity coupled with protocol-based device removal are another method that has demonstrated significant and sustained reductions in the number of catheter-days when compared to usual practice.[60,61] Similar multidisciplinary initiatives involving venous access teams to evaluate the need for CVCs and the selection of catheter type can lead to a reduction in the prevalence of CVCs, with a corresponding decrease in risk of catheter-associated bloodstream infections (CLABSIs).

Horizontal Versus Vertical Approaches to Infection Prevention

Historically, acute care hospitals have taken a "vertical approach" to infection control, intensively targeting specific high-burden MDRO pathogens, such as MRSA, VRE, and carbapenem-resistant *Enterobacteriaceae*, with methods of active surveillance, pathogen-directed contact precautions, and targeted decolonization.[62] Vertical strategies are designed to reduce colonization, infection, and potential transmission of these predetermined high-risk pathogens, but the impact of these interventions on other potential pathogens is limited. In contrast, horizontal interventions are designed to reduce overall infection risk, rather than target any specific pathogen. Examples of horizontal interventions include hand hygiene campaigns, antimicrobial stewardship programs, and programs to limit the use of indwelling devices.[62] As vertical infection strategies control are resource intensive, post–acute care facilities may favor horizontal interventions that can be focused on high-risk individuals with intensive, multifaceted approaches.[62,63]

Standard Precautions and Hand Hygiene

Standard precautions are the most basic set of prevention interventions that should be applied to all patient encounters to protect both patients and health care personnel from infection. Standard precautions include hand hygiene before and after any patient contact, respiratory hygiene, use of personal protective equipment when needed, safe injection practices, and safe handling of potentially contaminated equipment and surfaces.[64]

An essential aspect of standard precautions is effective hand hygiene, a priority area of outreach by the Centers for Disease Control and Prevention (CDC).[65] Emphasizing excellent hand hygiene is particularly important for nursing home personnel, because their hands are frequently colonized with pathogenic organisms, including gram-negative bacilli, *Candida* sp, *S aureus*, and VRE.[66] Despite the well-known benefits of this simple intervention, hand hygiene compliance in LTCFs is low, and several studies demonstrate limited understanding of standard precautions principles and the importance of hand hygiene for preventing HAIs.[66–68]

Contact Precautions

The most recent guidelines for infection control in LTCFs recommend instituting contact precautions based on clinical risk factors and general assessment of likelihood of transmitting MDRO pathogens. Several states passed legislation to mandate screening for MRSA colonization in hospitals and LTCFs.[69,70]

Despite these recommendations, implementing contact precautions for patients colonized with MDROs is controversial. Placement of patients in private rooms creates logistical challenges in long-term care, particularly for facilities with limited bed capacity.[18,30] Furthermore, use of contact precautions for prevention of some pathogens, such as MRSA and VRE, is increasingly a subject of debate.[71–75] Limited evidence suggests that cohabitation with an MRSA-colonized roommate does not significantly impact MRSA acquisition, possibly because of the nature of patient-patient and patient-provider interactions in skilled nursing facilities.[30] Residents in skilled nursing facilities are exposed to a spectrum of patients and environments; thus interventions that focus on limiting specific patient-to-patient interactions may be ineffective for reducing MDRO transmission.[30] From a practical standpoint, isolation may not be feasible, because of the need for residents to participate in various activities outside of their room, including physical therapy, social programs, meals, and other forms of rehabilitation.[42]

Further clouding the picture, recent studies suggest that placing patients, particularly older adults, into isolation is associated with adverse outcomes and measurable increased morbidity. Adverse impacts of contact precautions include less attention from staff and increased rates of delirium.[76–78] With these issues in mind, many acute care facilities continue to perform active surveillance of MDROs, which remains an area of ongoing research. Given these challenges, most community nursing homes are using standard precautions without additional contact isolation to care for residents colonized with MRSA.[79]

Bundled Approaches

In older adults with indwelling devices, the presence of comorbidities and functional disability makes infection prevention efforts more challenging. Prevention bundles, which include evidence-based sets of interventions designed to reduce infection, are one method of reducing DRIs. Implementation of prevention bundles has successfully reduced the rates of many DRIs, including CAUTIs and central line–associated bloodstream infections, among others.[80]

A randomized, controlled trial with the "bundle" of active surveillance, enhanced contact precautions, and intensive education programs of hand hygiene and infection prevention focused on indwelling devices found a significant reduction in the prevalence density rate of MDRO colonization, incident CAUTIs, and antibiotic use when compared with usual care. Study authors hypothesized that barrier precautions led to decreased new MDRO colonization, whereas staff education simultaneously led to decreased transmission of pathogens and subsequent development of CAUTIs.[17] Although the intervention required substantial effort, it was targeted at particularly high-risk individuals with indwelling devices and provided benefits to all facility residents.

Environmental Cleaning

Effective environmental cleaning can help to break the link between the pathogenic organisms and the health care environment in the chain of infection. Cleaning of health care facilities is associated with HAI reductions.[81] Direct cleansing and disinfection of contaminated surfaces and equipment is the primary method of these efforts. It relies on the training of staff to properly use cleaning supplies to ensure the maximum reduction of pathogen burden.[33,82] Enhanced educational programs directed at staff, including a system of performance feedback such as fluorescent markers or adenosine triphosphate measurement, are effective at improving the quality of cleaning.[83–88] Despite these findings, incomplete cleaning or the incorrect utilization of cleansing products occurs with frequency, leaving behind potentially pathogenic organisms on environmental surfaces.[89–92] As a result, there is great interest in the development and application of emerging technologies to augment the efforts of environmental services staff, including the use of UV radiation devices, hydrogen peroxide vapor, and self-disinfecting materials impregnated with heavy metals or germicides.[33]

Antimicrobial Stewardship

Improving antimicrobial use with an active antimicrobial stewardship program can reduce *Clostridium difficile* infection and antibiotic utilization and lower pharmacy costs.[93,94] Issues surrounding antimicrobial stewardship are covered in more detail in McElligott and colleagues' article, "Antibiotic Stewardship in Nursing Facilities," in this issue.

Because of limited staffing and diagnostic resources, many antibiotic prescriptions are dispensed empirically before evaluation by a trained clinician and without appropriate testing.[25,95] Given the high rates of bacterial colonization among older adults with devices, particularly bacteriuria with indwelling urinary catheters, improving antimicrobial use can improve outcomes by limiting selection of MDRO pathogens and reducing medication toxicity. Increases in antimicrobial use are also associated with increased density of VRE colonization in the stool of hospitalized patients. Thus, reduction in the use or duration of antimicrobial therapy may help to limit the burden of resistant organisms found in the environment, thereby potentially limiting exposures and ultimately DRIs.[96]

Targeting Specific Device-Related Infections

The following sections focus on specific infection-prevention practices for reducing infections associated with the 3 most common indwelling devices in older adults: urinary catheters, vascular catheters, and percutaneous feeding tubes.

Urinary catheters

Indwelling urinary catheters provide a portal of entry for pathogenic bacteria to invade a susceptible host. As such, they are a major risk factor for UTI. In catheterized patients, UTI incidence is 6.2 per 1000 patient-days, more than double the incidence of patients without indwelling catheters (2.8 per 1000 patient-days).[13] Furthermore, presence of an indwelling urinary catheter is associated with worsening UTI severity, including pyelonephritis, prostatitis, and bacteremia. CAUTIs are also associated with substantial cost, up to $896 per episode, that may not be reimbursed by insurance carriers, including CMS payers.[97] Nonreimbursement theoretically provides additional motivations to prevent these infections, but recent analyses suggest that this policy did not lead to significant reductions in infection rates.[98]

The most important prevention strategy for reducing CAUTIs is reducing exposure to urinary catheters. Thus, the Healthcare Infection Control Practices Advisory Committee guidelines emphasize that urinary catheters should only be used in circumstances of necessity, such as urinary retention, rather than routinely or for convenience.[99] Implementing a mandatory daily review of catheter necessity and leveraging the electronic medical record for evaluation are 2 strategies that reduce indwelling catheter days and are mainstays of prevention practices.[99] Nurse-driven protocols are another effective approach.[60,61] Of note, indwelling urinary catheters also predispose older adults to other adverse health care-associated conditions, including reduced mobility, falls, venous thromboembolism, pressure ulcers, and damage to the urethra and lower urinary tract.[100,101] Thus, reducing catheter use has additional benefits beyond CAUTI reduction.

If avoidance of a urinary catheter is not possible, several steps can be taken to reduce infection risk. Universal application of the most recent CDC guidelines for the prevention of CAUTIs, which focuses on the appropriate use of indwelling catheters, proper techniques for insertion and maintenance, and CAUTI surveillance, is estimated to reduce CAUTI by 20% to 70%.[53,99]

If an indwelling urinary catheter is unavoidable, efforts to prevent CAUTI include hand hygiene before and after device management, cleansing and performing care to the groin before insertion, using aseptic technique with sterile supplies, and securing the device to prevent movement of the catheter.[80,102] These interventions are designed to reduce pathogen exposure, potentially breaking the link between the bacterial pathogen and the portal of entry. Practice bundles for catheter placement and management also include maintaining a sterile, continuous, closed system and minimizing loops or kinks in the drainage tubing so as to prevent stasis or retrograde flow of urine and reduce the risk of bacteriuria.[80] Positioning of the collecting bag below the level of the bladder and emptying urine from the collecting bag regularly further limits contamination and colonization.[80]

Devices that do not enter the bladder, and therefore do not provide a direct portal of entry into the host, can be used instead of indwelling catheters in some patients, particularly if obstruction and retention are not the reason for the catheter. Examples of external urinary collection systems include condom catheters and the ReliaFit (Eloquest Healthcare, Ferndale, MI, USA) male urinary device.[103] When compared with indwelling urinary catheters, condom catheters reduce symptomatic UTI, bacteriuria, and death in older men, particularly those without dementia.[104,105] In patients where external devices are not an option, such as patients with neurogenic bladder, intermittent catheterization decreases symptomatic UTI and bacteriuria when compared with chronic indwelling catheters.[99,106–108]

In facilities with particularly high CAUTI incidence, additional more aggressive prevention strategies may be considered. Altering the design of the urinary catheter is an engineering approach that may reduce the incidence of CAUTI independent of health care personnel practices. Urinary catheters can be constructed of hydrophilic latex or silicone tubing and may be coated with antimicrobial substances, such as silver. Hydrophilic latex catheters are associated with improvements in patient satisfaction, pain, and decreased incidence of hematuria when compared with silicone, but a reduction in CAUTI has not been demonstrated.[99] Antimicrobial-impregnated and silver-coated catheters are designed to reduce catheter colonization, theoretically reducing biofilm formation and infections. In a large, multicenter trial, patients requiring indwelling catheterization were randomized to receive either a silver alloy–coated catheter, a nitrofural-impregnated catheter, or a control catheter; primary outcome was incidence of symptomatic CAUTI. The study authors found no difference in the rates of CAUTI between the intervention and control arms (−0.1% [95% confidence interval, CI, −2.4–2.2] and −2.1% [95% CI −4.2–0.1], respectively).[109] These findings were supported by a recent meta-analysis that found that silver alloy–coated catheters were not associated with a reduction in CAUTIs when compared with other catheter designs. Similarly, no significant difference in clinical outcomes was found between patients receiving nitrofural-impregnated catheters compared with standard catheters, although some studies suggested a lower rate of symptomatic CAUTI and bacteriuria.[110] Cost is another consideration: these coated catheters cost between 2.5- and 6.6-fold more than standard catheters, and large clinical trials have failed to demonstrate significant improvements.[111,112] Thus, their uptake into clinical practice has been limited. Nonetheless, they are a consideration in settings with high CAUTI rates where more standard interventions have been ineffective.

In particularly high-risk individuals with indwelling urinary catheters, for whom traditional methods of infection prevention have had limited success, bacterial interference has been attempted. Bacterial interference includes intentional colonization of low-virulence bacteria into an individual's urinary tract. The theory behind bacterial interference is that the low-virulence organisms will not cause clinical infections, but will out-compete potentially pathogenic strains, thereby limiting infections. Reducing infections, in turn, limits antimicrobial exposure, which then limits the emergence of antimicrobial resistance and adverse drug events that accompany prevention strategies that employ chronic antimicrobials.[113] Multiple small studies demonstrate that the use of nonpathogenic *Escherichia coli* strains to inoculate the bladder, through instillation of bacteria-laden normal saline solution, can lead to long-term asymptomatic colonization.[114–116] Although a reduction in rates of symptomatic CAUTIs has been found among patients colonized with these nonpathogenic strains, including a more than 2-fold reduction over a year in a randomized controlled trial of patients with neurogenic bladder, achieving long-term colonization can be challenging and resource intens, requiring patients to undergo repeated inoculation procedures.[113] As a result, adoption of bacterial interference has not been widespread.

Central venous catheters

CVCs are used in older adults for many reasons, including delivery of parenteral medications, administration of nutrition, and as a means of performing hemodialysis. However, CVCs also serve as a direct portal of entry for pathogenic bacteria. CLABSIs are a major cause of morbidity and mortality in the United States, with an estimated 41,000 cases in 2009. Mortalities following CLABSI approach 25%.[117,118]

Analogous to indwelling urinary catheters, the most effective means of limiting the risk of CLABSI is to minimize exposure to CVCs. The clinical indications and need for a CVC are often more apparent than those of a urinary catheter; however, the challenges of ensuring appropriate monitoring and prompt removal when no longer required are similar. Prompt discontinuation of CVCs when they are no longer clinically indicated is particularly challenging with older adults in post-acute care or long-term care settings, where limited resources and less frequent interactions with health care staff may inadvertently prolong the number of CVC days, particularly if a needs assessment is not integrated into routine patient care.[63,94] In the intensive care unit, the inclusion of process measures, such as the documentation of CVC presence and duration, contributes to CLABSI reduction.[119] In skilled nursing facilities and the home care environment, lack of consistent documentation concerning central catheter indication and planned duration is a frequent quality gap.[120,121]

CVCs can become colonized and serve as a portal of entry for potentially pathogenic bacteria via 2 major mechanisms: colonization at the insertion site with migration along the external surface of the catheter or direct inoculation of the connectors or hubs, leading to internal colonization.[122] Once contaminated, pathogens can migrate to the bloodstream and cause infection.

Because contamination is the first step in the pathway to infection, interventions targeted toward preventing device contamination at the time of placement can break the link between the pathogen and the portal of entry. Hand hygiene campaigns, use of chlorhexidine gluconate (CHG)-alcohol antiseptic for skin preparation (as compared with povidone-iodine preparation), and the use of sterile barrier precautions are basic prevention strategies that reduce bacterial contamination and thereby reduce CLABSI.[123–126] Because inoculation of catheter tubing and hubs is a mechanism of bacterial contamination, limiting the number of catheter lumens is also associated with reduced rates of bloodstream infections, particularly for PICCs.[127,128]

Antiseptic and antimicrobial impregnated CVCs, to reduce bacterial colonization and biofilm formation, are another consideration. Minocycline/rifampin-impregnated catheters are associated with reductions in bacterial colonization (7.9% vs 22.8%, $P<.001$) and CLABSI (3.4% vs 0.3%, $P<.002$).[129] A second-generation chlorhexidine/silver sulfadiazine catheter, with antiseptic coating both the internal and the external aspects of the device, demonstrates additional improvements.[130] Chlorhexidine-impregnated PICCs are also available, but studies demonstrate mixed results with these devices.[118,131] Clinically, impregnated and standard catheters have similar CLABSI risk during the first 10 days after placement, and a cost-effectiveness analysis suggested that minocycline/rifampin catheters are an attractive strategy only if the catheter is in place for 8 days or more.[132] Considering the higher costs associated with these interventions and the limited resources for infection prevention available at LTCFs, the decision to implement these additional infection prevention measures should be considered based on the risk of incident CLABSI and anticipated duration of CVC need.[133]

Once a CVC is placed, interventions that limit bacterial contamination reduce infections. Basic practices to reduce contamination include hand hygiene before device handling, disinfection of catheter hubs and connections before access, and minimizing unnecessary manipulation of the line, including for blood draws.[80,117] Alcohol-containing connector caps and CHG-containing device dressings are also effective.[134–137] Among particularly high-risk patients, such as those with long-term hemodialysis catheters, total parenteral nutrition requirements, or a history of recurrent CLABSIs, antibiotic or alcohol lock solutions may lead to additional reductions.[138]

Percutaneous feeding tubes

Although controversial, many older adults, particularly those with advanced dementia and difficulty swallowing, receive percutaneous feeding tubes. These feeding tubes are associated with many risks, including pneumonia, skin and soft tissue infections, and higher rates of *C difficile* infections. Teasing out the independent impact of the feeding tube from overall elevated infection risk in older adults is difficult, but a small observational study of 30 LTCF residents with feeding tubes found that 57% developed 23 distinct infections over 100 resident-months, most of which were pneumonias and UTIs.[13]

Among older adults with dementia, observational studies demonstrate higher rates of mortality due to pneumonia in tube-fed patients as compared with those who are fed orally; however, confounding by indication is a consideration.[139] Feeding tubes are associated with increased rates of reflux and aspiration of gastric contents, potentially leading to aspiration events and aspiration pneumonia.[140] Interventions that increase the incidence of pneumonia are concerning because pneumonia is the leading cause of mortality in the LTCF population and is also the primary indication for transfer to higher-acuity facilities. In the United States, 10% to 18% of all pneumonia hospitalizations are initiated as a transfer from LTCFs.[141]

Several steps can be taken to limit infection risk associated with feeding tube–related infections. Skin and soft tissue infections can be reduced with periprocedural antimicrobial prophylaxis, excellent wound care, and MRSA decolonization.[142,143] *C difficile* infections can be reduced through antimicrobial stewardship efforts.[144] Pneumonia prevention efforts may include aspiration and delirium precautions, elevating the head of the bed, and avoidance of unnecessary proton pump inhibitors.[145]

The "Quest for Zero"

Increasingly, health care organizations are striving toward a goal of eliminating all HAIs, including DRIs.[146] The prevailing notion of a "Quest for Zero" promotes aggressive DRI reduction measures, but the impact of these policies on health care quality is unclear.[147] Public reporting of facility-specific HAI rates is a nationwide strategy that was implemented to improve prevention practices. Beginning in 2011, hospitals were required to report CLABSIs acquired in the intensive care unit. CAUTI reporting was added in 2012.[80] Public reporting was expanded to include general medical and surgical units in 2015.[80] By requiring reporting and transparency, incentivized through additional funding, the mandate of these policies is to encourage and reinforce infection prevention. However, despite these goals, analysis of policies regarding CMS nonpayment for HAIs has not resulted in changes to provider behaviors or facility infection rates.[98,148] Beyond infection prevention, the implementation of public reporting policies to increase transparency has unfortunately worsened outcomes in other areas of clinical medicine, calling into question the benefits of this approach.[149,150] Another attempt to improve care through payment restructuring is The Improving Medicare Post-Acute Care Transformation Act of 2014, which aims to increase quality across post–acute care settings by aligning the measures of quality across all types of providers, thereby incentivizing appropriate use and care of indwelling devices in older adults.[151] The impact of better defining quality measures for providers in post-acute care settings on clinical outcomes is not yet known.

Resource Constraints and Economic Considerations

As a shift away from inpatient clinical care settings has occurred, older adults, with indwelling devices and increasingly complex comorbidities, are being cared for in lower acuity settings; 42% of Medicare recipients discharged from an acute care hospital were transferred to a subacute facility.[50,152,153] Many of these patients have indwelling devices, are often colonized with MDROs, and move between facilities. Frequent transfers increase the risk of horizontal transmission to other patients and health care personnel alike.[152]

As a result of frequent transitions between acute care facilities, post–acute care, rehabilitation, and home health care, older adults will often experience different and conflicting approaches to infection prevention and maintenance of indwelling devices.[25] Without clear consensus on how best to prevent and control bacterial colonization, it is left to individual facilities to determine how often to screen patients for MDROs, where to obtain specimens, and what forms of precautions are necessary, including isolation.[50] Heterogeneity in practice between different health care facilities results in practice variations in the management of possible infections.

Implementation of guidelines for prevention and management of HAIs in LTCFs is limited.[154] Although officially a requirement of CMS, a recent review found that failure to implement an infection prevention program was the most frequently cited health deficiency in these facilities.[6] Furthermore, even when programs are in place, less than 10% of infection preventionists working in LTCFs have specific training in the area.[155]

High leadership turnover is another challenge faced by post–acute care facilities. Turnover leads to limited support for educational and philosophic efforts to improve infection prevention practices. Without local leadership to encourage best practice, unclear perceptions and varying adherence persist.[12] Lack of an on-site physician can present additional challenges, because nurses and nursing assistants perform clinical evaluations and are tasked with early identification of infections, despite limited training.[94] Compounding the problem of limited training, nursing turnover at post–acute care facilities is high and also associated with increased risk of HAIs and hospitalizations due to infection.[63,156]

SUMMARY

DRIs are a major cause of morbidity and mortality among older adults. The frequent use of indwelling devices in this vulnerable population results in a significant burden to the health care system and is an important target for infection prevention and antimicrobial stewardship efforts. Fortunately, within the chain of infection that leads to DRIs in older adults, there are multiple opportunities to implement interventions to "break the links" and reduce MDRO colonization and infections and to improve antimicrobial use.

REFERENCES

1. Strausbaugh LJ, Joseph CL. The burden of infection in long-term care. Infect Control Hosp Epidemiol 2000;21(10):674–9.
2. Kunin CM, Douthitt S, Dancing J, et al. The association between the use of urinary catheters and morbidity and mortality among elderly patients in nursing homes. Am J Epidemiol 1992;135(3):291–301.
3. Kunin CM, Chin QF, Chambers S. Morbidity and mortality associated with indwelling urinary catheters in elderly patients in a nursing home–confounding due to the presence of associated diseases. J Am Geriatr Soc 1987;35(11): 1001–6.
4. Mamun K, Lim J. Role of nasogastric tube in preventing aspiration pneumonia in patients with dysphagia. Singapore Med J 2005;46(11):627–31.
5. Ortman JMV, Velkoff VA, Hogan H. An aging nation: the older population in the United States. Washington, DC: U.S. Department of Commerce, Economics and Statistics Administration, U.S Census Bureau; 2014.
6. Centers for Medicare and Medicaid Services. Nursing home data compendium 2015 edition. Washington, DC: Department of Health and Human Services; 2015.
7. Tsan L, Davis C, Langberg R, et al. Prevalence of nursing home-associated infections in the Department of Veterans Affairs nursing home care units. Am J Infect Control 2008;36(3):173–9.

8. Eikelenboom-Boskamp A, Cox-Claessens JH, Boom-Poels PG, et al. Three-year prevalence of healthcare-associated infections in Dutch nursing homes. J Hosp Infect 2011;78(1):59–62.

9. Rogers MA, Mody L, Kaufman SR, et al. Use of urinary collection devices in skilled nursing facilities in five states. J Am Geriatr Soc 2008;56(5):854–61.

10. Tsan L, Langberg R, Davis C, et al. Nursing home-associated infections in Department of Veterans Affairs community living centers. Am J Infect Control 2010;38(6):461–6.

11. Gorina Y, Schappert S, Bercovitz A, et al. Prevalence of incontinence among older Americans. Vital Health Stat 3 2014;(36):1–33.

12. Mody L, Meddings J, Edson BS, et al. Enhancing resident safety by preventing healthcare-associated infection: a national initiative to reduce catheter-associated urinary tract infections in nursing homes. Clin Infect Dis 2015; 61(1):86–94.

13. Wang L, Lansing B, Symons K, et al. Infection rate and colonization with antibiotic-resistant organisms in skilled nursing facility residents with indwelling devices. Eur J Clin Microbiol Infect Dis 2012;31(8):1797–804.

14. Mitchell SL, Teno JM, Roy J, et al. Clinical and organizational factors associated with feeding tube use among nursing home residents with advanced cognitive impairment. JAMA 2003;290(1):73–80.

15. Jones AL, Dwyer LL, Bercovitz AR, et al. The national nursing home survey: 2004 overview. Vital Health Stat 13 2009;(167):1–155.

16. Department of Health and Human Services. National action plan to prevent health care-associated infections: road map to elimination - long-term care facilities. Washington, DC: Department of Health and Human Services; 2013.

17. Mody L, Krein SL, Saint S, et al. A targeted infection prevention intervention in nursing home residents with indwelling devices: a randomized clinical trial. JAMA Intern Med 2015;175(5):714–23.

18. Smith PW, Bennett G, Bradley S, et al. SHEA/APIC guideline: infection prevention and control in the long-term care facility, July 2008. Infect Control Hosp Epidemiol 2008;29(9):785–814.

19. Gavazzi G, Krause KH. Ageing and infection. Lancet Infect Dis 2002;2(11): 659–66.

20. Castle SC. Clinical relevance of age-related immune dysfunction. Clin Infect Dis 2000;31(2):578–85.

21. Lord JM, Butcher S, Killampali V, et al. Neutrophil ageing and immunesenescence. Mech Ageing Dev 2001;122(14):1521–35.

22. Lesourd BM, Mazari L, Ferry M. The role of nutrition in immunity in the aged. Nutr Rev 1998;56(1 Pt 2):S113–25.

23. Constans T, Bacq Y, Brechot JF, et al. Protein-energy malnutrition in elderly medical patients. J Am Geriatr Soc 1992;40(3):263–8.

24. Lesourd B. Immune response during disease and recovery in the elderly. Proc Nutr Soc 1999;58(1):85–98.

25. Montoya A, Mody L. Common infections in nursing homes: a review of current issues and challenges. Aging Health 2011;7(6):889–99.

26. Nicolle LE, SHEA Long-Term-Care-Committee. Urinary tract infections in long-term-care facilities. Infect Control Hosp Epidemiol 2001;22(3):167–75.

27. Min L, Galecki A, Mody L. Functional disability and nursing resource use are predictive of antimicrobial resistance in nursing homes. J Am Geriatr Soc 2015;63(4):659–66.

28. Knol W, van Marum RJ, Jansen PA, et al. Antipsychotic drug use and risk of pneumonia in elderly people. J Am Geriatr Soc 2008;56(4):661–6.

29. Flannery EL, Wang L, Zollner S, et al. Wounds, functional disability, and indwelling devices are associated with cocolonization by methicillin-resistant Staphylococcus aureus and vancomycin-resistant enterococci in southeast Michigan. Clin Infect Dis 2011;53(12):1215–22.

30. Furuno JP, Shurland SM, Zhan M, et al. Comparison of the methicillin-resistant Staphylococcus aureus acquisition among rehabilitation and nursing home residents. Infect Control Hosp Epidemiol 2011;32(3):244–9.

31. Bhalla A, Pultz NJ, Gries DM, et al. Acquisition of nosocomial pathogens on hands after contact with environmental surfaces near hospitalized patients. Infect Control Hosp Epidemiol 2004;25(2):164–7.

32. Morgan DJ, Rogawski E, Thom KA, et al. Transfer of multidrug-resistant bacteria to healthcare workers' gloves and gowns after patient contact increases with environmental contamination. Crit Care Med 2012;40(4):1045–51.

33. Weber DJ, Anderson D, Rutala WA. The role of the surface environment in healthcare-associated infections. Curr Opin Infect Dis 2013;26(4):338–44.

34. Stiefel U, Cadnum JL, Eckstein BC, et al. Contamination of hands with methicillin-resistant Staphylococcus aureus after contact with environmental surfaces and after contact with the skin of colonized patients. Infect Control Hosp Epidemiol 2011;32(2):185–7.

35. Weinstein RA. Epidemiology and control of nosocomial infections in adult intensive care units. Am J Med 1991;91(3B):179S–84S.

36. Hota B. Contamination, disinfection, and cross-colonization: are hospital surfaces reservoirs for nosocomial infection? Clin Infect Dis 2004;39(8):1182–9.

37. Kramer A, Schwebke I, Kampf G. How long do nosocomial pathogens persist on inanimate surfaces? A systematic review. BMC Infect Dis 2006;6:130.

38. Murphy CR, Eells SJ, Quan V, et al. Methicillin-resistant Staphylococcus aureus burden in nursing homes associated with environmental contamination of common areas. J Am Geriatr Soc 2012;60(6):1012–8.

39. Vendrell E, Capdevila JA, Barrufet P, et al. Mortality among methicillin-resistant Staphylococcus aureus carriers in long-term care facilities. Rev Esp Quimioter 2015;28(2):92–7.

40. Mendy A, Vieira ER, Albatineh AN, et al. Staphylococcus aureus colonization and long-term risk for death, United States. Emerg Infect Dis 2016;22(11): 1966–9.

41. Gibson KE, McNamara SE, Cassone M, et al. Methicillin-resistant Staphylococcus aureus: site of acquisition and strain variation in high-risk nursing home residents with indwelling devices. Infect Control Hosp Epidemiol 2014; 35(12):1458–65.

42. Mody L, Maheshwari S, Galecki A, et al. Indwelling device use and antibiotic resistance in nursing homes: identifying a high-risk group. J Am Geriatr Soc 2007;55(12):1921–6.

43. Costerton JW, Stewart PS, Greenberg EP. Bacterial biofilms: a common cause of persistent infections. Science 1999;284(5418):1318–22.

44. Donlan RM. Biofilms and device-associated infections. Emerg Infect Dis 2001; 7(2):277–81.

45. Romling U, Kjelleberg S, Normark S, et al. Microbial biofilm formation: a need to act. J Intern Med 2014;276(2):98–110.

46. Brown MR, Allison DG, Gilbert P. Resistance of bacterial biofilms to antibiotics: a growth-rate related effect? J Antimicrob Chemother 1988;22(6):777–80.

47. Smith PW, Seip CW, Schaefer SC, et al. Microbiologic survey of long-term care facilities. Am J Infect Control 2000;28(1):8–13.
48. Hooton TM, Bradley SF, Cardenas DD, et al. Diagnosis, prevention, and treatment of catheter-associated urinary tract infection in adults: 2009 International Clinical Practice Guidelines from the Infectious Diseases Society of America. Clin Infect Dis 2010;50(5):625–63.
49. Nicolle LE, Bentley DW, Garibaldi R, et al. Antimicrobial use in long-term-care facilities. SHEA Long-Term-Care Committee. Infect Control Hosp Epidemiol 2000;21(8):537–45.
50. Mody L, Bradley SF, Galecki A, et al. Conceptual model for reducing infections and antimicrobial resistance in skilled nursing facilities: focusing on residents with indwelling devices. Clin Infect Dis 2011;52(5):654–61.
51. Heinze KG, Gibson KE, Cassone M, et al;. Species distribution and risk factors for carbapenem resistance among beta-lactam and fluoroquinolone-resistant Enterobacteriaceae isolated from high-risk nursing home residents. Paper presented at: SHEA Spring 2017. St Louis, March 29-31, 2017.
52. McNulty CA, Bowen J, Foy C, et al. Urinary catheterization in care homes for older people: self-reported questionnaire audit of catheter management by care home staff. J Hosp Infect 2006;62(1):29–36.
53. Fink R, Gilmartin H, Richard A, et al. Indwelling urinary catheter management and catheter-associated urinary tract infection prevention practices in Nurses Improving Care for Healthsystem Elders hospitals. Am J Infect Control 2012; 40(8):715–20.
54. Mody L, Saint S, Galecki A, et al. Knowledge of evidence-based urinary catheter care practice recommendations among healthcare workers in nursing homes. J Am Geriatr Soc 2010;58(8):1532–7.
55. Trinkoff AM, Han K, Storr CL, et al. Turnover, staffing, skill mix, and resident outcomes in a national sample of US nursing homes. J Nurs Adm 2013;43(12): 630–6.
56. Dubbert PM, Dolce J, Richter W, et al. Increasing ICU staff handwashing: effects of education and group feedback. Infect Control Hosp Epidemiol 1990;11(4): 191–3.
57. Naikoba S, Hayward A. The effectiveness of interventions aimed at increasing handwashing in healthcare workers - a systematic review. J Hosp Infect 2001; 47(3):173–80.
58. Saint S, Olmsted RN, Fakih MG, et al. Translating health care-associated urinary tract infection prevention research into practice via the bladder bundle. Jt Comm J Qual Patient Saf 2009;35(9):449–55.
59. Saint S, Greene MT, Kowalski CP, et al. Preventing catheter-associated urinary tract infection in the United States: a national comparative study. JAMA Intern Med 2013;173(10):874–9.
60. Leis JA, Corpus C, Rahmani A, et al. Medical directive for urinary catheter removal by nurses on general medical wards. JAMA Intern Med 2016;176(1): 113–5.
61. Fakih MG, Rey JE, Pena ME, et al. Sustained reductions in urinary catheter use over 5 years: bedside nurses view themselves responsible for evaluation of catheter necessity. Am J Infect Control 2013;41(3):236–9.
62. Septimus E, Weinstein RA, Perl TM, et al. Approaches for preventing healthcare-associated infections: go long or go wide? Infect Control Hosp Epidemiol 2014; 35(Suppl 2):S10–4.

63. Mody L. Infection control issues in older adults. Clin Geriatr Med 2007;23(3): 499–514, vi.

64. APIC. Follow all Posted Precaution Signs. Available at: http://professionals.site. apic.org/10-ways-to-protect-patients/follow-the-rules-for-isolation-precautions/. Accessed April 10, 2017.

65. Boyce JM, Pittet D, Healthcare Infection Control Practices Advisory Committee, Society for Healthcare Epidemiology of America, Association for Professionals in Infection Control, Infectious Diseases Society of America, Hand Hygiene Task Force. Guideline for hand hygiene in health-care settings: recommendations of the Healthcare Infection Control Practices Advisory Committee and the HIC-PAC/SHEA/APIC/IDSA Hand Hygiene Task Force. Infect Control Hosp Epidemiol 2002;23(12 Suppl):S3–40.

66. Mody L, McNeil SA, Sun R, et al. Introduction of a waterless alcohol-based hand rub in a long-term-care facility. Infect Control Hosp Epidemiol 2003;24(3): 165–71.

67. Thompson BL, Dwyer DM, Ussery XT, et al. Handwashing and glove use in a long-term-care facility. Infect Control Hosp Epidemiol 1997;18(2):97–103.

68. Albrecht JS, Croft L, Morgan DJ, et al. Perceptions of gown and glove use to prevent methicillin-resistant Staphylococcus aureus transmission in nursing homes. J Am Med Dir Assoc 2017;18(2):158–61.

69. Weber SG, Huang SS, Oriola S, et al. Legislative mandates for use of active surveillance cultures to screen for methicillin-resistant Staphylococcus aureus and vancomycin-resistant enterococci: position statement from the Joint SHEA and APIC Task Force. Am J Infect Control 2007;35(2):73–85.

70. Diekema DJ, Climo M. Preventing MRSA infections: finding it is not enough. JAMA 2008;299(10):1190–2.

71. Morgan DJ, Murthy R, Munoz-Price LS, et al. Reconsidering contact precautions for endemic methicillin-resistant Staphylococcus aureus and vancomycin-resistant enterococcus. Infect Control Hosp Epidemiol 2015;36(10):1163–72.

72. Martin EM, Russell D, Rubin Z, et al. Elimination of routine contact precautions for endemic methicillin-resistant Staphylococcus aureus and vancomycin-resistant Enterococcus: a retrospective quasi-experimental study. Infect Control Hosp Epidemiol 2016;37(11):1323–30.

73. Gandra S, Barysauskas CM, Mack DA, et al. Impact of contact precautions on falls, pressure ulcers and transmission of MRSA and VRE in hospitalized patients. J Hosp Infect 2014;88(3):170–6.

74. Almyroudis NG, Osawa R, Samonis G, et al. Discontinuation of systematic surveillance and contact precautions for vancomycin-resistant Enterococcus (VRE) and its impact on the incidence of VRE faecium bacteremia in patients with hematologic malignancies. Infect Control Hosp Epidemiol 2016;37(4):398–403.

75. Edmond MB, Masroor N, Stevens MP, et al. The impact of discontinuing contact precautions for VRE and MRSA on device-associated infections. Infect Control Hosp Epidemiol 2015;36(8):978–80.

76. McCusker J, Cole M, Abrahamowicz M, et al. Environmental risk factors for delirium in hospitalized older people. J Am Geriatr Soc 2001;49(10):1327–34.

77. Stelfox HT, Bates DW, Redelmeier DA. Safety of patients isolated for infection control. JAMA 2003;290(14):1899–905.

78. Saint S, Higgins LA, Nallamothu BK, et al. Do physicians examine patients in contact isolation less frequently? A brief report. Am J Infect Control 2003; 31(6):354–6.

79. Ye Z, Mukamel DB, Huang SS, et al. Healthcare-associated pathogens and nursing home policies and practices: results from a national survey. Infect Control Hosp Epidemiol 2015;36(7):759–66.
80. Septimus EJ, Moody J. Prevention of device-related healthcare-associated infections. F1000Res 2016;5 [pii:F1000 Faculty Rev-65].
81. Donskey CJ. Does improving surface cleaning and disinfection reduce health care-associated infections? Am J Infect Control 2013;41(5 Suppl):S12–9.
82. Kundrapu S, Sunkesula V, Sitzlar BM, et al. More cleaning, less screening: evaluation of the time required for monitoring versus performing environmental cleaning. Infect Control Hosp Epidemiol 2014;35(2):202–4.
83. Eckstein BC, Adams DA, Eckstein EC, et al. Reduction of Clostridium difficile and vancomycin-resistant Enterococcus contamination of environmental surfaces after an intervention to improve cleaning methods. BMC Infect Dis 2007;7:61.
84. Goodman ER, Platt R, Bass R, et al. Impact of an environmental cleaning intervention on the presence of methicillin-resistant Staphylococcus aureus and vancomycin-resistant enterococci on surfaces in intensive care unit rooms. Infect Control Hosp Epidemiol 2008;29(7):593–9.
85. Luick L, Thompson PA, Loock MH, et al. Diagnostic assessment of different environmental cleaning monitoring methods. Am J Infect Control 2013;41(8):751–2.
86. Huang YS, Chen YC, Chen ML, et al. Comparing visual inspection, aerobic colony counts, and adenosine triphosphate bioluminescence assay for evaluating surface cleanliness at a medical center. Am J Infect Control 2015;43(8):882–6.
87. Boyce JM, Havill NL, Dumigan DG, et al. Monitoring the effectiveness of hospital cleaning practices by use of an adenosine triphosphate bioluminescence assay. Infect Control Hosp Epidemiol 2009;30(7):678–84.
88. Branch-Elliman W, Robillard E, McCarthy G Jr, et al. Direct feedback with the ATP luminometer as a process improvement tool for terminal cleaning of patient rooms. Am J Infect Control 2014;42(2):195–7.
89. Alfa MJ, Dueck C, Olson N, et al. UV-visible marker confirms that environmental persistence of Clostridium difficile spores in toilets of patients with C. difficile-associated diarrhea is associated with lack of compliance with cleaning protocol.e. BMC Infect Dis 2008;8:64.
90. Boyce JM. Measuring healthcare worker hand hygiene activity: current practices and emerging technologies. Infect Control Hosp Epidemiol 2011;32(10):1016–28.
91. Cadnum JL, Hurless KN, Kundrapu S, et al. Transfer of Clostridium difficile spores by nonsporicidal wipes and improperly used hypochlorite wipes: practice + product = perfection. Infect Control Hosp Epidemiol 2013;34(4):441–2.
92. Manian FA, Griesenauer S, Senkel D, et al. Isolation of Acinetobacter baumannii complex and methicillin-resistant Staphylococcus aureus from hospital rooms following terminal cleaning and disinfection: can we do better? Infect Control Hosp Epidemiol 2011;32(7):667–72.
93. Standiford HC, Chan S, Tripoli M, et al. Antimicrobial stewardship at a large tertiary care academic medical center: cost analysis before, during, and after a 7-year program. Infect Control Hosp Epidemiol 2012;33(4):338–45.
94. Rhee SM, Stone ND. Antimicrobial stewardship in long-term care facilities. Infect Dis Clin North Am 2014;28(2):237–46.
95. Warren JW, Palumbo FB, Fitterman L, et al. Incidence and characteristics of antibiotic use in aged nursing home patients. J Am Geriatr Soc 1991;39(10):963–72.

96. Donskey CJ, Chowdhry TK, Hecker MT, et al. Effect of antibiotic therapy on the density of vancomycin-resistant enterococci in the stool of colonized patients. N Engl J Med 2000;343(26):1925–32.

97. Zimlichman E, Henderson D, Tamir O, et al. Health care-associated infections: a meta-analysis of costs and financial impact on the US health care system. JAMA Intern Med 2013;173(22):2039–46.

98. Lee GM, Kleinman K, Soumerai SB, et al. Effect of nonpayment for preventable infections in U.S. hospitals. N Engl J Med 2012;367(15):1428–37.

99. Gould CV, Umscheid CA, Agarwal RK, et al, Healthcare Infection Control Practices Advisory Committee. Guideline for prevention of catheter-associated urinary tract infections 2009. Infect Control Hosp Epidemiol 2010;31(4):319–26.

100. Saint S, Lipsky BA, Goold SD. Indwelling urinary catheters: a one-point restraint? Ann Intern Med 2002;137(2):125–7.

101. Hollingsworth JM, Rogers MA, Krein SL, et al. Determining the noninfectious complications of indwelling urethral catheters: a systematic review and meta-analysis. Ann Intern Med 2013;159(6):401–10.

102. Fasugba O, Koerner J, Mitchell BG, et al. Systematic review and meta-analysis of the effectiveness of antiseptic agents for meatal cleaning in the prevention of catheter-associated urinary tract infections. J Hosp Infect 2017;95(3):233–42.

103. Lucas LMI, Iseler J, Gale L. Evaluation of a new, novel male external urinary management device. Paper presented at: Cleveland Clinic Spring 2013 WOC Nursing Symposium. Cleveland (OH), April 12, 2013.

104. Saint S, Kaufman SR, Rogers MA, et al. Risk factors for nosocomial urinary tract-related bacteremia: a case-control study. Am J Infect Control 2006;34(7):401–7.

105. Saint S, Kaufman SR, Rogers MA, et al. Condom versus indwelling urinary catheters: a randomized trial. J Am Geriatr Soc 2006;54(7):1055–61.

106. Vickrey BG, Shekelle P, Morton S, et al. Prevention and management of urinary tract infections in paralyzed persons. Evid Rep Technol Assess (Summ) 1999;(6):1–3.

107. Tang MW, Kwok TC, Hui E, et al. Intermittent versus indwelling urinary catheterization in older female patients. Maturitas 2006;53(3):274–81.

108. Turi MH, Hanif S, Fasih Q, et al. Proportion of complications in patients practicing clean intermittent self-catheterization (CISC) vs indwelling catheter. J Pak Med Assoc 2006;56(9):401–4.

109. Pickard R, Lam T, MacLennan G, et al. Antimicrobial catheters for reduction of symptomatic urinary tract infection in adults requiring short-term catheterisation in hospital: a multicentre randomised controlled trial. Lancet 2012;380(9857): 1927–35.

110. Lam TB, Omar MI, Fisher E, et al. Types of indwelling urethral catheters for short-term catheterisation in hospitalised adults. Cochrane Database Syst Rev 2014;(9):CD004013.

111. Karchmer TB, Giannetta ET, Muto CA, et al. A randomized crossover study of silver-coated urinary catheters in hospitalized patients. Arch Intern Med 2000; 160(21):3294–8.

112. Pickard R, Lam T, Maclennan G, et al. Types of urethral catheter for reducing symptomatic urinary tract infections in hospitalised adults requiring short-term catheterisation: multicentre randomised controlled trial and economic evaluation of antimicrobial- and antiseptic-impregnated urethral catheters (the CATHETER trial). Health Technol Assess 2012;16(47):1–197.

113. Darouiche RO, Green BG, Donovan WH, et al. Multicenter randomized controlled trial of bacterial interference for prevention of urinary tract infection in patients with neurogenic bladder. Urology 2011;78(2):341–6.

114. Hull R, Rudy D, Donovan W, et al. Urinary tract infection prophylaxis using Escherichia coli 83972 in spinal cord injured patients. J Urol 2000;163(3):872–7.

115. Sunden F, Hakansson L, Ljunggren E, et al. Escherichia coli 83972 bacteriuria protects against recurrent lower urinary tract infections in patients with incomplete bladder emptying. J Urol 2010;184(1):179–85.

116. Trautner BW, Hull RA, Thornby JI, et al. Coating urinary catheters with an avirulent strain of Escherichia coli as a means to establish asymptomatic colonization. Infect Control Hosp Epidemiol 2007;28(1):92–4.

117. O'Grady NP, Alexander M, Burns LA, et al. Guidelines for the prevention of intravascular catheter-related infections. Clin Infect Dis 2011;52(9):e162–93.

118. Storey S, Brown J, Foley A, et al. A comparative evaluation of antimicrobial coated versus nonantimicrobial coated peripherally inserted central catheters on associated outcomes: a randomized controlled trial. Am J Infect Control 2016;44(6):636–41.

119. Higuera F, Rosenthal VD, Duarte P, et al. The effect of process control on the incidence of central venous catheter-associated bloodstream infections and mortality in intensive care units in Mexico. Crit Care Med 2005;33(9):2022–7.

120. Chopra V, Montoya A, Joshi D, et al. Peripherally inserted central catheter use in skilled nursing facilities: a pilot study. J Am Geriatr Soc 2015;63(9):1894–9.

121. Baumgarten K, Hale Y, Messonnier M, et al. Bridging the gap: a collaborative to reduce peripherally inserted central catheter infections in the home care environment. Ochsner J 2013;13(3):352–8.

122. Crnich CJ, Maki DG. The promise of novel technology for the prevention of intravascular device-related bloodstream infection. II. Long-term devices. Clin Infect Dis 2002;34(10):1362–8.

123. Johnson L, Grueber S, Schlotzhauer C, et al. A multifactorial action plan improves hand hygiene adherence and significantly reduces central line-associated bloodstream infections. Am J Infect Control 2014;42(11):1146–51.

124. Chaiyakunapruk N, Veenstra DL, Lipsky BA, et al. Chlorhexidine compared with povidone-iodine solution for vascular catheter-site care: a meta-analysis. Ann Intern Med 2002;136(11):792–801.

125. Mimoz O, Lucet JC, Kerforne T, et al. Skin antisepsis with chlorhexidine-alcohol versus povidone iodine-alcohol, with and without skin scrubbing, for prevention of intravascular-catheter-related infection (CLEAN): an open-label, multicentre, randomised, controlled, two-by-two factorial trial. Lancet 2015;386(10008):2069–77.

126. Raad II, Hohn DC, Gilbreath BJ, et al. Prevention of central venous catheter-related infections by using maximal sterile barrier precautions during insertion. Infect Control Hosp Epidemiol 1994;15(4 Pt 1):231–8.

127. Szeinbach SL, Pauline J, Villa KF, et al. Evaluating catheter complications and outcomes in patients receiving home parenteral nutrition. J Eval Clin Pract 2015;21(1):153–9.

128. Ratz D, Hofer T, Flanders SA, et al. Limiting the number of lumens in peripherally inserted central catheters to improve outcomes and reduce cost: a simulation study. Infect Control Hosp Epidemiol 2016;37(7):811–7.

129. Darouiche RO, Raad II, Heard SO, et al. A comparison of two antimicrobial-impregnated central venous catheters. Catheter Study Group. N Engl J Med 1999;340(1):1–8.

130. Rupp ME, Lisco SJ, Lipsett PA, et al. Effect of a second-generation venous catheter impregnated with chlorhexidine and silver sulfadiazine on central catheter-related infections: a randomized, controlled trial. Ann Intern Med 2005;143(8):570–80.

131. Rutkoff GS. The influence of an antimicrobial peripherally inserted central catheter on central line-associated bloodstream infections in a hospital environment. J Assoc Vasc Access 2014;19:172–9.

132. Marciante KD, Veenstra DL, Lipsky BA, et al. Which antimicrobial impregnated central venous catheter should we use? Modeling the costs and outcomes of antimicrobial catheter use. Am J Infect Control 2003;31(1):1–8.

133. National Nosocomial Infections Surveillance System. National Nosocomial Infections Surveillance (NNIS) System Report, data summary from January 1992 through June 2004, issued October 2004. Am J Infect Control 2004; 32(8):470–85.

134. Sweet MA, Cumpston A, Briggs F, et al. Impact of alcohol-impregnated port protectors and needleless neutral pressure connectors on central line-associated bloodstream infections and contamination of blood cultures in an inpatient oncology unit. Am J Infect Control 2012;40(10):931–4.

135. Wright MO, Tropp J, Schora DM, et al. Continuous passive disinfection of catheter hubs prevents contamination and bloodstream infection. Am J Infect Control 2013;41(1):33–8.

136. Timsit JF, Schwebel C, Bouadma L, et al. Chlorhexidine-impregnated sponges and less frequent dressing changes for prevention of catheter-related infections in critically ill adults: a randomized controlled trial. JAMA 2009;301(12):1231–41.

137. Timsit JF, Mimoz O, Mourvillier B, et al. Randomized controlled trial of chlorhexidine dressing and highly adhesive dressing for preventing catheter-related infections in critically ill adults. Am J Respir Crit Care Med 2012;186(12):1272–8.

138. Zacharioudakis IM, Zervou FN, Arvanitis M, et al. Antimicrobial lock solutions as a method to prevent central line-associated bloodstream infections: a meta-analysis of randomized controlled trials. Clin Infect Dis 2014;59(12):1741–9.

139. Finucane TE, Christmas C, Travis K. Tube feeding in patients with advanced dementia: a review of the evidence. JAMA 1999;282(14):1365–70.

140. Kitamura T, Nakase H, Iizuka H. Risk factors for aspiration pneumonia after percutaneous endoscopic gastrostomy. Gerontology 2007;53(4):224–7.

141. El-Solh AA, Niederman MS, Drinka P. Management of pneumonia in the nursing home. Chest 2010;138(6):1480–5.

142. Lipp A, Lusardi G. Systemic antimicrobial prophylaxis for percutaneous endoscopic gastrostomy. Cochrane Database Syst Rev 2013;(11):CD005571.

143. Horiuchi A, Nakayama Y, Kajiyama M, et al. Nasopharyngeal decolonization of methicillin-resistant Staphylococcus aureus can reduce PEG peristomal wound infection. Am J Gastroenterol 2006;101(2):274–7.

144. Yokoe DS, Anderson DJ, Berenholtz SM, et al. A compendium of strategies to prevent healthcare-associated infections in acute care hospitals: 2014 updates. Infect Control Hosp Epidemiol 2014;35(8):967–77.

145. Klompas M, Branson R, Eichenwald EC, et al. Strategies to prevent ventilator-associated pneumonia in acute care hospitals: 2014 update. Infect Control Hosp Epidemiol 2014;35(8):915–36.

146. Cardo D, Dennehy PH, Halverson P, et al. Moving toward elimination of healthcare-associated infections: a call to action. Am J Infect Control 2010; 38(9):671–5.

147. Malani PN. Bundled approaches for surgical site infection prevention: the continuing quest to get to zero. JAMA 2015;313(21):2131–2.
148. Morgan DJ, Meddings J, Saint S, et al. Does nonpayment for hospital-acquired catheter-associated urinary tract infections lead to overtesting and increased antimicrobial prescribing? Clin Infect Dis 2012;55(7):923–9.
149. Joynt KE, Blumenthal DM, Orav EJ, et al. Association of public reporting for percutaneous coronary intervention with utilization and outcomes among medicare beneficiaries with acute myocardial infarction. JAMA 2012;308(14):1460–8.
150. Waldo SW, McCabe JM, O'Brien C, et al. Association between public reporting of outcomes with procedural management and mortality for patients with acute myocardial infarction. J Am Coll Cardiol 2015;65(11):1119–26.
151. Centers for Medicare and Medicaid Services. IMPACT act of 2014 data standardization & cross setting measures. Washington, DC: Services Department of Health and Human Services; 2014.
152. Crossley K. Long-term care facilities as sources of antibiotic-resistant nosocomial pathogens. Curr Opin Infect Dis 2001;14(4):455–9.
153. Crosson FJ. Report to the congress: Medicare and the health care delivery system. Washington, DC: Commission MPA; 2016.
154. McGeer A, Campbell B, Emori TG, et al. Definitions of infection for surveillance in long-term care facilities. Am J Infect Control 1991;19(1):1–7.
155. Roup BJ, Scaletta JM. How Maryland increased infection prevention and control activity in long-term care facilities, 2003-2008. Am J Infect Control 2011;39(4):292–5.
156. Zimmerman S, Gruber-Baldini AL, Hebel JR, et al. Nursing home facility risk factors for infection and hospitalization: importance of registered nurse turnover, administration, and social factors. J Am Geriatr Soc 2002;50(12):1987–95.

Urinary Tract Infection and Asymptomatic Bacteriuria in Older Adults

Nicolas W. Cortes-Penfield, MD[a], Barbara W. Trautner, MD, PhD[a,b],
Robin L.P. Jump, MD, PhD[c,d],*

KEYWORDS

- Older adults • Urinary tract infection • Asymptomatic bacteriuria

KEY POINTS

- Differentiating urinary tract infection (UTI) from asymptomatic bacteriuria (ASB) helps health care providers avoid harming older adults with inappropriate antibiotic therapy.
- Testing for UTI should be ordered only when suggestive clinical symptoms are present because laboratory tests alone cannot differentiate ASB from infection.
- The role of testing for UTI is primarily to exclude the diagnosis. With rare exceptions, treatment of UTI should not be given when a patient has a negative urinalysis or urine culture.
- In a clinically stable older adult without genitourinary tract symptoms, active monitoring and oral hydration may obviate antibiotic use.

INTRODUCTION

Urinary tract infections (UTIs) are responsible for an estimated 7 million office visits, 1 million emergency room visits, and 100,000 hospitalizations each year, accounting for some 25% of all infections in geriatric patients.[1] Health care providers often confuse asymptomatic bacteriuria (ASB), defined as bacteria in the urine without any symptoms, with UTI, and unnecessary antibiotic treatment of ASB in older adults is common.[2] In the United States, the prevalence of antimicrobial resistance in urinary organisms in the

Disclosure Statement: Zambon Pharmaceuticals, Grant investigator or recipient (B.W. Trautner). Pfizer: Grant recipient. Steris: Grant recipient (R.L.P. Jump).
[a] Section of Infectious Diseases, Department of Medicine, Baylor College of Medicine, 1 Baylor Plaza, Houston, TX 77030, USA; [b] Center for Innovations in Quality, Effectiveness, and Safety, Michael E. DeBakey Veterans Affairs Medical Center, 2002 Holcombe Boulevard (152), Houston, TX 77030, USA; [c] Division of Infectious Diseases and HIV Medicine, Department of Medicine, Case Western Reserve University, 11100 Euclid Avenue, Cleveland, OH 44195-5029, USA; [d] Geriatric Research, Education, and Clinical Center (GRECC), Specialty Care Center of Innovation, Louis Stokes Cleveland Veterans Affairs Medical Center, 111C(W), 10701 East Boulevard, Cleveland, OH 44106, USA
* Corresponding author. Geriatric Research, Education, and Clinical Center (GRECC), Specialty Care Center of Innovation, Louis Stokes Cleveland Veterans Affairs Medical Center, 111C(W), 10701 East Boulevard, Cleveland, OH 44106.
E-mail address: robinjump@gmail.com

Infect Dis Clin N Am 31 (2017) 673–688
http://dx.doi.org/10.1016/j.idc.2017.07.002
0891-5520/17/Published by Elsevier Inc.

id.theclinics.com

community is increasing, including in older adults.[3–5] In nursing home settings, colonization with multidrug-resistant organisms (MDROs) is high, and these organisms spread to other settings along with the colonized patients.[6] Multidrug-resistant bacteria implicated in UTIs include extended-spectrum beta-lactamase (ESBL)–producing organisms, carbapenem-resistant *Enterobacteriaceae*, and now colistin-resistant gram-negative bacilli.[7–9] At the same time, the severe and sometimes life-threatening adverse events associated with commonly prescribed antibiotics increasingly recognize.[10] These trends highlight the need for a renewed emphasis on antimicrobial stewardship in the treatment of UTIs, which includes increased recognition of ASB.

Confusion about several key issues complicates the approach to the spectrum of syndromes included in the broad category of UTI. Particularly among older adults, these issues include:

- Poorly defined clinical criteria to diagnose UTIs
- Reliance on laboratory criteria rather than clinical symptoms to define infection
- Limited guidance regarding the use and interpretation of diagnostic tests
- Challenges for selecting empiric antimicrobial therapy
- Difficulty distinguishing ASB from UTI, particularly in older adults with dementia
- Increased risk of adverse events and drug interactions related to antibiotic use.

This article summarizes the epidemiology, microbiology, and pathogenesis of UTI in older adults; provides clinically applicable definitions; discusses the approach to diagnostic testing for UTIs in this population; and offers guidance regarding optimal treatment of UTIs in elderly patients when treatment is indicated. UTI in the older adult is framed as a diagnosis of exclusion throughout. Much of inappropriate antibiotic prescribing for UTIs comes from diagnoses based on nonspecific findings, such as leukocytosis, weakness, and malaise.[11] Given that the risk of harm in delaying UTI treatment in clinically stable patients is low,[12] in general, the risk-benefit balance favors a cautious approach to diagnosing and prescribing antibiotics for UTIs in the absence of localizing signs and symptoms.

EPIDEMIOLOGY, MICROBIOLOGY, AND PATHOGENESIS OF URINARY TRACT INFECTIONS
Epidemiology

Among patients older than 65 years, UTIs cause 15.5% of hospitalizations and 6.2% of deaths attributable to an infectious disease.[13] UTIs are the most common type of infection among institutionalized adults and make up more than one-third of all infections in this population.[14,15] Estimates suggest the overall incidence of UTIs in elderly men and women is in the range of 1 infection per 14 to 20 person-years (0.05–0.07 infections per person-year).[16,17] These estimates, however, are based on administrative data that are limited by variations in what the practitioners considered to be a UTI.

Increasing age is itself a risk factor for UTIs. This risk is likely multifactorial, with increasing rates of urinary incontinence and urinary retention, hospitalizations and accompanying urinary catheterizations, long-term medical institutionalization, and immune senescence all contributing. Potentially modifiable factors contributing to UTIs include anatomic abnormalities of the urinary tract, particularly those that produce incontinence or urinary retention (eg, prostatic hyperplasia), uncontrolled diabetes mellitus, treatment with the sodium-glucose cotransporter 2 inhibitors (eg, canagliflozin and dapagliflozin), vaginal atrophy in postmenopausal women, sexual intercourse, which is a risk factor for both men and women, and, most critically in the elderly population, urinary catheterization.[18–24]

Microbiology

Epidemiologic surveillance of outpatient urine cultures offers important insights into the changing prevalence and antibiotic susceptibilities of specific uropathogens. Among patients older than 65 years with uncomplicated cystitis, *Escherichia coli* remains the predominant pathogen, causing nearly two-thirds of cases, followed by *Klebsiella oxytoca* (~ 15% of cases), and *Proteus mirabilis* (~ 7% of cases). Taken together, gram-negative bacteria are present in more than 90% of cases of cystitis in older adults.[4] The microbiology of catheter-associated UTI (CAUTI) is more much diverse. In a review of multicenter data on CAUTIs reported to the National Healthcare Safety Network between 2011 and 2014, *E coli* was still the most common pathogen but made up only 23.9% of cases, whereas rates of *Candida* spp (17.8%), *Enterococcus* spp (13.8%), and *Pseudomonas aeruginosa* (10.3%) were significantly higher than those reported in uncatheterized patients.[25]

Colonization and infection with antibiotic-resistant bacteria increases with age, though the degree to which resistance increases varies by antibiotic class, likely reflecting variation in rates of antibiotic prescribing. For example, among female outpatients in 2012, susceptibility to ceftriaxone among urinary isolates was similar between girls aged 0 to 17 and women older than 65 years (83.4% and 84.3%), whereas for ciprofloxacin the rates of susceptibility dropped from 95.4% to 75% between those groups.[4,26] A limitation to these surveillance data is that, in the outpatient setting, a significant proportion of women may receive treatment of cystitis without a urine culture. Consequently, antimicrobial resistance patterns in the community may differ somewhat from the results based on surveillance data.[27] In the case of older adults with UTI, particular attention should be paid to any history of colonization or infection (including infections other than UTIs) with MDROs, as well the patient's history of antibiotic exposure (ie, which antibiotics the patient received in the past several months). Both prior carriage of MDROs and prior receipt of antimicrobials, the latter producing selective pressure for MDROs, are risk factors for infections with resistant bacteria. Special attention should also be paid to the local susceptibilities of *E coli*, which is responsible for most infections in uncatheterized patients. The resistance profile of *E coli* in the community, which providers may assess using their local antibiogram, will help inform the selection of antibiotics likely to be effective when empiric treatment of UTIs is necessary.

Pathogenesis

Several recent genomic sequencing-based studies of human urine demonstrate that the urinary tract is not sterile even when urine cultures are negative; instead, the healthy urinary tract is host to a unique community of bacteria and viruses.[28–30] Notably, the bladder microbiome of patients with ASB is ecologically distinct from that of healthy patients with negative cultures.[31] Disruption of the urinary microbiota correlates with several genitourinary diseases, including urinary urgency and incontinence, chronic prostatitis, and symptom flares in chronic pelvic pain.[32–34]

The urinary microbiota may also mediate susceptibility to UTIs.[35,36] In theory, constituents of the healthy urinary microbiome may play a role in preventing UTIs by occupying attachment sites at the genitourinary epithelium, competing for limited nutrients, and limiting the proliferation of uropathogens via bacteriophage infection. Persistent urinary dysbiosis may compromise host defenses and lead to recurrent UTIs much in the same way that persistent disruption of intestinal microbiota predispose people to recurrence of *Clostridium difficile* infections. This model challenges the assumption that ASB is necessarily a prelude to symptomatic UTI and further suggests a role for nonantibiotic approaches to managing recurrent UTI. So far, probiotic supplementation has not shown consistent benefit in preventing UTIs, though the quantity and quality of evidence is limited.[37]

Bacterial adhesion to the uroepithelium is a critical step in the pathogenesis of UTIs and thus a potential drug target. Cranberry proanthocyanidins inhibit adherence of *E coli* P-fimbria to uroepithelial cells and have provoked a longstanding interest in the use of various cranberry products for the prevention of UTI. However, multiple investigations on this topic have failed to show a consistent and clinically relevant benefit of cranberries in UTI prevention, and a recent randomized controlled trial showed no benefit of cranberry supplementation in preventing pyuria plus bacteriuria among older women in a nursing home setting.[38,39]

Urinary catheters, the most important risk factor for UTIs, function as portals for bacteria that are not part of the healthy urinary microbiome to enter the urinary tract. The catheter serves as a pathway for bacterial immigration into the ecological niche of the bladder such that bacterial colonization is ubiquitous in catheterized individuals. Although antibiotics can render the urine temporarily sterile, colonization invariably recurs days after antibiotic cessation. Because a persistently sterile urine culture is not a realistic goal for the patient with an indwelling urinary catheter, attempting to eliminate bacteriuria in such a patient with repeated antibiotic prescription merely selects for antibiotic-resistant organisms that may cause the patient future harm.[40]

DEFINING CLINICAL AND LABORATORY CRITERIA FOR URINARY TRACT INFECTION

As a clinical descriptor, UTI encompasses several clinical syndromes, including cystitis, pyelonephritis, and renal or perinephric abscess. Any of these conditions may be accompanied by systemic illness, including bacteremia and sepsis, and any of them can occur in the context of urinary catheterization, referred to as CAUTI. Providers' diagnostic uncertainty in differentiating UTI from ASB contributes to antibiotic overprescribing, and bacteriuria is a risk factor for both receipt of antibiotics for UTI and isolation of multidrug-resistant gram-negative rods in the urine of nursing home residents.[41,42] The authors propose definitions for ASB, which is generally not a clinical condition that merits treatment in older adults, and for the spectrum of conditions that comprise UTI. These definitions are used to differentiate older adults who are likely to benefit from receiving antibiotics from those who are not (**Fig. 1**). Note that this figure is intended to be used in clinical diagnosis and management of UTI. This criteria for UTI differs from the revised McGeer criteria, which are intended for surveillance for UTI in long-term care.[43]

ASB is defined as the presence of bacteria in the urine, with or without pyuria, in the absence of clinical symptoms indicating a UTI. ASB is common in older adults; in 1 study of nursing home residents, 25% to 50% of subjects had bacteriuria at any given time.[44] After adjusting for other comorbidities, older adults with ASB do not experience increases in mortality.[2,45] Antibiotics administered for ASB do not reduce the rates of subsequent complication and perversely, may increase the risk for a subsequent symptomatic UTI.[46] Furthermore, unnecessary antibiotic treatment is associated with acquisition of drug-resistant pathogens, *C difficile* infection, and other drug-related adverse events.[46–48] Guidelines from the Infectious Diseases Society of America recommend treating ASB only in pregnant women or immediately before a urologic procedure likely to involve mucosal injury.[2]

UTIs are defined by 3 components. First, the patient should have clinical symptoms suggesting infection of the urinary tract. In older adults, accepted clinical

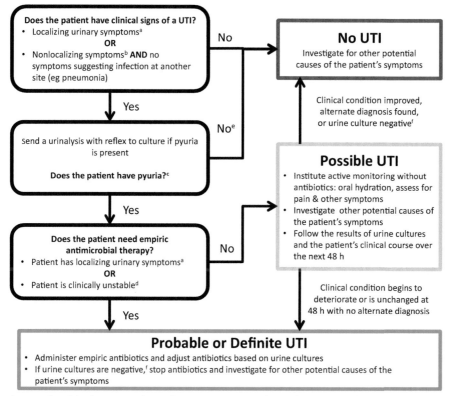

Fig. 1. Algorithmic approach to diagnosing ASB and possible, probable, or definite UTI.
[a] Dysuria, frequency, suprapubic pain, gross hematuria, costovertebral angle tenderness, or new or worsening urgency or urinary incontinence. [b] Fever, rigors, or clear-cut delirium. [c] Greater than 10 white blood cells per high-powered field on microscopy or positive leukocyte esterase. [d] Fever, sepsis or acute illness requiring care within an intensive care unit. [e] UTI can still be considered in patients with neutropenia or other conditions that might cause the absence of pyuria. [f] Urine cultures may be negative if obtained after the patient has received antibiotics; in such cases, stop antibiotics given specifically for UTI if the patient's clinical condition is not improving.

criteria include dysuria alone or fever accompanied by frequency, suprapubic pain, gross hematuria, costovertebral angle tenderness, or new or worsening urgency or urinary incontinence.[49] For those with an indwelling urinary catheter or who had 1 removed in the previous 48 hours, fever, rigors, or delirium alone (all of which are nonspecific); or new costovertebral tenderness, may herald a CAUTI.[49] Note that the revised McGeer criteria for UTI, which were developed for epidemiologic surveillance of UTI, differ slightly in their definitions for UTI and CAUTI (eg, leukocytosis and acute functional decline with no alternate diagnosis in the criteria for CAUTI) than the criteria we propose, which are intended to guide antibiotic prescribing in clinical practice.

Determining whether a change in behavior or mental status is present can be particularly challenging, as evinced by documentation of interobserver variability among nursing home staff for these criteria in 5 nursing homes.[50] Fortunately, dysuria was identified reliably. The presence of dysuria appears to be among strongest predictors of bacteriuria plus pyuria in nursing home residents, and new dysuria is the most helpful clinical finding in identifying UTI in older adults.[51,52]

Other signs and symptoms can be misleading and are often misinterpreted as an indication for urinary testing. Falls are often considered a reason to test a nursing home resident for UTI, but the association of falls and UTI is controversial. A prospective study in these same 5 nursing homes included 397 suspected episodes of UTI and did not find an association between falls and the presence of bacteriuria plus pyuria.[53] Urine turbidity, sediment color, and odor do not reliably correlate with the presence of infection and are not in themselves symptoms of UTI; they are, however, associated with antibiotic overprescribing.[54–56] Such changes in urine may suggest a need for increased oral hydration, reflecting a decreased thirst response in older adults, or may be due to their medications (eg, multivitamins) or diet (eg, asparagus).

Second, laboratory evidence should demonstrate both pyuria and bacteriuria. Pyuria, which indicates an inflammatory reaction in the urinary tract, is generally defined as a positive leukocyte esterase on urine dipstick or greater than or equal to 10 white blood cells per high-powered field (WBCs/HPF), a threshold selected based on offering a negative predictive value for urine culture positivity and clinical UTI.[57] The accepted criteria for bacteriuria is at least 10^5 colony-forming units (CFUs) per 1 mL of a single organism in the urine of an uncatheterized patient or 10^3 CFU/mL greater than or equal to 1 bacterial species in the urine of a catheterized patient.[2,24]

Laboratory testing is primarily useful for excluding UTIs. Pyuria is sensitive but not specific for UTI, particularly among catheterized patients in whom its presence is ubiquitous. Reliance on pyuria alone for the diagnosis of UTI would lead to widespread antibiotic overtreatment, particularly because pyuria accompanies ASB.[2,58] Indeed, CAUTI is overdiagnosed, with retrospective studies showing that only 30% to 50% patients given the clinical diagnosis of CAUTI meet standardized criteria for CAUTI treatment.[59] Studies of the diagnostic value of the urinalysis for UTI have shown that it is an effective rule-out test but that poor specificity limits its value in ruling in UTI.[60,61] In this regard, the clinical utility of the urinalysis for diagnosing UTI is akin to that of the D-dimer for the diagnosis of a pulmonary embolism; a negative result is of great value for patients with all but the highest pretest probabilities of disease, whereas a positive result is necessary but not sufficient to establish the diagnosis.

Finally, the authors define UTI as a diagnosis that can only be made after a thorough search for other causes to explain the patient's symptoms and laboratory findings. This third criterion intends to avoid delays in appropriate therapy due to premature diagnosis of UTI and diagnostic closure. This is particularly relevant for older adults, in whom symptoms attributed to UTI are often not specific to the urinary tract (eg, fever, lethargy and confusion) and may belie infection at another site (eg, pneumonia), systemic infection (eg, influenza), or another cause entirely (eg, heart failure exacerbation).

The clinical presentation of UTI in older adults varies. In a multicenter evaluation of clinical features of UTI in nursing home patients, dysuria and change in mentation were 2 of the most frequently identified characteristics, with the important limitation that in this study UTI was defined by bacteriuria and pyuria alone, without consideration of clinical symptoms.[51] Factors that may complicate the diagnostic impression include urinary catheterization (which can obscure symptoms such as urinary frequency, urgency, or dysuria), baseline urologic comorbidities producing chronic urinary urgency or frequency, and a higher incidence of baseline cognitive impairments (ie, dementia) that can prevent the patient from effectively conveying their symptoms to the provider. In such cases, a careful history from caregivers, thorough physical examination of the patient, and prudent laboratory testing may help differentiate UTI from other conditions.

For older adults especially, specific and clear criteria to diagnose UTIs are critical. First, recognition of ASB reduces unnecessary antibiotic exposure in a population rendered vulnerable to adverse drug events by comorbid conditions and polypharmacy.[62] Second, attributing clinical changes to a UTI without consideration of alternative diagnoses risks patient harm by delaying recognition and response to other medical problems. For example, a nursing home resident with a chronic indwelling urinary catheter who develops an acute change in mental status may be diagnosed with a UTI based on a urine dipstick showing pyuria. Providers may reflexively prescribe antibiotics, without considering other reasons for a clinical change, such as an acute cardiac event or ischemic stroke. This may delay appropriate interventions and lead to patient harm. Recognizing the high prevalence of ASB and the potential for misdiagnosis of UTIs based on laboratory findings, both The Society for Post-Acute Care and Long-Term Care Medicine and the American Geriatrics Society caution against ordering urine cultures in patients without urinary symptoms.[63,64]

QUALITY AND INTERPRETATION OF URINE SPECIMEN COLLECTION

Obtaining an adequate quality urine sample is frequently the first major barrier to appropriately diagnosing UTI in older adults. Guidelines specific to long-term care residents recommend collecting a midstream clean-catch urine specimen for urine studies.[65] In reality, such a collection is an often laborious process requiring the patient to possess not only urinary continence but a degree of cognition, coordination, and mobility that many older adults, particularly those who are institutionalized, may lack. For patients who cannot provide such a specimen, recommendations are to place an external condom catheter in men or perform in-out urinary catheterization in women, which can cause significant discomfort. Staff collecting urine specimens may use approaches that are not recommended by guidelines, such as obtaining the urine from a chronic urinary catheter or urine collection bag, both of which become contaminated with bacteria within hours of urinary catheter placement.[24] Finally, the person who interprets the results of urine studies may or may not be the same person who ordered the tests and is most certainly not the person who collected the sample.

Clinical symptoms that localize to the genitourinary tract should prompt testing urine for possible infection (see **Fig. 1**). In such patients, the diagnostic test of choice is a urinalysis with reflex to urine culture for specimens with pyuria (≥ 10 WBCs/HPF or positive leukocyte esterase). The urinalysis has a negative predictive value for growth of bacteria in urine culture approaching 100%.[66] In patients who lack pyuria, attention should be turned away from UTI and toward other diagnostic considerations, except in rare cases in which neutropenia or other conditions may prevent pyuria. This algorithmic approach combining the urinalysis and urine culture offers both excellent sensitivity and specificity for UTI, with the reflex criteria averting inappropriate urine culture orders, a primary driver of unnecessary antibiotic prescription in patients with ASB.[56,57]

Because of older patients' higher burden of comorbidity and consequent risk of adverse events due to antibiotic therapy, we recommend active monitoring without antibiotics for older adults with possible UTI symptoms who are clinically stable (ie, no evidence of sepsis) until the results of the urinalysis and reflex culture are available. Active monitoring includes frequent assessment of vital signs for early detection of sepsis, parameters for hydration, and criteria for notifying the physician or other provider if the patient's condition worsens.[67] If a patient spontaneously improves while waiting for the results of urine tests, a positive urine culture likely reflects ASB and the provider should consider other reasons for the patient's symptoms. If the patient deteriorates during a period of active monitoring, then providers should consider empiric antibiotic therapy until culture results become available or, depending on the clinical symptoms, consider other diagnoses. Order sets that support monitoring off antibiotics can help standardize active monitoring interventions.[67] When it is necessary to start antibiotics before culture results are known, facility antibiograms should inform selection of empiric treatment, if available.

Urine cultures should not be obtained in older adults unless clinical symptoms suggest a UTI and the accompanying urinalysis demonstrates pyuria (or the patient is neutropenic). Inappropriate ordering of urine cultures is harmful because, just as with a urinalysis, a urine culture does not distinguish between UTI and ASB. Detection of bacteriuria may lead to inappropriate antibiotic therapy, particularly when the patient has a peripheral leukocytosis or when the urine is colonized by a typical or multidrug-resistant uropathogen.[11] In older adults with both pyuria and clinical symptoms consistent with a UTI, obtaining a urine culture permits selecting antibiotics informed by microbiological results. Especially for older adults, we recommend against prescribing antibiotics for UTIs without first obtaining urine cultures to guide the choice of agent because the presence of antibiotic-resistant bacteria increases with age.[4]

TREATMENT OF URINARY TRACT INFECTIONS

For patients with a UTI, antibiotics provide symptomatic relief and may help prevent complications such as pyelonephritis, perinephric abscess, and bacteremia. The 2010 Infectious Diseases Society of America guidelines recommend 4 agents for the treatment of uncomplicated cystitis in women: nitrofurantoin; fosfomycin; pivmecillinam; and, where resistance rates are less than 20%, trimethoprim-sulfamethoxazole.[68] No recommendations have been made for UTI in men or empiric treatment of complicated UTI. However, when choosing empiric treatment in these settings, the provider should refer to the results of prior urine cultures. A study done in predominantly older men with UTI caused by MDROs found that prior urine culture results, even those collected as long ago as 2 years from the index case, were useful at predicting the causative pathogen and its susceptibilities.[69]

Currently, pivmecillinam is not available in the Unites States. Resistance to trimethoprim-sulfamethoxazole now exceeds 20% nationally among common uropathogens in older adults, emphasizing the importance of local antibiogram data in determining whether this agent remains an appropriate empiric agent in a provider's region of practice.[4] Nitrofurantoin is well-tolerated, and susceptibility of uropathogens to this agent remains high in older adults. However, nitrofurantoin achieves poor levels in tissue and serum and thus is only appropriate in patients who have cystitis without suspicion for upper tract disease. A retrospective study of male veterans with UTI treated with nitrofurantoin showed a clinical cure rate of 77% rate, which is comparable to other agents.[70] Decreased creatinine clearance predicted clinical failure in this study; however, 2 additional studies in older adults, 1 limited to women, refuted the concern that nitrofurantoin is less effective in treating UTI in patients with reduced creatinine clearance.[71,72] Particularly in older adults, for whom adverse event profile and collateral damage to the microbiome are important considerations, nitrofurantoin is a good choice for uncomplicated UTIs, including in men with preserved renal function.

Fosfomycin is administered as a single-dose oral packet (sachet) that is mixed with water then consumed. Fosfomycin is effective in the treatment of UTI, but its use is limited by availability, cost, and lack of standardized susceptibility testing. Furthermore, similar to nitrofurantoin, fosfomycin has poor tissue penetration, precluding its use in patients known or suspected to have upper urinary tract disease. In addition, this agent is among few remaining oral agents with reliable activity against ESBL-producing uropathogens, suggesting that its use might be justifiably reserved for people known to have these organisms.

Considered a second-line therapy, tetracycline antibiotics achieve therapeutic levels in urine, are well-tolerated, and may have an emerging role as an oral option for UTIs caused by ESBL-producing and carbapenem-resistant organisms. Most laboratories, however, do not routinely test urinary isolates for susceptibility to tetracyclines. Furthermore, uropathogens that are MDROs may also be resistant to tetracyclines, and only limited clinical data support using tetracyclines to treat UTIs.[73,74]

Other second-line therapies for uncomplicated UTIs include fluoroquinolones, aminoglycosides, β-lactam/β-lactamase inhibitor combinations, and extended-spectrum cephalosporins. Although narrow-spectrum β-lactams and first-generation cephalosporins have historically played a minor role in the treatment of uncomplicated UTI due to concerns about inferior efficacy versus other agents, they are effective in treating urinary isolates known to be susceptible.[68] Using fluoroquinolones to treat UTIs has become commonplace, in part due to their high oral bioavailability and broad spectrum. In May 2016, however, the US Food and Drug Administration (FDA) advised that the risks of these medications generally outweigh their benefits for uncomplicated cystitis when other treatment options are available.[10] Beyond the prevalence of resistant organisms, fluoroquinolones increase the risk of several adverse events to which older adults are particularly vulnerable: QT prolongation, tendonitis and tendon rupture, seizures, delirium, and *C difficile* colitis.[48,75–78] Susceptibility to aminoglycosides remains high among most uropathogens. However, the lack of oral formulations of these drugs, the need to monitor serum drug levels, and the risk of major adverse events, including nephrotoxicity, vestibular toxicity, and ototoxicity, limit the role of this class in treating UTIs outside of the inpatient setting. β-lactam/β-lactamase inhibitor combinations and extended-spectrum cephalosporins are broad-spectrum agents, which may lead to increased collateral damage to the patient's microbiome and selection of ESBL-producing organisms.

For patients with severe or systemic infections arising from the urinary tract, including pyelonephritis or bacteremia, empiric therapy with broad-spectrum agents is appropriate.[68] In these cases, fluoroquinolones, β-lactam/β-lactamase inhibitor combinations, such as piperacillin-tazobactam, and extended-spectrum cephalosporins represent reasonable choices until culture results permit identification of an appropriate narrow-spectrum agent.

The duration of treatment of acute nonsevere UTI is best established in women, for whom the recommended duration of therapy varies by drug from 1 to 5 days.[68] Fosfomycin is given in a single dose, trimethoprim-sulfamethoxazole is given over 3 days, and nitrofurantoin requires a 5-day course of therapy. No clinical trial has demonstrated the superiority of extended (7–14 day) courses of therapy in male UTI or CAUTI versus shorter courses, whereas the harms of unnecessary antibiotic therapy are clear. In older adults, who are particularly susceptible to antibiotic-related adverse events, the risk-benefit calculus of antibiotic treatment favors shorter lengths of therapy. Mounting evidence demonstrates that clinical cure can be effective achieved for CAUTI using a short course of antibiotics ($\leq$7 days) when the catheter is removed if the patient is responding rapidly to initial therapy.[79–81] Similarly, longer lengths of therapy (>7 days) do not prevent recurrent UTIs and instead are associated with increased *C difficile* infection.[18]

Until more data are available, longer duration antibiotic therapy (ie, 10–14 days) remains reasonable for patients with severe urinary tract disease, including pyelonephritis and perinephric abscess, bacteremia, or need for hospitalization due to unstable clinical condition. However, we have intentionally chosen to avoid the labels uncomplicated UTI and complicated UTI in this discussion. We find the latter term problematic because it encompasses a heterogeneous group of conditions, some of which lack strong data supporting the need for extended courses of therapy (eg, UTI in men and diabetic women) and others for which extended antibiotic therapy alone may be inadequate (eg, UTI in the setting of urinary obstruction requiring mechanical intervention). Instead, we advocate that UTIs be classified by the extent of urinary tract and systemic involvement, and that potentially complicating factors, such as diabetes and urinary obstruction, be identified and addressed separately, tailoring the antibiotic duration to the complication and the patient's response to therapy.

PREVENTION OF URINARY TRACT INFECTION
Effective Approaches to Catheter-Associated Urinary Tract Infection Prevention in Long-Term Care

Removing indwelling urinary catheters is key to managing CAUTI because this both prevents further bacterial influx into the urinary tract and eliminates the reservoir of bacteria in biofilms that adhere to the catheter. Practically speaking, CAUTI prevention hinges on routine reevaluation of catheterized patients to determine whether they continue to have an indication for an indwelling urinary catheter, as well as identifying and treating the underlying comorbidities necessitating the catheter, and replacing indwelling catheters with clean intermittent catheterization when appropriate.

Removing catheters that are no longer necessary is an example of a technical intervention, defined as providing professional development and training in urinary catheter utilization, care, and maintenance. More recently, CAUTI prevention efforts have also included a socioadaptive component, specifically encouraging improvements in attitudes and behavior concerning patient safety. Two large-scale studies of CAUTI prevention in acute care and long-term care suggest that interventions that combine both cultural change and technical training can be successful at decreasing CAUTI.[82,83]

Ineffective Approaches to Catheter-Associated Urinary Tract Infection Prevention

Long-term indwelling urinary catheters need be exchanged only when clinically indicated (eg, obstructed catheter flow, leakage from around the catheter insertion site, physical defect in the catheter, or CAUTI) rather than routinely because there is inadequate evidence that the latter practice reduces rates of CAUTI.[84] Attempts to decrease rates of CA UTI and bacteriuria by coating catheters with antibiotics or antiseptic materials have been largely unsuccessful, with either no or limited reductions in clinical outcome at the expense of increased patient discomfort and higher costs.[85] Systemic antibiotic prophylaxis for patients with long-term urinary catheters does not reduce rates of bacteriuria, CAUTI, or death.[84]

SUMMARY

UTIs cause significant morbidity and mortality among older adults. Unfortunately, inappropriate or unnecessary antibiotics prescribed to older adults to treat suspected

UTI based on nonspecific symptoms or positive urine studies also leads to adverse events. The authors favor an approach to diagnosing UTIs rooted in the recognition of clinical signs and symptoms localizing to the genitourinary tract. Furthermore, we emphasize the value of the urinalysis as an exclusionary rather a confirmatory tools for UTIs. For instances when long-term care residents exhibit nonspecific changes, active monitoring, including hydration, treating pain, and reviewing medications, offers the possibility of avoiding unnecessary antibiotics while assuring residents and their family members that the health care team is responding to their concerns. Posting criteria for ordering urine studies, reviewing methods to collect good-quality urine specimens, implementing active monitoring order sets, and offering clinical decision support all represent systems-based approaches that may help curb inappropriate orders for urine studies and for antibiotics.

Developing technologies, such as colonizing the bladder with nonpathogenic bacteria or using catheters impregnated with bacteriophage cocktails are intriguing; however, currently, the most important means to prevent UTIs is by identifying and addressing modifiable risk factors. When older adults develop UTIs, providers should give preference to narrow-spectrum agents and short courses of therapy in most cases, with empiric antibiotic selections informed by local antibiogram data. Treatment and overtreatment of UTIs represents a significant proportion of antibiotic prescribing for older adults, driving the proliferation of resistant organisms in the community. Also, because older adults are particularly susceptible to adverse events associated with antibiotic treatment, whereas the harms associated with delays in appropriate antimicrobial therapy for UTI are small for most clinically stable patients, providers should take an approach to the diagnosis and treatment of UTIs that balances the potential benefit for the individual patient with both the risk of harm to that individual and the provider's duty as an antibiotic steward to protect the health of the larger community.

REFERENCES

1. Ruben FL, Dearwater SR, Norden CW, et al. Clinical infections in the noninstitutionalized geriatric age group: methods utilized and incidence of infections. The Pittsburgh good health study. Am J Epidemiol 1995;141(2):145–57.
2. Nicolle LE, Bradley S, Colgan R, et al. Infectious Diseases Society of America guidelines for the diagnosis and treatment of asymptomatic bacteriuria in adults. Clin Infect Dis 2005;40(5):643–54.
3. Gupta K, Scholes D, Stamm WE. Increasing prevalence of antimicrobial resistance among uropathogens causing acute uncomplicated cystitis in women. JAMA 1999;281(8):736–8.
4. Sanchez GV, Babiker A, Master RN, et al. Antibiotic resistance among urinary isolates from female outpatients in the United States in 2003 and 2012. Antimicrob Agents Chemother 2016;60(5):2680–3.
5. Swami SK, Liesinger JT, Shah N, et al. Incidence of antibiotic-resistant *Escherichia coli* bacteriuria according to age and location of onset: a population-based study from Olmsted County, Minnesota. Mayo Clin Proc 2012;87(8):753–9.
6. Mitchell SL, Shaffer ML, Loeb MB, et al. Infection management and multidrug-resistant organisms in nursing home residents with advanced dementia. JAMA Intern Med 2014;174(10):1660–7.
7. Lob SH, Nicolle LE, Hoban DJ, et al. Susceptibility patterns and ESBL rates of *Escherichia coli* from urinary tract infections in Canada and the United States, SMART 2010-2014. Diagn Microbiol Infect Dis 2016;85(4):459–65.

8. Thaden JT, Lewis SS, Hazen KC, et al. Rising rates of carbapenem-resistant enterobacteriaceae in community hospitals: a mixed-methods review of epidemiology and microbiology practices in a network of community hospitals in the southeastern United States. Infect Control Hosp Epidemiol 2014;35(8):978–83.

9. Mediavilla JR, Patrawalla A, Chen L, et al. Colistin- and carbapenem-resistant *Escherichia coli* harboring mcr-1 and blaNDM-5, causing a complicated urinary tract infection in a patient from the United States. MBio 2016;7(4) [pii:e01191-16].

10. FDA Drug Safety Communication: FDA advises restricting fluoroquinolone antibiotic use for certain uncomplicated infections; warns about disabling side effects that can occur together. 2016. Available at: https://www.fda.gov/Drugs/DrugSafety/ucm500143.htm. Accessed April 12, 2017.

11. Trautner BW, Bhimani RD, Amspoker AB, et al. Development and validation of an algorithm to recalibrate mental models and reduce diagnostic errors associated with catheter-associated bacteriuria. BMC Med Inform Decis Mak 2013;13:48.

12. Knottnerus BJ, Geerlings SE, Moll van charante EP, et al. Women with symptoms of uncomplicated urinary tract infection are often willing to delay antibiotic treatment: a prospective cohort study. BMC Fam Pract 2013;14:71.

13. Curns AT, Holman RC, Sejvar JJ, et al. Infectious disease hospitalizations among older adults in the United States from 1990 through 2002. Arch Intern Med 2005; 165(21):2514–20.

14. Tsan L, Davis C, Langberg R, et al. Prevalence of nursing home-associated infections in the Department of Veterans Affairs nursing home care units. Am J Infect Control 2008;36(3):173–9.

15. Cotter M, Donlon S, Roche F, et al. Healthcare-associated infection in Irish long-term care facilities: results from the First National Prevalence Study. J Hosp Infect 2012;80(3):212–6.

16. Jackson SL, Boyko EJ, Scholes D, et al. Predictors of urinary tract infection after menopause: a prospective study. Am J Med 2004;117(12):903–11.

17. Griebling TL. Urologic diseases in America project: trends in resource use for urinary tract infections in women. J Urol 2005;173(4):1281–7.

18. Drekonja DM, Rector TS, Cutting A, et al. Urinary tract infection in male veterans: treatment patterns and outcomes. JAMA Intern Med 2013;173(1):62–8.

19. Boyko EJ, Fihn SD, Scholes D, et al. Diabetes and the risk of acute urinary tract infection among postmenopausal women. Diabetes Care 2002;25(10):1778–83.

20. Li D, Wang T, Shen S, et al. Urinary tract and genital infections in patients with type 2 diabetes treated with sodium-glucose co-transporter 2 inhibitors: a meta-analysis of randomized controlled trials. Diabetes Obes Metab 2017; 19(3):348–55.

21. Rahn DD, Carberry C, Sanses TV, et al. Vaginal estrogen for genitourinary syndrome of menopause: a systematic review. Obstet Gynecol 2014;124(6): 1147–56.

22. Moore EE, Hawes SE, Scholes D, et al. Sexual intercourse and risk of symptomatic urinary tract infection in post-menopausal women. J Gen Intern Med 2008; 23(5):595–9.

23. David LM, Natin D, Walzman M, et al. Urinary symptoms, sexual intercourse and significant bacteriuria in male patients attending STD clinics. Genitourin Med 1996;72(4):266–8.

24. Hooton TM, Bradley SF, Cardenas DD, et al. Diagnosis, prevention, and treatment of catheter-associated urinary tract infection in adults: 2009 International clinical practice guidelines from the Infectious Diseases Society of America. Clin Infect Dis 2010;50(5):625–63.

25. Weiner LM, Webb AK, Limbago B, et al. Antimicrobial-resistant pathogens associated with healthcare-associated infections: summary of data reported to the National Healthcare Safety Network at the centers for disease control and prevention, 2011-2014. Infect Control Hosp Epidemiol 2016;37(11):1288–301.
26. Cortes-penfield NW, Trautner BW. Nitrofurantoin, an excellent empiric choice for outpatient cystitis. Antimicrob Agents Chemother 2016;60(12):7535.
27. Gupta K, Hooton TM, Miller L. Managing uncomplicated urinary tract infection–making sense out of resistance data. Clin Infect Dis 2011;53(10):1041–2.
28. Lewis DA, Brown R, Williams J, et al. The human urinary microbiome; bacterial DNA in voided urine of asymptomatic adults. Front Cell Infect Microbiol 2013; 3:41.
29. Siddiqui H, Nederbragt AJ, Lagesen K, et al. Assessing diversity of the female urine microbiota by high throughput sequencing of 16S rDNA amplicons. BMC Microbiol 2011;11:244.
30. Malki K, Sible E, Cooper A, et al. Seven bacteriophages isolated from the female urinary microbiota. Genome Announc 2016;4(6) [pii:e01003-16].
31. Fouts DE, Pieper R, Szpakowski S, et al. Integrated next-generation sequencing of 16S rDNA and metaproteomics differentiate the healthy urine microbiome from asymptomatic bacteriuria in neuropathic bladder associated with spinal cord injury. J Transl Med 2012;10:174.
32. Karstens L, Asquith M, Davin S, et al. Does the urinary microbiome play a role in urgency urinary incontinence and its severity? Front Cell Infect Microbiol 2016;6:78.
33. Shoskes DA, Altemus J, Polackwich AS, et al. The urinary microbiome differs significantly between patients with chronic prostatitis/chronic pelvic pain syndrome and controls as well as between patients with different clinical phenotypes. Urology 2016;92:26–32.
34. Nickel JC, Stephens A, Landis JR, et al. Assessment of the lower urinary tract microbiota during symptom flare in women with urologic chronic pelvic pain syndrome: a MAPP Network Study. J Urol 2016;195(2):356–62.
35. Nienhouse V, Gao X, Dong Q, et al. Interplay between bladder microbiota and urinary antimicrobial peptides: mechanisms for human urinary tract infection risk and symptom severity. PLoS One 2014;9(12):e114185.
36. Horwitz D, Mccue T, Mapes AC, et al. Decreased microbiota diversity associated with urinary tract infection in a trial of bacterial interference. J Infect 2015;71(3): 358–67.
37. Schwenger EM, Tejani AM, Loewen PS. Probiotics for preventing urinary tract infections in adults and children. Cochrane Database Syst Rev 2015;(12):CD008772.
38. Jepson RG, Williams G, Craig JC. Cranberries for preventing urinary tract infections. Cochrane Database Syst Rev 2012;(10):CD001321.
39. Juthani-mehta M, Van ness PH, Bianco L, et al. Effect of cranberry capsules on bacteriuria plus pyuria among older women in nursing homes: a randomized clinical trial. JAMA 2016;316(18):1879–87.
40. Warren JW, Anthony WC, Hoopes JM, et al. Cephalexin for susceptible bacteriuria in afebrile, long-term catheterized patients. JAMA 1982;248(4):454–8.
41. Lee MJ, Kim M, Kim NH, et al. Why is asymptomatic bacteriuria overtreated?: a tertiary care institutional survey of resident physicians. BMC Infect Dis 2015; 15:289.
42. Das R, Towle V, Van ness PH, et al. Adverse outcomes in nursing home residents with increased episodes of observed bacteriuria. Infect Control Hosp Epidemiol 2011;32(1):84–6.

43. Stone ND, Ashraf MS, Calder J, et al. Surveillance definitions of infections in long-term care facilities: revisiting the McGeer criteria. Infect Control Hosp Epidemiol 2012;33(10):965–77.

44. Nicolle LE. Asymptomatic bacteriuria in the elderly. Infect Dis Clin North Am 1997; 11(3):647–62.

45. Nicolle LE. Urinary tract infections in the older adult. Clin Geriatr Med 2016;32(3): 523–38.

46. Cai T, Nesi G, Mazzoli S, et al. Asymptomatic bacteriuria treatment is associated with a higher prevalence of antibiotic resistant strains in women with urinary tract infections. Clin Infect Dis 2015;61(11):1655–61.

47. Wagenlehner FM, Naber KG, Weidner W. Asymptomatic bacteriuria in elderly patients: significance and implications for treatment. Drugs Aging 2005;22(10): 801–7.

48. Werner NL, Hecker MT, Sethi AK, et al. Unnecessary use of fluoroquinolone antibiotics in hospitalized patients. BMC Infect Dis 2011;11:187.

49. Loeb M, Bentley DW, Bradley S, et al. Development of minimum criteria for the initiation of antibiotics in residents of long-term-care facilities: results of a consensus conference. Infect Control Hosp Epidemiol 2001;22(2):120–4.

50. Juthani-mehta M, Tinetti M, Perrelli E, et al. Interobserver variability in the assessment of clinical criteria for suspected urinary tract infection in nursing home residents. Infect Control Hosp Epidemiol 2008;29(5):446–9.

51. Juthani-mehta M, Quagliarello V, Perrelli E, et al. Clinical features to identify urinary tract infection in nursing home residents: a cohort study. J Am Geriatr Soc 2009;57(6):963–70.

52. Mody L, Juthani-mehta M. Urinary tract infections in older women: a clinical review. JAMA 2014;311(8):844–54.

53. Rowe T, Towle V, Van ness PH, et al. Lack of positive association between falls and bacteriuria plus pyuria in older nursing home residents. J Am Geriatr Soc 2013;61(4):653–4.

54. Foley A, French L. Urine clarity inaccurate to rule out urinary tract infection in women. J Am Board Fam Med 2011;24(4):474–5.

55. Midthun SJ, Paur R, Lindseth G. Urinary tract infections. Does the smell really tell? J Gerontol Nurs 2004;30(6):4–9.

56. Sloane PD, Kistler CE, Reed D, et al. Urine culture testing in community nursing homes: gateway to antibiotic overprescribing. Infect Control Hosp Epidemiol 2017;38(5):524–31.

57. Pfaller M, Ringenberg B, Rames L, et al. The usefulness of screening tests for pyuria in combination with culture in the diagnosis of urinary tract infection. Diagn Microbiol Infect Dis 1987;6(3):207–15.

58. Tambyah PA, Maki DG. The relationship between pyuria and infection in patients with indwelling urinary catheters: a prospective study of 761 patients. Arch Intern Med 2000;160(5):673–7.

59. Armbruster CE, Prenovost K, Mobley HL, et al. How often do clinically diagnosed catheter-associated urinary tract infections in nursing homes meet standardized criteria? J Am Geriatr Soc 2017;65(2):395–401.

60. Devillé WL, Yzermans JC, Van duijn NP, et al. The urine dipstick test useful to rule out infections. A meta-analysis of the accuracy. BMC Urol 2004;4:4.

61. St john A, Boyd JC, Lowes AJ, et al. The use of urinary dipstick tests to exclude urinary tract infection: a systematic review of the literature. Am J Clin Pathol 2006; 126(3):428–36.

62. Faulkner CM, Cox HL, Williamson JC. Unique aspects of antimicrobial use in older adults. Clin Infect Dis 2005;40(7):997–1004.

63. Society for Post-Acute Care and Long-Term Care Medicine. Choosing wisely: ten things physicians and patients should question. 2015. Available at: http://www.choosingwisely.org/wp-content/uploads/2015/02/AMDA-Choosing-Wisely-List.pdf. Accessed April 19, 2017.

64. American Geriatrics Society. Choosing wisely: ten things clinicians and patients should question. 2015. Available at: http://www.choosingwisely.org/societies/american-geriatrics-society/. Accessed May 5, 2017.

65. High KP, Bradley SF, Gravenstein S, et al. Clinical practice guideline for the evaluation of fever and infection in older adult residents of long-term care facilities: 2008 update by the Infectious Diseases Society of America. Clin Infect Dis 2009;48(2):149–71.

66. Kayalp D, Dogan K, Ceylan G, et al. Can routine automated urinalysis reduce culture requests? Clin Biochem 2013;46(13–14):1285–9.

67. Nace DA, Drinka PJ, Crnich CJ. Clinical uncertainties in the approach to long term care residents with possible urinary tract infection. J Am Med Dir Assoc 2014;15(2):133–9.

68. Gupta K, Hooton TM, Naber KG, et al. International clinical practice guidelines for the treatment of acute uncomplicated cystitis and pyelonephritis in women: a 2010 update by the Infectious Diseases Society of America and the European Society for Microbiology and Infectious Diseases. Clin Infect Dis 2011;52(5):e103–20.

69. Linsenmeyer K, Strymish J, Gupta K. Two simple rules for improving the accuracy of empiric treatment of multidrug-resistant urinary tract infections. Antimicrob Agents Chemother 2015;59(12):7593–6.

70. Ingalsbe ML, Wojciechowski AL, Smith KA, et al. Effectiveness and safety of nitrofurantoin in outpatient male veterans. Ther Adv Urol 2015;7(4):186–93.

71. Santos JM, Batech M, Pelter MA, et al. Evaluation of the risk of nitrofurantoin lung injury and its efficacy in diminished kidney function in older adults in a large integrated healthcare system: a matched cohort study. J Am Geriatr Soc 2016;64(4):798–805.

72. Singh N, Gandhi S, Mcarthur E, et al. Kidney function and the use of nitrofurantoin to treat urinary tract infections in older women. CMAJ 2015;187(9):648–56.

73. Cunha BA. Oral doxycycline for non-systemic urinary tract infections (UTIs) due to P. aeruginosa and other Gram negative uropathogens. Eur J Clin Microbiol Infect Dis 2012;31(11):2865–8.

74. Livermore DM, Warner M, Mushtaq S, et al. What remains against carbapenem-resistant Enterobacteriaceae? Evaluation of chloramphenicol, ciprofloxacin, colistin, fosfomycin, minocycline, nitrofurantoin, temocillin and tigecycline. Int J Antimicrob Agents 2011;37(5):415–9.

75. Arabyat RM, Raisch DW, Mckoy JM, et al. Fluoroquinolone-associated tendon-rupture: a summary of reports in the Food and Drug Administration's adverse event reporting system. Expert Opin Drug Saf 2015;14(11):1653–60.

76. Liu HH. Safety profile of the fluoroquinolones: focus on levofloxacin. Drug Saf 2010;33(5):353–69.

77. Slimings C, Riley TV. Antibiotics and hospital-acquired Clostridium difficile infection: update of systematic review and meta-analysis. J Antimicrob Chemother 2014;69(4):881–91.

78. Lim CJ, Cheng AC, Kennon J, et al. Prevalence of multidrug-resistant organisms and risk factors for carriage in long-term care facilities: a nested case-control study. J Antimicrob Chemother 2014;69(7):1972–80.

79. Darouiche RO, Al mohajer M, Siddiq DM, et al. Short versus long course of anti-biotics for catheter-associated urinary tract infections in patients with spinal cord injury: a randomized controlled noninferiority trial. Arch Phys Med Rehabil 2014; 95(2):290–6.

80. Jarrell AS, Wood GC, Ponnapula S, et al. Short-duration treatment for catheter-associated urinary tract infections in critically ill trauma patients. J Trauma Acute Care Surg 2015;79(4):649–53.

81. Dinh A, Toumi A, Blanc C, et al. Management of febrile urinary tract infection among spinal cord injured patients. BMC Infect Dis 2016;16:156.

82. Saint S, Greene MT, Krein SL, et al. A program to prevent catheter-associated urinary tract infection in acute care. N Engl J Med 2016;374(22):2111–9.

83. Mody L, Green T, Meddings J, et al. A national program to prevent catheter-associated urinary tract infection in nursing home residents. JAMA Intern Med, in press 2017;177(8):1154–62.

84. Cooper FP, Alexander CE, Sinha S, et al. Policies for replacing long-term indwelling urinary catheters in adults. Cochrane Database Syst Rev 2016;(7):CD011115.

85. Lam TB, Omar MI, Fisher E, et al. Types of indwelling urethral catheters for short-term catheterisation in hospitalised adults. Cochrane Database Syst Rev 2014;(9):CD004013.

Bacterial Pneumonia in Older Adults

Oryan Henig, MD, Keith S. Kaye, MD, MPH*

KEYWORDS

- Pneumonia ● Older adults ● Long-term care facility ● Multidrug-resistant organisms
- Empiric treatment

KEY POINTS

- The incidence of pneumonia increases with age, and is particularly high in patients who reside in long-term care facilities (LTCFs).
- Despite diagnostic and therapeutic advances, mortality rates for pneumonia in the elderly are high and have not decreased in the last decade.
- Atypical symptoms such as confusion, general clinical deterioration, new onset of recurrent falls, and exacerbation of underlying illness should trigger clinical suspicion and evaluation for pneumonia.
- Decisions regarding the site of care for older adults with pneumonia should take into account scoring systems of pneumonia severity, patient wishes regarding intensity of care, supportive environment, and clinical judgment.
- Empiric treatment of pneumonia should be based on clinical assessment of illness severity and risk factors for multidrug-resistant organisms, which are more common in older adults and LTCF residents.

OVERVIEW AND EPIDEMIOLOGY

Pneumonia is a serious infection that occurs when a pathogen's virulence overcomes a person's host defenses. Aging is associated with general deterioration of organ function in a way that dictates not only an individual's risk of developing pneumonia, but also clinical manifestations and outcomes. In addition to increased complexity of clinical presentation and more rapid progression of disease, older patients are at higher risk to have pneumonia owing to resistant organisms including Gram-negative bacilli, and therefore empiric as well as definitive treatment can be challenging. The incidence of pneumonia increases with age, as does the impact of pneumonia on morbidity and mortality.

Disclosure: All authors report no conflicts of interest relevant to this article.

Division of Infectious Diseases, Department of Medicine, University of Michigan, 1150 West Medical Center Drive, Ann Arbor, MI 48109-5680, USA

* Corresponding author. Division of Infectious Diseases, University of Michigan Medical School, 5510A MSRB I, SPC 5680, 1150 West Medical Center Drive, Ann Arbor, MI 48109-5680.

E-mail address: keithka@med.umich.edu

Infect Dis Clin N Am 31 (2017) 689–713

http://dx.doi.org/10.1016/j.idc.2017.07.015

id.theclinics.com

0891-5520/17/© 2017 Elsevier Inc. All rights reserved.

In the 19th century, before the antimicrobial era, pneumonia was described by Sir William Osler as a fatal disease in older adults. Mortality rates are still high, particularly in elderly patients. Pneumonia, together with influenza, is the eighth leading cause of death in the United States and accounts for 2.3% of all death cases in patients older than 65 years.[1]

Risk factors for pneumonia among older adults include underlying comorbid conditions, such as cardiovascular and lung disease, diabetes mellitus, and malignancy, all of which are more prevalent in advanced age. Male gender and smoking have been identified as independent risk factors for community-acquired pneumonia (CAP) in older adults,[2–4] as has reduced functional capacity, and residence in an institution (long-term care facility [LTCF] or nursing home).[5–7]

Polypharmacy is a common finding in older patients, and several drugs are associated with higher risk of pneumonia, including antipsychotic and anticholinergic drugs, both used to treat symptoms that are more common in elderly patients. These drugs are used to treat dementia symptoms, urinary incontinence, depression, pain, and insomnia.[8] Some of the anticholinergic side effects include sedation and altered mental status, which increase the risk of pneumonia, and can also be symptoms of pneumonia.[9] In addition, inhaled corticosteroids have been associated with recurrent pneumonia.[10]

The burden of pneumonia on health care resources is enormous owing to both hospitalization costs and long-term outcomes, particularly in elderly patients.[11] With the anticipated growth of the population of older adults, the burden of pneumonia, both community acquired and health care associated, is anticipated to increase.[11,12]

PATHOGENESIS: WHAT MAKES ELDERLY PATIENTS PRONE TO DEVELOPING PNEUMONIA?

In general, regardless of age, pneumonia occurs when an organism's ability to penetrate and infect the lung parenchyma overcomes the host's defense mechanisms.[6] Several factors common in the elderly contribute to breaches in their defense systems, making elderly patients not only more vulnerable to infection, but also more vulnerable to severe infection associated with prolonged recovery and poor outcomes.

Structural and functional changes across the respiratory system lead to reduced host defenses. These factors include (1) impaired function of mucociliary clearance, an important defense mechanism against pathogen entrance to the upper airways and respiratory tree. Slower and less efficient clearance of secretions by the mucociliary system in the elderly has been shown to correlate with pneumonia.[13] (2) Chest wall mobility and compliance decrease with aging owing to costovertebral joint alteration, rib cartilage calcification, loss of muscle strength, and changes in the shape of rib cage such as kyphosis or scoliosis. (3) Lung compliance is reduced owing to changes in lung parenchyma, which affect the lung's elastic recoil.[6] These alterations in the chest wall and lung compliance lead to increased air trapping, reduced ability to clear secretions, and an increase in the workload of respiratory muscles. In older age, a further increase in the work of breathing, as occurs in cases of pneumonia and particularly in the presence of underlying diseases such as cardiovascular and lung diseases, compromise functionality during infection and may lead to respiratory failure.[14]

Neurologic changes predisposing older adults to "silent aspiration" include reduced ability to cough owing to gag reflex dysfunction as well as changes in mental status.[15] In one study, oropharyngeal dysphagia was strongly associated with CAP in the elderly (occurring in 91% of patients with CAP; odds ratio, 16.3; 95% CI, 4.6–58.2).[16] In addition, pneumonia has been estimated to occur in about 10% to 30% of patients after a stroke.[17,18] In a study that followed patients older than 65 years with infarcts, patients with bilateral basal ganglia infarcts had the highest incidence of pneumonia compared with those with no infarct or less extensive lesions.[19] The response to infection is altered in the elderly owing to lower sensitivity of the respiratory centers to hypoxia and hypercapnia. Altered mentation and absence of cough or appropriate ventilator response also modify clinical presentation in the elderly, delay diagnosis and treatment, and consequently impact clinical outcomes.[20,21] The increased frequency of respiratory tract colonization in older adults[22–24] leads to an increased likelihood of chemical aspiration developing into aspiration pneumonia.[25]

The alterations in the immune system that occur with aging are not well-defined. Several animal and human observations have demonstrated immune dysregulation in both innate and adaptive immune components.[26] However, some studies demonstrate prolonged low-grade inflammation, and some levels of proinflammatory cytokines are higher in patients older than 70 years compared with patients younger than 60 years.[27–29] Some authors propose that low-grade inflammation, called "inflammaging" may contribute to blunted immune response to respiratory tract infection.[21,30] Further research is needed to understand the magnitude and the role of alterations in the immune system associated with pneumonia in elderly patients.

Comorbid conditions also contribute to increased risk. Most elderly persons with pneumonia have 1 or more comorbid conditions.[31] Fry and colleagues[5] compared 2 cohorts of patients who were hospitalized with CAP and showed that the proportion of patients with 1 or more comorbid conditions increased with age, as well as during the study period (77% in the group of 2000–2002 vs 66% in the group of 1988–1990).

DIFFERENT EPIDEMIOLOGIC CATEGORIES OF PNEUMONIA IN OLDER ADULTS

Pneumonia has traditionally been epidemiologically categorized by the site of onset, for example, CAP, nursing home–acquired pneumonia, and hospital-acquired pneumonia. CAP is defined as pneumonia that occurs in patients who are not hospitalized or who are admitted to the hospital for less than 48 hours.[32] Within the spectrum CAP, patients can be categorized to patients who are at risk of acquiring CAP owing to multidrug-resistant organisms (CAP-MDRO), and patients without risk factors of MDROs.

In the 2005 guidelines for hospital-acquired pneumonia the term health care–associated pneumonia (HCAP) was introduced to identify patients who develop pneumonia outside of the hospital but owing to health care exposures were at increased risk for MDRO pathogens. The criteria for HCAP included patients who were hospitalized in an acute care hospital for 2 or more days within the 90 days before infection; had recently resided in a nursing home or a LTCF; had received recent intravenous antibiotic therapy, chemotherapy, or wound care within the 30 days before the current infection; or had recently attended a hospital or hemodialysis clinics.[33]

Owing to concerns regarding how effective HCAP was in identifying patients with MDRO pneumonia and concerns that the guidelines in some instances promoted unnecessary broad-spectrum antimicrobial use for HCAP patients,[34] recently published 2016 hospital-acquired pneumonia guidelines did not include the category HCAP.[35] This issue is pertinent to this article, because between 2005 and 2016, pneumonia acquired in a LTCF was considered to be HCAP, but now would be categorized as CAP, and in many instances CAP with risk factors for MDRO pathogens.

In the current review, we categorize CAP in the unique population of elderly persons into 3 subgroups: CAP in elderly patients who are not at risk for acquiring pneumonia owing to MDRO (referred to as CAP), CAP in elderly patients who are at risk for acquiring pneumonia owing to MDRO (referred to as CAP-MDRO), and CAP among LTCF residents (**Fig. 1**).[36,37] Many, but not all persons who fit into the CAP among LTCF residents category also fit into the CAP owing to MDRO category (see **Fig. 1**). This article does not discuss pneumonia occurring in persons who are ventilator dependent or have hospital-acquired pneumonia.

EPIDEMIOLOGY

CAP is a relatively common infection in older adults, accounting for more than 30% to 40% of the hospitalizations in this age group, and is associated with an increased risk of morbidity and mortality.[10,38]

In a prospective study that included more than 25,000 men in the United States, the risk of CAP in patients older than 65 years was 4.17 times higher than in patients younger than 45 years of age.[39] In another surveillance study in 4 European countries, the incidence of CAP in 2009 was 10.8-fold higher in those aged greater than 85 years compared with adults aged 50 to 64 years.[40] The incidence of CAP ranges from 8 to 18.2 episodes per 1000 persons who were older than 65 years and remained stable across various studies from different geographic areas between 1981 and 2011.[2,41–43]

In general, approximately 30% of the patients with CAP (of all ages) require admission to the hospital.[44] Elderly patients' hospitalization rates are much higher. In the Patient Outcomes Research Team (PORT) study in 1991, of 693 patients with CAP who were older than 65 years, more than 80% of patients were treated as inpatients.[45] In a large prospective US study (Etiology of Pneumonia in the Community [EPIC]) from 2010 to 2012, the annual incidence of hospitalization for CAP was 24.8 cases per 10,000 adults and increased with age: patients in the age group of 65 to 79 years, and those in the age group of 80 years and older had 9 and 25 times higher incidences of hospitalization, respectively, compared with patients between 18 to 40 years of age.[46]

Fry and colleagues[5] analyzed data from the National Hospital Discharge Survey (NHDS) to explore the factors that contribute to increased rates of hospitalization among elderly persons with pneumonia from 1988 to 2002. Of 173 million hospitalizations, 9.1% had a pneumonia discharge diagnosis. The rate of hospitalization among patients older than 85 years was 2 to 4 times than the younger groups (65–74, 75–84 years). Underlying diseases (cardiovascular disease, chronic lung disease, and diabetes mellitus) were associated with high rates of hospitalization in this study.

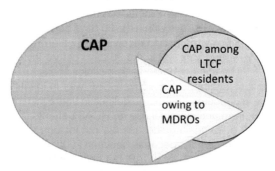

Fig. 1. Distribution of community-acquired pneumonia (CAP) and subsets of CAP, including CAP among long-term care facility residents (LTCF), and CAP owing to multidrug-resistant organisms (MDROs).

Pneumonia Among Lon-term Care Facility Residents

Nursing home–acquired pneumonia constitutes the largest proportion of CAP among LTCF patients.[37] In 2014 in the United States, about 1.4 million people were cared for in nursing homes and more than 90% were older than 65 years.[47,48]

The incidence of pneumonia among residents of LTCFs is higher than among elderly persons who live at home. The median reported annual incidence of pneumonia among LTCF residents is 365 cases per 1000 persons (range, 99–912),[49] approximately 11 times the incidence reported among patients from the community older than 75 years of age (34 per 1000 persons).[41,50]

Pneumonia is the most common infectious reason for transfer of a person from the nursing home residence to the hospital, accounting for 21.6% of admissions.[49] Marrie[51] reported a hospitalization rate among nursing home residents with pneumonia that was nearly 30 times higher than that among elderly patients living at home with CAP (33:1000 persons vs 1.14:1000 persons).

Patients who acquire pneumonia in an LTCF often have multiple comorbid diseases (eg, cardiovascular, respiratory, and neurologic) and poor functional status. In addition, risk factors for aspiration among LTCF residents (eg, nasogastric feeding, difficulty swallowing, receiving sedative agents, and poor functional status) increase risk for the development of pneumonia.[52–54]

MICROBIOLOGY

In general, despite technological diagnostic improvements, the causative pathogen is not identified in nearly one-half of pneumonia episodes across all ages,[32,55] and in up to 77% of pneumonia episodes that occur in elderly patients.[56] Cough reflex dysfunction and altered mentation often preclude the availability of sputum, and only 30% to 40% of patients are able to provide sputum for analysis.[6,44] In addition, elderly patients tend to receive antibiotic treatment before attempts at diagnostic procedures, particularly in persons residing in LTCFs.[57]

Common Causes of Pneumonia Among Elderly Patients in the Community, Including Long-term Care Facilities

Streptococcus pneumoniae is by far the most common pathogen detected in CAP, and accounts for 20% to 85% of cases in the elderly. *Haemophilus influenza* is the second most common detected pathogen (2.9%–29.4%),[6,56,58] followed by respiratory viruses, in particular influenza, coronavirus, and rhinovirus (**Table 1**).[46,56]

Legionella is detected in 1.0% to 17.5%[57–59] of cases and in some studies is considered to be the second or third commonest cause of pneumonia in the elderly, particularly in cases of severe CAP.[60] Other atypical organisms (including *Mycoplasma pneumoniae* and *Chlamydia* spp) are infrequently identified in adults aged over 65 years.[6,42]

Coinfection with bacterial and viral pathogens has been reported in 3% to 40% of cases of CAP,[4,44] and detection of coinfection has increased with the use of improved diagnostic tests. Bacterial coinfection complicates approximately 2.5% of influenza cases in older patients and those with comorbid conditions. In the 2009 H1N1 pandemic, bacterial coinfection complicated 18% to 34% of intensive care unit (ICU) cases, and more than one-half of the fatal cases.[61]

In 6 studies that evaluated pneumonia among LTCF residents, *S pneumoniae* (12.9%) was identified as the most common cause of pneumonia, followed by *H influenza* (6.4%), *Staphylococcus aureus* (6.4%), and *Moraxella catarrhalis* (4.4%). Enteric Gram-negative bacteria accounted for 4.2% to 14.3% of cases.[51] The role of atypical

Table 1
Epidemiology of bacterial pathogens causing CAP among elderly patients and residents of LTCF, and risk factors for each organism

	CAP in the Elderly (Range of Prevalence), % [36,49,56-58,60,66,81,105,138]	CAP Among LTCF Residents (Range of Prevalence), % [45,55,99,133,139]	Risk Factors for Pneumonia Owing to Each Organism [65,71,72,75,77,119,140]
Streptococcus pneumonia	20–85	9–55	Risk for pneumonia owing to nonsusceptible *S pneumoniae*[a] Use of β-lactam, fluoroquinolones or macrolides within the past 90 d COPD Probable aspiration Previous episode of pneumonia within the past 12 mo
Staphylococcus aureus	0–7	0–33	Risk for pneumonia owing to MRSA: Hospitalization for ≥2 d within the past 90 d Use of antibiotics within the past 90 d LTCF residence Chronic dialysis during the preceding 30 d Exposure to previous intravenous treatment within the past 30 d Positive MRSA history within the past 90 d Comorbidities: congestive heart failure, diabetes mellitus, dementia, cerebrovascular disease Severe illness at presentation: altered mental status, bilateral or cavitary disease Use of gastric acid suppressive agents
Haemophilus influenza	2.9–29.4	2–22	Risk for pneumonia owing to resistant *H influenza*[b] Use of prior antibiotic within the past 90 d
Legionella	1–17.5	0–6	N/A

Enteric GNB	0–12	4.2–14.3	Risk for pneumonia owing to enteric GNB: LTCF residence; Nonambulatory status; Probable aspiration; Tube feedings; Comorbid conditions: pulmonary disease, heart failure, cerebrovascular diseases, dementia; Use of gastric acid suppression agents
Pseudomonas aeruginosa	2–17.1	0–6	Risk for pneumonia owing to *P aeruginosa*: Hospitalization for ≥2 d within the past 90 d; Use of antibiotics within the previous 90 d; Probable aspiration; Impaired swallowing; Use of gastric acid suppression agents; Prior history of severe structural lung disease, either severe COPD or bronchiectasis; Prior respiratory culture positive for *P aeruginosa* within the past 12 mo; Severe illness on admission (need for ICU admission or ventilator assistance)
Atypical pathogens: *Chlamydia spp, Mycoplasma pneumonia*	1–32	0–19	N/A

Abbreviations: CAP, community-acquired pneumonia; COPD, chronic obstructive pulmonary disease; GNB, Gram-negative bacilli; ICU, intensive care unit; LTCF, long term care facilities; MRSA, methicillin-resistant *S aureus*; N/A, not applicable.

[a] Nonsusceptible *S pneumoniae* includes resistance to one or more of the following classes of antibiotics: penicillins, cephalosporins, macrolides, and fluoroquinolones.

[b] Resistant *H influenza* includes resistance to penicillin, typically owing to β-lactamase production.

pathogens (*Chlamydia spp*, *M pneumoniae*, *Legionella*) as a cause of pneumonia among LTCF patients is less defined.[62]

Pneumonia Owing to less Common Pathogens, Including Multidrug-resistant Pathogens, Among Older Adults in the Community and in Long-term Care Facilities

Gram-negative bacilli
Gram-negative bacilli are detected in 2.8% to 14.0% of CAP cases, and may colonize the respiratory tract of elderly patients with oropharyngeal dysphagia,[63] particularly those admitted to the hospital from LTCFs.[50,58] Among LTCF patients with severe aspiration pneumonia, enteric Gram-negative bacilli were detected as the predominant cause in 49% of cases.[64]

In the Competence Network for Community-Acquired Pneumonia (CAPNETZ) study, predictors of CAP owing to *Enterobacteriaceae* included age greater than 65 years, heart failure and cerebrovascular disease.[65] *Pseudomonas aeruginosa* was reported in 2.0% to 17.1% of patients, and was associated with impaired swallowing, chronic obstructive pulmonary disease, bronchiectasis, severe disease, admission from nursing homes, and presence of a feeding tube.[36,60,63,65,66] Although there are no data that support empiric anti-*Pseudomonas* treatment in elderly patients, this pathogen should be considered in severe infection in the presence of structural lung disease and known prior colonization.

Resistant Streptococcus pneumoniae
The introduction of pneumococcal conjugated vaccine PCV7 in 2000 (PCV7) and then PCV13 (2010) was followed by a 45% decrease nonsusceptible invasive pneumococcal disease (IPD) in elderly patients.[67] Data from the Centers for Disease Control and Prevention's active bacterial core surveillance demonstrated a large decrease in the multidrug–nonsusceptible IPD (*S pneumoniae* nonsusceptible to ≥3 antimicrobial classes), from 4.2 to 1.8 cases per 100,000 adults older than 65 years. Among cases of nonsusceptible IPD, the frequency of nonsusceptibility patterns of *S pneumoniae* strains was as follows: 86.6% nonsusceptible to macrolides, 47.7% to cephalosporins, 43.6% to tetracycline, and 32.1% to penicillin. No fluoroquinolone or glycopeptide resistance was found.[68] These patterns of resistance should be considered when treating IPD in the post–PCV-13 era.

Staphylococcus aureus including methicillin-resistant Staphylococcus aureus
S aureus has been identified in 1% to 25.5% of CAP cases.[36,46,60,66,69,70] The AWARE study, a surveillance study that evaluated more than 2000 samples of hospitalized patients from 65 medical centers in the United States, including respiratory tract samples, demonstrated that among patients older than 65 years, 52.6% of *S aureus* were methicillin-resistant *Staphylococcus aureus* (MRSA), and the resistance rates to erythromycin, clindamycin, and levofloxacin were substantially higher in this age group as well.[71] Shorr and colleagues[72] assessed risk factors for MRSA among patients hospitalized with CAP (cultures were taken within 48 hours of admission). MRSA was the second most common pathogen in the cohort (14%) after *S pneumoniae* (17.5%). In this study, age greater than 79 years was identified as a predictor of MRSA, as were prior health care exposure, severe illness, and comorbidities (dementia, cerebrovascular, and, for females, diabetes mellitus).

Community-acquired MRSA was first described in 1999 in the United States and became a significant pathogen by 2005.[73] Community-acquired MRSA pneumonia is a recognized complication of influenza and typically presents as a severe disease. Although MRSA is an important cause of pneumonia in elderly, particularly among

LTCF residents, community-acquired MRSA has not been reported to be a significant cause of pneumonia in elderly patients.[74]

Risk factors for community-acquired pneumonia owing to multidrug-resistant organisms

Several scores were developed in the past decade to evaluate patients who are at risk for CAP owing to MDROs. **Table 1** shows risk factors associated with CAP owing to MDRO.[72,75,76] No consensus exists as to which is the most reliable combination of risk factors predicting the likelihood of patients hospitalized for CAP owing to MDROs. Brito and Niederman[77] reviewed several studies that evaluated patients with HCAP and proposed an algorithm that combined severity of illness and number of risk factors. In general, most of the studies included patients who were recently hospitalized, or arrived from LTCFs with severe CAP (ie, were admitted to the ICU). The most common resistant pathogens described in these studies were MRSA and P aeruginosa, as well as other gram-negative bacilli. Risk factors included in this algorithm were recent antibiotic therapy in the past 6 months, recent hospitalization in the past 3 months, the presence of immune suppression, and poor functional status as defined by inability to perform activities of daily living.[77] According to the authors, patients with severe CAP and 1 risk factor should receive empiric broad spectrum antibiotic treatment, whereas patients who have nonsevere CAP needed to have 2 or more risk factors before broad spectrum therapy would be indicated. This algorithm might be useful as a supplement to clinical judgment when managing patients with pneumonia.

CLINICAL PRESENTATION AND DIAGNOSIS

Pneumonia in elderly patients was described by William Osler as a painless and fatal disease. The disease was described as latent, without chills, with mild cough, and sometimes without sputum. Physical examination was marked owing to the lack of classic evidence of consolidation, and mental status changes might be the only signs of pneumonia.[25]

Not much has changed in our knowledge regarding pneumonia manifestations in the elderly. Fever may be absent in 25% to 55% of pneumonia cases in older adults,[20,25,78] and a similar proportion of elderly patients present with altered mental status.[57] Of 48 patients older than 65 years in a veteran's administration medical center who were diagnosed with pneumonia based on new pulmonary infiltrates and symptoms, only 35% presented with fever and cough. The absence of classic symptoms was more common in patients with reduced baseline functional capacity.[79] A study that evaluated 1812 patients from 4 US hospitals demonstrated that, as patients became older, the number of reported symptoms of pneumonia decreased.[20]

Among patients who reside in LTCFs, pneumonia-related signs and symptoms were demonstrated to be subtler than in CAP patients from the same age group.[80] As many as 73% of these LTCF cases present with confusion. Fever and respiratory symptoms were less common than in other CAP patients.[49] In residents of LTCFs, diagnosis of pneumonia based on symptoms and physical examination has low sensitivity and specificity (47%–69% and 58%–75%, respectively).[51] In addition, owing to the presence of other comorbid conditions, there is often a broad and nonspecific differential diagnosis, which can lead to diagnostic challenges and delays. An association between latent pneumonia and poor outcomes was described by Osler William, who stressed that fever may actually be a positive predictor of outcome, a notion that was later supported by other researchers.[81–84]

The diagnosis of pneumonia in the elderly depends on a high index of suspicion and should be considered in the presence of one of the following atypical signs and symptoms: confusion, delirium, disorientation,[25] or loss of appetite. Particularly in an older adult with dementia, urinary incontinence may sometimes be an early indicator of debility caused by pneumonia.[79] These atypical symptoms should not be automatically attributed to a patient's baseline dementia.[81,85] Unexplained deterioration in general health, weakness, new onset of recurrent falls, and functional decline (ie, general deterioration) may also be important manifestations of pneumonia in older adults, as well as exacerbation of underlying illnesses, such as congestive heart failure, chronic pulmonary lung disease, and impaired diabetic control.[25]

Simple physical examination findings, including respiratory rate (>25 breathes per minute) and pulse oximetry (oxygen saturation <90%) have a high sensitivity for pneumonia and, if present, indicate the need for further evaluation of pneumonia, potentially including imaging, testing, and referral to an acute care hospital.[86,87] In 1 study of LTFC subjects with pneumonia, an oxygen saturation of less than 94% was sensitive and specific for the diagnosis of pneumonia (80% and 91%, respectively).[88]

Imaging

Evaluating imaging findings in elderly persons with suspected pneumonia is challenging. The classic pulmonary opacity used as part of the gold standard for diagnosis of pneumonia may not be identified by a regular chest radiograph owing to poor film quality. Poor quality might be owing in part to the patient's poor cognitive status, poor muscle strength, and inability to maintain posture.[86] In addition, lung disease (chronic obstructive pulmonary disease, malignancies, interstitial lung disease) and chest wall abnormalities, which are more frequent in the elderly, may complicate the interpretation of chest radiographs. In several studies of elderly patients, computed tomography (CT) scan detected pneumonia in up to 47% of cases that were not identified by using chest radiographs.[89,90] There are also interobserver discrepancies in the interpretation of chest radiographs, which may be particularly problematic when portable chest radiographs are used.[91]

Among residents of LTCFs, imaging has an important role in the diagnosis of pneumonia, as well as in identifying other high-risk conditions that warrant the transfer to an acute care facility. Often, LTCFs have contracted services that provide portable chest radiographs; these portable chest radiographs have similar limitations to standard chest radiographs, as described. Further complicating the usefulness of chest radiographs in LTCFs is a lack of previous films for comparison.[86] Nevertheless, several studies have reported that 75% to 90% of chest radiographs taken for evaluation of suspected pneumonia among LTCF residents showed evidence of pneumonia. Thus, chest radiograph should be conducted as part of the evaluation of pneumonia in LTCF residents.[86,92]

Although CT scan is the gold standard for diagnosis of pneumonia, limitations such as cost, radiation exposure, availability, and identification of incidental findings, which are particularly common in the elderly,[93] limit its usefulness. Chest CT should be limited to cases where chest radiograph findings are inconclusive, pneumonia complications might be present (eg, lung abscess), or when there is suspicion for pathologies that cannot be diagnosed by chest radiograph (eg, pulmonary embolism, tumor, etc).

Lung ultrasound (LUS) imaging was recently evaluated for the diagnosis of CAP in the elderly, when the chest radiograph findings were inconclusive. In a cohort of 169 elderly frail patients, the sensitivity of LUS imaging was 91% and of chest radiograph was 47% (gold standard was considered to be clinical diagnosis, with or without CT scan).[94] Recent metaanalyses that evaluated LUS imaging for the diagnosis of pneumonia reported a pooled sensitivity of 94% to 95% and specificity of 90% to 96% when LUS imaging findings were compared with diagnosis of pneumonia by clinical signs and/or chest radiograph or CT findings, and a high correlation between LUS imaging and CT findings was reported (Spearman correlation coefficient of 0.87).[95,96] Radiographic resolution lags behind clinical resolution of pneumonia, but older age was not found to be associated with delayed resolution compared with younger age groups.[97]

Laboratory Evaluation

As in other age groups, blood tests are indicated to support the diagnosis of pneumonia by evaluating inflammatory markers (white blood cell counts), and to evaluate organ damage and severity of illness (creatinine level, liver enzymes, platelet counts, etc).

In elderly persons, inflammatory responses may be subtle, and white blood cell counts may be normal or low. Several studies of elderly patients who were diagnosed with pneumonia reported that the absence of leukocytosis, as well as leukopenia, was associated with increased mortality (29% vs 4% in patients without vs patients with leukocytosis).[83,98] Among patients who reside in LTCFs, neutrophil percentage of greater than 90% and left shift (neutrophil band percentage of >6%) were associated with high likelihood of bacterial infection.[86]

Recently, extensive discussion occurred pertaining to the value of inflammatory markers such as C-reactive protein (CRP) and procalcitonin (PCT) in discriminating bacterial pneumonia from other inflammatory and infectious processes. The usefulness of PCT in differentiating bacterial pneumonia from other acute illnesses in the real world is controversial.[99,100] In addition, the role of PCT in elderly persons is unclear, because this population group is usually excluded from clinical studies. A recent retrospective study in Italy evaluated the role of CRP in elderly patients who presented to the emergency department with respiratory symptoms and were discharged with or without a final diagnosis of pneumonia. This study reported an association between high CRP levels and pneumonia, even after adjusting for confounders, with a cutoff of 61 mg/L providing the best sensitivity and specificity (odds ratio, 3.59; 95% CI, 2.35–5.48). In the same study, PCT levels were not significantly associated with pneumonia.[90] The use of CRP and PCT was evaluated for severity of pneumonia in elderly patients, and was not found to predict mortality.[101,102]

Low serum albumin levels are associated with poor prognosis in CAP patients.[103] In 1 study that compared clinical manifestations of pneumonia among CAP patients and LTCF residents, the albumin level was much lower among LTCF residents with pneumonia than in non-LTCF CAP patients.[104] In another study, low serum albumin levels and lymphocytes (both of which represent poor nutritional status) were associated with mortality.[80]

Microbiologic Diagnosis

The current recommendations are to search for a pathogenic etiology only in patients where the results might lead to a change in management and may reduce treatment failure. These types of patients include high-risk patients, with either severe pneumonia, or who have multiple comorbid conditions.[32] In patients who are ill enough to be hospitalized with severe pneumonia, 2 sets of blood cultures should be obtained, in addition to sputum cultures and urinary antigen tests for *Streptococcus pneumonia* and *Legionella pneumophila*. ICU patients with severe pneumonia often require more extensive evaluation, including bronchoalveolar lavage for microbiologic diagnosis of viruses and bacterial pathogens. These recommendations and clinical guidance are not specific for elderly patients. Clinical judgment should be used to consider the yield of a particular test and the impact of its results on clinical management.

Among LTCF residents, the yield from blood cultures is low when patients are treated in the LTCF. However, when an LTCF resident acquires pneumonia severe enough to be transferred to an acute care facility, blood cultures are recommended.[86] In addition, because of the poor functional capacity of many LTCF residents, sputum examination is often not performed, even when residents are admitted to an acute care facility (<30% of the patients have sputum examined). When sputum is obtained, frequently samples are not adequate for diagnostic evaluation. Thus, sputum sampling is not recommended for initial assessment, except for cases of severe pneumonia.[86,105] Urine antigen testing may be used to detect *S pneumoniae* or *L pneumophila*. Although the prevalence of Legionella pneumonia in LTCF residents is not greater than in other elderly patients (0.0%–6.5%),[86,104,106] in outbreak settings, urinary antigen diagnostics might play an important role in diagnosis and infection control. During the appropriate season, rapid antigen and polymerase chain reaction tests for influenza and respiratory syncytial virus are often useful.

MANAGEMENT
Site of Care

Severity assessment and site-of-care decisions are critical when managing elderly patients who present with CAP. Various useful severity of illness scores have been published, aiming to predict risk of mortality and assist in decisions regarding site of care (eg, admission to the hospital vs care as outpatient at home). In both the Pneumonia Severity Index score and CURB-65 score (Confusion, Urea, Respiratory rate, Blood pressure, age >65 years), age is a significant component of severity scoring highlighting the poor outcomes associated with pneumonia in elderly patients.[4] According to these scores, Pneumonia Severity Index score class of IV or more, or CURB-65 score of 2 or more indicate the need for a patient with pneumonia to be hospitalized.

Parameters that may compromise the success of home care include homelessness, need for oxygen, an impaired ability to take and/or swallow oral medications, poor social support for persons who are frail, and substance abuse. These factors increase the risk of treatment failure, and hence need for hospital admission, and should be part of the clinical decision making regarding need for hospital admission.[21]

Admission to the ICU is appropriate in many patients with severe CAP who require high level of care. The Infectious Diseases Society of America/American Thoracic Society guidelines for CAP management from 2007 proposed criteria for severe CAP. Major criteria include mechanical ventilation and septic shock. There are nine minor criteria, including CURB components, as well as hypothermia, Pao_2:Fio_2 ratio of 250 or less, bilateral or multilobar infiltrates, leukopenia, and thrombocytopenia. One major criteria or 3 minor criteria indicate the need for ICU admission. In addition, a CURB-65 of greater than 3 may indicate severe pneumonia and the potential need for intensive care.[32]

For LTCF residents, most mild to moderate pneumonia can be treated in the LTCF, and the decision to transfer the patient to an acute care facility is based on both clinical assessment, LTCF management availability (chest radiograph availability, intravenous treatment, physician availability), and social considerations. Loeb and colleagues[107] demonstrated that an intervention that included initial assessment of patient eligibility to be treated in the LTCF, followed by early imaging, oral antibiotic treatment, as well as intensive maintenance of hydration and oxygenation in, resulted in reduced hospitalization rate (18% compared with 30% in the usual care group) and costs, and did not impact mortality rates. According to expert panel recommendations from the Infectious Diseases Society of America in 2008, LTCF residents who have suspected pneumonia and an increased respiratory rate (>25/min) as well as hypoxemia (pulse oximetry <90%) should be transferred to the hospital, as should persons with imaging findings that require more intensive management (pleural effusion, heart failure). Residents should also be transferred to an acute care facility when critical diagnostic tests or necessary therapies are not available in the LTCF. In addition to these considerations, when considering site of care for LTCF residents, the patient's desire to be transferred to an acute care facility and intensively treated is another factor to consider.[51,86]

Antibiotic Treatment

The principles of pneumonia treatment are valid for both CAP in older community-dwelling adults and CAP among LTCF residents and are discussed as a single entity. Treating CAP, including CAP among LTCF residents, is empiric in most cases, and choosing an antibiotic is based on several factors that guide the clinician to the most likely pathogens in different scenarios. These factors include site of care, severity of disease, the patient's risk for resistant organisms, and local epidemiology.

In general, because the most common pathogens causing CAP in the elderly are S pneumoniae, H influenza, and Legionella spp, these organisms need to be routinely covered, regardless of whether the patient is treated as an outpatient, inpatient, or in an ICU. In addition, enteric Gram-negative bacilli and resistant organisms should be treated according to the patient's risk factors to acquire these organisms (see **Table 1**), whether the patient resides at home (CAP) or at an LTCF (CAP among LTCF residents). **Table 2** lists treatment options based on the latest Infectious Diseases Society of America/American Thoracic Society guidelines.[32] These guidelines do not specifically address elderly patients.

Considerations in Community-acquired Pneumonia Treatment

The Infectious Diseases Society of America guidelines recommend treating patients admitted to a medical ward (moderate to severe CAP) with either a respiratory fluoroquinolone, or a combination of a β-lactam plus a macrolide. For patients admitted to the ICU, combination of either β-lactam plus a macrolide or fluoroquinolone is recommended, as well as assessing risk factors to determine the need for coverage of P aeruginosa and MRSA.

Several studies have reported conflicting results regarding the potential advantage of combination treatment over monotherapy in patients with moderate to severe CAP. The CAP-START study, which evaluated treatment of inpatient, nonsevere CAP patients treated with either monotherapy (a β-lactam or a fluoroquinolone), or combination therapy (a β-lactam plus a macrolide) reported noninferiority of β-lactam monotherapy in terms of 90-day mortality.[108] Another study that evaluated treatment of moderate to severe CAP demonstrated worse outcomes with β-lactam monotherapy (compared with combination therapy with a β-lactam plus a macrolide), with regard to time to clinical stability and readmission within 30 days, particularly in patients older than 65 years.[109] A systematic review of 28 observational studies demonstrated a relative decrease of 18% in mortality when a macrolide-containing regimen was administered in critically ill CAP patients, compared with other nonmacrolide regimens.[110] Other studies have reported an advantage of combining a β-lactam with a macrolide as compared with combining a β-lactam with a respiratory fluoroquinolone, in terms of duration of stay[111] and ICU mortality.[112] A potential explanation for these findings relates to the immunomodulatory effects of macrolides.[113]

In contrast, in a recent metaanalysis, monotherapy with fluoroquinolones for moderate to severe CAP had an advantage over both the combination of a β-lactam with a

Table 2
Empiric antimicrobial treatment for community-acquired pneumonia among elderly patients, LTCF residence, with or without risk factors for multidrug-resistant organisms

	Elderly, Home, No Risk Factors for eGNB, MRSA or *P aeruginosa*	Elderly, LTCF, No Risk Factors for MRSA or *P aeruginosa*	Elderly, Home or LTCF, Risk Factors for MRSA or *P aeruginosa*
Mild pneumonia (outpatient *or* inpatient owing to other reasons)	Macrolide[d] Alternative: doxycycline Combine β-lactam and macrolide if macrolide resistance is common	β-Lactam[a] + macrolide or Respiratory fluoroquinolone[e]	Consider local susceptibilities for inpatient vs outpatient decision
Moderate pneumonia, in-patient, medical ward	β-Lactam[b] + macrolide or Respiratory fluoroquinolone	β-Lactam[b] + macrolide or Respiratory fluoroquinolone	β-Lactam + macrolide or Respiratory fluoroquinolone *P aeruginosa* risk: Use antipseudomonal β-lactam[c] MRSA risk: add vancomycin or linezolid or clindamycin
Severe pneumonia, inpatient, ICU	β-Lactam[c] + macrolide or β-Lactam[c] + respiratory fluoroquinolone	β-Lactam[c] + macrolide or β-Lactam[c] + respiratory fluoroquinolone	β-Lactam[c] + macrolide or β-Lactam[c] + respiratory fluoroquinolone with or without vancomycin or linezolid

Abbreviations: eGNB, enteric gram-negative bacilli; ICU, intensive care unit; LTCF, long-term care facility; MRSA, methicillin-resistant *Staphylococcus aureus*; *P aeruginosa*, *Pseudomonas aeruginosa*.

[a] β-Lactam choices: high-dose amoxicillin, amoxicillin with clavulanate. Alternatives for penicillin allergy: respiratory fluoroquinolone.

[b] β-Lactam: Ceftriaxone, cefotaxime, Ampicillin/sulbactam. Alternative for penicillin allergy: respiratory fluoroquinolone.

[c] β-Lactam with antipseudomonal activity: piperacillin plus tazobactam, cefepime, carbapenems (consider local *P aeruginosa* susceptibility patterns). Alternative for penicillin allergy: aztreonam plus respiratory fluoroquinolone.

[d] Macrolide included: azithromycin, clarithromycin.

[e] Respiratory fluoroquinolones include levofloxacin (750 mg), moxifloxacin.

macrolide and the combination of β-lactam with a fluoroquinolone in terms of treatment failure, antimicrobial discontinuation, and adverse events.[114] The explanation of these results suggesting an advantage of quinolone monotherapy is unclear, and additional study is needed to further clarify the role of quinolone monotherapy as compared with β-lactam–based combination therapy in moderate to severe CAP.

In summary, there are no solid data to support one guideline-recommended therapy over another. Monotherapy with a β-lactam is not recommended for inpatient treatment. Choosing between the combination of a β-lactam with either a respiratory fluoroquinolones or a macrolide for treatment of severe CAP should be guided in part by local patterns of epidemiology and resistance. For patients treated in the ICU, a β-lactam combined with either a macrolide or fluoroquinolone is recommended.

The duration of treatment for CAP is based on the level of severity at the time of presentation, the presence of infectious complications (empyema, extrapulmonary complications), and the time required to reach clinical stability. In general, for many patients with CAP who become afebrile and reach clinical stability within 3 days, a course of 5 to 7 days of treatment is appropriate. In certain clinical scenarios (such as patients with severe or complicated pneumonia or patients who do not reach clinical stability within 3 days) and for certain pathogens (eg, *Legionella pneumonia*, *P aeruginosa*, MRSA) longer courses of treatment (7–14 days) are recommended.[32,115]

Corticosteroids in Community-acquired Pneumonia

Even with appropriate empiric treatment, mortality rates in CAP remain high, particularly in patients with severe CAP, approaching 45% for patients admitted to ICU. This is owing in part to a strong proinflammatory response and dysregulation of the immune system. Antiinflammatory drugs, in particular corticosteroids, have been used in attempts to improve patient outcomes.

A randomized, controlled trial evaluated addition of methylprednisolone (0.5 mg/kg every 12 hours for 5 days started within 36 hours of admission) to standard therapy for patients with severe CAP and a vigorous inflammatory response, defined as a CRP of greater than 150 mg/L. In this study, treatment failure rates (mostly late, defined as progressive pulmonary infiltrates) were higher in the placebo group, whereas no difference in mortality was demonstrated between the groups. Several metaanalyses have been conducted in the last decade and have reported a benefit of using corticosteroids, particularly in severe CAP, including decreased duration of stay in ICU, lower rates of acute respiratory distress syndrome, and a shorter time to clinical stability. Of note, these studies have not demonstrated a clear impact on mortality. Studies have not demonstrated an increased rate of adverse events, including gastrointestinal hemorrhage, in the groups receiving corticosteroids.[116–118]

Prina and colleagues[119] proposed an algorithm for the use of corticosteroids, where patients with severe CAP are evaluated for degree of inflammation based on CRP level. If not contraindicated, the authors recommend that patients with a high degree of inflammation should be treated with methylprednisolone 0.5 mg/kg every 12 hours for 5 days.

Studies that have evaluated corticosteroids in CAP did not specifically study elderly patients or patients in LTCFs. In addition, patients who were at high risk for adverse events (ie, recent gastrointestinal bleeding, immunocompromised patients) were excluded from some of the trials included in the metaanalyses mentioned. Although it may be reasonable to use corticosteroids in some severe cases of CAP, based on currently available data, corticosteroids are not recommended for routine CAP management in elderly patients.

Other Considerations in the Management of Community-acquired Pneumonia in Elderly Patients

Supportive treatment of sepsis has an important role in the management of CAP regardless of age, and is beyond the scope of this review. However, careful monitoring of oxygen saturation and appropriate hydration are extremely important factors to consider in elderly patients, given the considerably high rate of underlying illnesses that might be present and impacted.

Adverse events and drug–drug interactions are more prevalent in older adults and should be considered when choosing an antibiotic as well as in follow-up evaluations. Tendon rupture, in particular Achilles tendon rupture, has been described in association with fluoroquinolone treatment.[120] Drug–drug interactions (such as those leading to a prolonged QT interval occurring with administration of fluoroquinolones or macrolides) and prolongation of the prothrombin time and International Normalized Ratio (when fluoroquinolones and warfarin are coadministered) are examples of potential adverse events associated with CAP treatment. Renal dose adjustment is important to avoid renal toxicity as well as other adverse reactions.[6]

OUTCOMES

Mortality rates in pneumonia remain high despite effective treatment options, increased vaccination rates, and increased availability of diagnostic tests.[11] Rates of mortality range from 4.9% to 48%, increasing with age and severity of illness.[50,57,121] Age was found as an independent predictor for mortality, even after adjusting for comorbidities.[59] In a cohort of 173,145 patients who were hospitalized with CAP in 2000 to 2002, the in-hospital mortality rate among patients older than 75 years was twice the mortality rate of patients aged 65 to 74 years (10.6% vs 4.9%, respectively).[5] Other predictors of mortality in the elderly included residence status (residence in a nursing home or other chronic care institution), cerebrovascular disease, chronic liver disease, treatment failure, immune suppression, malnutrition, and severe pneumonia according to the CURB-65 index.[7,50,84,122] In addition, admission to the hospital was associated with increased mortality compared with patients who were treated as an outpatient.[2,11]

A long-term follow-up study reported high rates of 1-year mortality among patients older than 65 years (22.4%–33.6%) and patients older than 90 years (67%).[31,85,123] Among 428 patients who survived hospitalization for CAP, independent predictors for 1-year mortality included male gender, severe undernutrition (measured as mid arm circumference), recurrent admission for pneumonia, and frailty.[123] Studies conducting longer-term follow-up of 5 years or greater reported mortality rates of 30.3% to 53.0%.[124,125] Other complications in the LTCF population include acute coronary syndrome, congestive heart failure, empyema, nosocomial infection, and venous thromboembolism.[98,126,127]

The mean duration of stay of elderly patients hospitalized with CAP ranges between 5.6 and 11.2 days.[3,38,43,50,57] The Centers for Disease Control and Prevention reported a decrease in duration of stay between 1990 and 2009 in patients aged 65 to 74 from 9.8 days to 5.8 days, and from 10.4 to 6.0 days in patients aged 75 to 84 years.[128]

In a systematic review of patients who were discharged after CAP, all-cause 30-day readmission rates ranged from 16.8% to 20.1%, and pneumonia was one of the main reasons for readmissions, accounting for 17.9% to 29.4% of early readmissions.[129] Risk factors for readmission include age, chronic obstructive pulmonary disease, smoking, increased Pneumonia Severity Index score, and previous ICU admission.[11] In addition, nursing miscommunication with patients about their illness and treatment recommendations at time of discharge was also associated with a higher risk for readmission.[130] Outpatient visits associate with CAP are also more frequent among patients older than 65 years, reported as annual rate of visits of 45 visits per 1000 patients (compared with an average rate of 12.5–15.7 visits per 1000 patients).[131]

In several US studies, the cost of inpatient care for pneumonia ranges between $3000 and $18,600 per episode, is higher among patients older than 65 years, and accounts for 80% to 95% of the total cost for pneumonia care in this age group.[11,132] For patients who have CAP treated as outpatient, the costs of single episode range from $130 to $4500.[98] Most of the costs in the outpatient setting are due to subsequent hospitalization.[133] The time to return to usual activities was reported to be up to 8 weeks in patients with CAP who were hospitalized, and may be longer in elderly patients.[98]

Outcomes of Pneumonia Among Residents of Long-term Care Facilities

Pneumonia is the leading cause of death among nursing home residents.[49] The mortality rate of LTCF residents with pneumonia is close to that of patients with hospital-acquired pneumonia (20% to 40%), and is higher than is seen in elderly persons with CAP. In 1 study that compared 71 hospitalized subjects with pneumonia who were admitted from nursing homes with 93 hospitalized patients with CAP who were admitted from home (median aged, 77 years), the in-hospital mortality rate, as well as the 1-year mortality rate of the hospitalized patients from LTCFs with CAP, was twice the mortality rate CAP patients admitted from home (in-hospital mortality rates of 32% vs 14%, and 1-year mortality rates of 58% vs 33%).[51]

Mortality rates are higher for patients who require hospitalization than for patients who are treated in the nursing home (17.6%–53% and 8.8%–28%, respectively). The most important predictor of both in-hospital and long-term mortality in nursing home patients with lower respiratory tract infection is functional status, measured as independence with activities of daily living.[134,135] A poor activities of daily living score is also more common in patients with recurrent pneumonia,[52] as well as those who require admission to the hospital for diseases other than pneumonia. Functional deterioration may also be a long term consequence of pneumonia in LTCF patients.[136]

The costs of pneumonia in nursing home patients were prospectively evaluated in 36 nursing homes in Missouri. The estimated mean total cost per episode treated in the hospital was $10,408, whereas an episode treated in the nursing home cost approximately $3789.[137]

SUMMARY

Managing elderly patients with pneumonia, in particular LTCF residents, is complex. Recent guidelines do not discuss LTCF residents. Guidelines for management of pneumonia in older adults, and particularly LTCF residents would be very useful to clinicians. Ideally, such guidelines would address not only the challenges in the diagnosis and treatment of elderly, but would address issues that have ethical implications, such where to treat older adults, and in end-of-life situations, how to best manage older adults with pneumonia. Whether pneumonia is the old man's friend or enemy depends on the clinical situation and the patient's perspective.

REFERENCES

1. Heron M. Deaths: leading causes for 2014. Natl Vital Stat Rep 2016;65(5):1–96.
2. Jackson ML, Neuzil KM, Thompson WW, et al. The burden of community-acquired pneumonia in seniors: results of a population-based study. Clin Infect Dis 2004;39(11):1642–50.

3. Ochoa-Gondar O, Vila-Corcoles A, de Diego C, et al. The burden of community-acquired pneumonia in the elderly: the Spanish EVAN-65 study. BMC Public Health 2008;8:222.

4. Marrie TJ, File TM Jr. Bacterial pneumonia in older adults. Clin Geriatr Med 2016;32(3):459–77.

5. Fry AM, Shay DK, Holman RC, et al. Trends in hospitalizations for pneumonia among persons aged 65 years or older in the United States, 1988-2002. JAMA 2005;294(21):2712–9.

6. Donowitz GR, Cox HL. Bacterial community-acquired pneumonia in older patients. Clin Geriatr Med 2007;23(3):515–34, vi.

7. Koivula I, Sten M, Makela PH. Risk factors for pneumonia in the elderly. Am J Med 1994;96(4):313–20.

8. Gambassi G, Sultana J, Trifiro G. Antipsychotic use in elderly patients and the risk of pneumonia. Expert Opin Drug Saf 2015;14(1):1–6.

9. Paul KJ, Walker RL, Dublin S. Anticholinergic medications and risk of community-acquired pneumonia in elderly adults: a population-based case-control study. J Am Geriatr Soc 2015;63(3):476–85.

10. Eurich DT, Lee C, Marrie TJ, et al. Inhaled corticosteroids and risk of recurrent pneumonia: a population-based, nested case-control study. Clin Infect Dis 2013;57(8):1138–44.

11. File TM Jr, Marrie TJ. Burden of community-acquired pneumonia in North American adults. Postgrad Med 2010;122(2):130–41.

12. World Population Aging 2015. Available at: http://www.un.org/en/development/desa/population/publications/pdf/ageing/WPA2015_Report.pdf. Accessed August 12, 2017.

13. Ho JC, Chan KN, Hu WH, et al. The effect of aging on nasal mucociliary clearance, beat frequency, and ultrastructure of respiratory cilia. Am J Respir Crit Care Med 2001;163(4):983–8.

14. Janssens JP, Pache JC, Nicod LP. Physiological changes in respiratory function associated with ageing. Eur Respir J 1999;13(1):197–205.

15. Kikuchi R, Watabe N, Konno T, et al. High incidence of silent aspiration in elderly patients with community-acquired pneumonia. Am J Respir Crit Care Med 1994;150(1):251–3.

16. Cabre M, Serra-Prat M, Palomera E, et al. Prevalence and prognostic implications of dysphagia in elderly patients with pneumonia. Age Ageing 2010;39(1):39–45.

17. Westendorp WF, Nederkoorn PJ, Vermeij JD, et al. Post-stroke infection: a systematic review and meta-analysis. BMC Neurol 2011;11:110.

18. Walker AE, Robins M, Weinfeld FD. The National Survey of Stroke. Clinical findings. Stroke 1981;12(2 Pt 2, Suppl 1):I13–44.

19. Nakagawa T, Sekizawa K, Arai H, et al. High incidence of pneumonia in elderly patients with basal ganglia infarction. Arch Intern Med 1997;157(3):321–4.

20. Metlay JP, Schulz R, Li YH, et al. Influence of age on symptoms at presentation in patients with community-acquired pneumonia. Arch Intern Med 1997;157(13):1453–9.

21. Metlay JP, Fine MJ. Testing strategies in the initial management of patients with community-acquired pneumonia. Ann Intern Med 2003;138(2):109–18.

22. Chang KH, Liou TH, Chen CI, et al. Pathogen colonization in patients with acute cerebral stroke. Disabil Rehabil 2013;35(8):662–7.

23. Valenti WM, Trudell RG, Bentley DW. Factors predisposing to oropharyngeal colonization with gram-negative bacilli in the aged. N Engl J Med 1978; 298(20):1108–11.
24. Sveinbjornsdottir S, Gudmundsson S, Briem H. Oropharyngeal colonization in the elderly. Eur J Clin Microbiol Infect Dis 1991;10(11):959–63.
25. Berk SL. Bacterial pneumonia in the elderly: the observations of Sir William Osler in retrospect. J Am Geriatr Soc 1984;32(9):683–5.
26. Castle SC. Clinical relevance of age-related immune dysfunction. Clin Infect Dis 2000;31(2):578–85.
27. Bruunsgaard H, Skinhoj P, Qvist J, et al. Elderly humans show prolonged in vivo inflammatory activity during pneumococcal infections. J Infect Dis 1999;180(2): 551–4.
28. Kelly E, MacRedmond RE, Cullen G, et al. Community-acquired pneumonia in older patients: does age influence systemic cytokine levels in community-acquired pneumonia? Respirology 2009;14(2):210–6.
29. Glynn P, Coakley R, Kilgallen I, et al. Circulating interleukin 6 and interleukin 10 in community acquired pneumonia. Thorax 1999;54(1):51–5.
30. Boe DM, Boule LA, Kovacs EJ. Innate immune responses in the ageing lung. Clin Exp Immunol 2017;187(1):16–25.
31. Kaplan V, Clermont G, Griffin MF, et al. Pneumonia: still the old man's friend? Arch Intern Med 2003;163(3):317–23.
32. Mandell LA, Wunderink RG, Anzueto A, et al. Infectious Diseases Society of America/American Thoracic Society consensus guidelines on the management of community-acquired pneumonia in adults. Clin Infect Dis 2007;44(Suppl 2):S27–72.
33. American Thoracic Society, Infectious Diseases Society of America. Guidelines for the management of adults with hospital-acquired, ventilator-associated, and healthcare-associated pneumonia. Am J Respir Crit Care Med 2005;171(4): 388–416.
34. Park SC, Kang YA, Park BH, et al. Poor prediction of potentially drug-resistant pathogens using current criteria of health care-associated pneumonia. Respir Med 2012;106(9):1311–9.
35. Kalil AC, Metersky ML, Klompas M, et al. Executive summary: management of adults with hospital-acquired and ventilator-associated pneumonia: 2016 clinical practice guidelines by the Infectious Diseases Society of America and the American Thoracic Society. Clin Infect Dis 2016;63(5):575–82.
36. Kollef MH, Shorr A, Tabak YP, et al. Epidemiology and outcomes of health-care-associated pneumonia: results from a large US database of culture-positive pneumonia. Chest 2005;128(6):3854–62.
37. Polverino E, Dambrava P, Cilloniz C, et al. Nursing home-acquired pneumonia: a 10 year single-centre experience. Thorax 2010;65(4):354–9.
38. DeFrances CJ, Lucas CA, Buie VC, et al. 2006 National hospital discharge survey. Natl Health Stat Rep 2008;(5):1–20.
39. Baik I, Curhan GC, Rimm EB, et al. A prospective study of age and lifestyle factors in relation to community-acquired pneumonia in US men and women. Arch Intern Med 2000;160(20):3082–8.
40. Tichopad A, Roberts C, Gembula I, et al. Clinical and economic burden of community-acquired pneumonia among adults in the Czech Republic, Hungary, Poland and Slovakia. PLoS One 2013;8(8):e71375.
41. Jokinen C, Heiskanen L, Juvonen H, et al. Incidence of community-acquired pneumonia in the population of four municipalities in eastern Finland. Am J Epidemiol 1993;137(9):977–88.

42. Jokinen C, Heiskanen L, Juvonen H, et al. Microbial etiology of community-acquired pneumonia in the adult population of 4 municipalities in eastern Finland. Clin Infect Dis 2001;32(8):1141–54.

43. Rozenbaum MH, Mangen MJ, Huijts SM, et al. Incidence, direct costs and duration of hospitalization of patients hospitalized with community acquired pneumonia: a nationwide retrospective claims database analysis. Vaccine 2015; 33(28):3193–9.

44. Janssens JP. Pneumonia in the elderly (geriatric) population. Curr Opin Pulm Med 2005;11(3):226–30.

45. Fine MJ, Stone RA, Singer DE, et al. Processes and outcomes of care for patients with community-acquired pneumonia: results from the Pneumonia Patient Outcomes Research Team (PORT) cohort study. Arch Intern Med 1999;159(9): 970–80.

46. Jain S, Self WH, Wunderink RG, et al. Community-acquired pneumonia requiring hospitalization. N Engl J Med 2015;373(24):2382.

47. Smith PW, Bennett G, Bradley S, et al. SHEA/APIC guideline: infection prevention and control in the long-term care facility. Am J Infect Control 2008;36(7): 504–35.

48. Harris-Kojetin L, Sengupta M, Park-Lee E, et al. Long-term care providers and services users in the United States: data from the National Study of long-Term care providers, 2013–2014. Vital Health Stat 3 2016;(38):x–xii, 1–105.

49. Muder RR. Pneumonia in residents of long-term care facilities: epidemiology, etiology, management, and prevention. Am J Med 1998;105(4):319–30.

50. Kaplan V, Angus DC, Griffin MF, et al. Hospitalized community-acquired pneumonia in the elderly: age- and sex-related patterns of care and outcome in the United States. Am J Respir Crit Care Med 2002;165(6):766–72.

51. Marrie TJ. Pneumonia in the long-term-care facility. Infect Control Hosp Epidemiol 2002;23(3):159–64.

52. Vergis EN, Brennen C, Wagener M, et al. Pneumonia in long-term care: a prospective case-control study of risk factors and impact on survival. Arch Intern Med 2001;161(19):2378–81.

53. Mylotte JM. Nursing home-associated pneumonia. Clin Geriatr Med 2007;23(3): 553–65, vi-vii.

54. Alvarez S, Shell CG, Woolley TW, et al. Nosocomial infections in long-term facilities. J Gerontol 1988;43(1):M9–17.

55. Prina E, Ranzani OT, Torres A. Community-acquired pneumonia. Lancet 2015; 386(9998):1097–108.

56. Torres A, Blasi F, Peetermans WE, et al. The aetiology and antibiotic management of community-acquired pneumonia in adults in Europe: a literature review. Eur J Clin Microbiol Infect Dis 2014;33(7):1065–79.

57. Zalacain R, Torres A, Celis R, et al. Community-acquired pneumonia in the elderly: Spanish multicentre study. Eur Respir J 2003;21(2):294–302.

58. Fernandez-Sabe N, Carratala J, Roson B, et al. Community-acquired pneumonia in very elderly patients: causative organisms, clinical characteristics, and outcomes. Medicine (Baltimore) 2003;82(3):159–69.

59. Kothe H, Bauer T, Marre R, et al. Outcome of community-acquired pneumonia: influence of age, residence status and antimicrobial treatment. Eur Respir J 2008;32(1):139–46.

60. El-Solh AA, Sikka P, Ramadan F, et al. Etiology of severe pneumonia in the very elderly. Am J Respir Crit Care Med 2001;163(3 Pt 1):645–51.

61. Chertow DS, Memoli MJ. Bacterial coinfection in influenza: a grand rounds review. JAMA 2013;309(3):275–82.

62. Meyer-Junco L. Role of atypical bacteria in hospitalized patients with nursing home-acquired pneumonia. Hosp Pharm 2016;51(9):768–77.

63. Almirall J, Rofes L, Serra-Prat M, et al. Oropharyngeal dysphagia is a risk factor for community-acquired pneumonia in the elderly. Eur Respir J 2013;41(4): 923–8.

64. El-Solh AA, Pietrantoni C, Bhat A, et al. Microbiology of severe aspiration pneumonia in institutionalized elderly. Am J Respir Crit Care Med 2003;167(12): 1650–4.

65. von Baum H, Welte T, Marre R, et al, CAPNETZ Study Group. Community-acquired pneumonia through Enterobacteriaceae and pseudomonas aeruginosa: diagnosis, incidence and predictors. Eur Respir J 2010;35(3):598–605.

66. Vila-Corcoles A, Ochoa-Gondar O, Rodriguez-Blanco T, et al. Epidemiology of community-acquired pneumonia in older adults: a population-based study. Respir Med 2009;103(2):309–16.

67. Dagan R. Impact of pneumococcal conjugate vaccine on infections caused by antibiotic-resistant Streptococcus pneumoniae. Clin Microbiol Infect 2009; 15(Suppl 3):16–20.

68. Tomczyk S, Lynfield R, Schaffner W, et al. Prevention of antibiotic-nonsusceptible invasive pneumococcal disease with the 13-valent pneumococcal conjugate vaccine. Clin Infect Dis 2016;62(9):1119–25.

69. Stralin K, Soderquist B. Staphylococcus aureus in community-acquired pneumonia. Chest 2006;130(2):623.

70. File TM Jr, Low DE, Eckburg PB, et al. FOCUS 1: a randomized, double-blinded, multicentre, phase III trial of the efficacy and safety of ceftaroline fosamil versus ceftriaxone in community-acquired pneumonia. J Antimicrob Chemother 2011; 66(Suppl 3):iii19–32.

71. Sader HS, Flamm RK, Farrell DJ, et al. Activity analyses of staphylococcal isolates from pediatric, adult, and elderly patients: AWARE ceftaroline surveillance program. Clin Infect Dis 2012;55(Suppl 3):S181–6.

72. Shorr AF, Myers DE, Huang DB, et al. A risk score for identifying methicillin-resistant Staphylococcus aureus in patients presenting to the hospital with pneumonia. BMC Infect Dis 2013;13:268.

73. Planet PJ. Life after USA300: the rise and fall of a superbug. J Infect Dis 2017; 215(suppl 1):S71–7.

74. Dean N. Methicillin-resistant Staphylococcus aureus in community-acquired and health care-associated pneumonia: incidence, diagnosis, and treatment options. Hosp Pract (1995) 2010;38(1):7–15.

75. Aliberti S, Di Pasquale M, Zanaboni AM, et al. Stratifying risk factors for multidrug-resistant pathogens in hospitalized patients coming from the community with pneumonia. Clin Infect Dis 2012;54(4):470–8.

76. Jeong BH, Koh WJ, Yoo H, et al. Risk factors for acquiring potentially drug-resistant pathogens in immunocompetent patients with pneumonia developed out of hospital. Respiration 2014;88(3):190–8.

77. Brito V, Niederman MS. Healthcare-associated pneumonia is a heterogeneous disease, and all patients do not need the same broad-spectrum antibiotic therapy as complex nosocomial pneumonia. Curr Opin Infect Dis 2009;22(3): 316–25.

78. Marrie TJ, Haldane EV, Faulkner RS, et al. Community-acquired pneumonia requiring hospitalization. Is it different in the elderly? J Am Geriatr Soc 1985; 33(10):671–80.
79. Harper C, Newton P. Clinical aspects of pneumonia in the elderly veteran. J Am Geriatr Soc 1989;37(9):867–72.
80. Maruyama T, Gabazza EC, Morser J, et al. Community-acquired pneumonia and nursing home-acquired pneumonia in the very elderly patients. Respir Med 2010;104(4):584–92.
81. Riquelme R, Torres A, el-Ebiary M, et al. Community-acquired pneumonia in the elderly. Clinical and nutritional aspects. Am J Respir Crit Care Med 1997;156(6): 1908–14.
82. Venkatesan P, Gladman J, Macfarlane JT, et al. A hospital study of community acquired pneumonia in the elderly. Thorax 1990;45(4):254–8.
83. Ahkee S, Srinath L, Ramirez J. Community-acquired pneumonia in the elderly: association of mortality with lack of fever and leukocytosis. South Med J 1997; 90(3):296–8.
84. Fang GD, Fine M, Orloff J, et al. New and emerging etiologies for community-acquired pneumonia with implications for therapy. A prospective multicenter study of 359 cases. Medicine (Baltimore) 1990;69(5):307–16.
85. Johnson JC, Jayadevappa R, Baccash PD, et al. Nonspecific presentation of pneumonia in hospitalized older people: age effect or dementia? J Am Geriatr Soc 2000;48(10):1316–20.
86. High KP, Bradley SF, Gravenstein S, et al. Clinical practice guideline for the evaluation of fever and infection in older adult residents of long-term care facilities: 2008 update by the Infectious Diseases Society of America. Clin Infect Dis 2009; 48(2):149–71.
87. Mylotte JM, Naughton B, Saludades C, et al. Validation and application of the pneumonia prognosis index to nursing home residents with pneumonia. J Am Geriatr Soc 1998;46(12):1538–44.
88. Kaye KS, Stalam M, Shershen WE, et al. Utility of pulse oximetry in diagnosing pneumonia in nursing home residents. Am J Med Sci 2002;324(5):237–42.
89. Haga T, Fukuoka M, Morita M, et al. Computed tomography for the diagnosis and evaluation of the severity of community-acquired pneumonia in the elderly. Intern Med 2016;55(5):437–41.
90. Nouvenne A, Ticinesi A, Folesani G, et al. The association of serum procalcitonin and high-sensitivity C-reactive protein with pneumonia in elderly multimorbid patients with respiratory symptoms: retrospective cohort study. BMC Geriatr 2016;16:16.
91. Albaum MN, Hill LC, Murphy M, et al. Interobserver reliability of the chest radiograph in community-acquired pneumonia. PORT Investigators. Chest 1996; 110(2):343–50.
92. Medina-Walpole AM, McCormick WC. Provider practice patterns in nursing home-acquired pneumonia. J Am Geriatr Soc 1998;46(2):187–92.
93. Gould MK, Tang T, Liu IL, et al. Recent trends in the identification of incidental pulmonary nodules. Am J Respir Crit Care Med 2015;192(10):1208–14.
94. Ticinesi A, Lauretani F, Nouvenne A, et al. Lung ultrasound and chest x-ray for detecting pneumonia in an acute geriatric ward. Medicine (Baltimore) 2016; 95(27):e4153.
95. Chavez MA, Shams N, Ellington LE, et al. Lung ultrasound for the diagnosis of pneumonia in adults: a systematic review and meta-analysis. Respir Res 2014; 15:50.

96. Ye X, Xiao H, Chen B, et al. Accuracy of lung ultrasonography versus chest radiography for the diagnosis of adult community-acquired pneumonia: review of the literature and meta-analysis. PLoS One 2015;10(6):e0130066.

97. Bruns AH, Oosterheert JJ, El Moussaoui R, et al. Pneumonia recovery: discrepancies in perspectives of the radiologist, physician and patient. J Gen Intern Med 2010;25(3):203–6.

98. Fine MJ, Smith MA, Carson CA, et al. Prognosis and outcomes of patients with community-acquired pneumonia. A meta-analysis. JAMA 1996;275(2):134–41.

99. Hirakata Y, Yanagihara K, Kurihara S, et al. Comparison of usefulness of plasma procalcitonin and C-reactive protein measurements for estimation of severity in adults with community-acquired pneumonia. Diagn Microbiol Infect Dis 2008; 61(2):170–4.

100. Steichen O, Bouvard E, Grateau G, et al. Diagnostic value of procalcitonin in acutely hospitalized elderly patients. Eur J Clin Microbiol Infect Dis 2009; 28(12):1471–6.

101. Thiem U, Niklaus D, Sehlhoff B, et al. C-reactive protein, severity of pneumonia and mortality in elderly, hospitalised patients with community-acquired pneumonia. Age Ageing 2009;38(6):693–7.

102. Kim JH, Seo JW, Mok JH, et al. Usefulness of plasma procalcitonin to predict severity in elderly patients with community-acquired pneumonia. Tuberc Respir Dis (Seoul) 2013;74(5):207–14.

103. Viasus D, Garcia-Vidal C, Simonetti A, et al. Prognostic value of serum albumin levels in hospitalized adults with community-acquired pneumonia. J Infect 2013; 66(5):415–23.

104. Umeki K, Tokimatsu I, Yasuda C, et al. Clinical features of healthcare-associated pneumonia (HCAP) in a Japanese community hospital: comparisons among nursing home-acquired pneumonia (NHAP), HCAP other than NHAP, and community-acquired pneumonia. Respirology 2011;16(5):856–61.

105. Marrie TJ, Durant H, Kwan C. Nursing home-acquired pneumonia. A case-control study. J Am Geriatr Soc 1986;34(10):697–702.

106. Micek ST, Kollef KE, Reichley RM, et al. Health care-associated pneumonia and community-acquired pneumonia: a single-center experience. Antimicrob Agents Chemother 2007;51(10):3568–73.

107. Loeb M, Carusone SC, Goeree R, et al. Effect of a clinical pathway to reduce hospitalizations in nursing home residents with pneumonia: a randomized controlled trial. JAMA 2006;295(21):2503–10.

108. Postma DF, van Werkhoven CH, van Elden LJ, et al. Antibiotic treatment strategies for community-acquired pneumonia in adults. N Engl J Med 2015;372(14): 1312–23.

109. Garin N, Genne D, Carballo S, et al. beta-Lactam monotherapy vs beta-lactam-macrolide combination treatment in moderately severe community-acquired pneumonia: a randomized noninferiority trial. JAMA Intern Med 2014;174(12): 1894–901.

110. Sligl WI, Asadi L, Eurich DT, et al. Macrolides and mortality in critically ill patients with community-acquired pneumonia: a systematic review and meta-analysis. Crit Care Med 2014;42(2):420–32.

111. Wilson BZ, Anzueto A, Restrepo MI, et al. Comparison of two guideline-concordant antimicrobial combinations in elderly patients hospitalized with severe community-acquired pneumonia. Crit Care Med 2012;40(8):2310–4.

112. Martin-Loeches I, Lisboa T, Rodriguez A, et al. Combination antibiotic therapy with macrolides improves survival in intubated patients with community-acquired pneumonia. Intensive Care Med 2010;36(4):612–20.
113. Nie W, Li B, Xiu Q. β-Lactam/macrolide dual therapy versus beta-lactam monotherapy for the treatment of community-acquired pneumonia in adults: a systematic review and meta-analysis. J Antimicrob Chemother 2014;69(6):1441–6.
114. Raz-Pasteur A, Shasha D, Paul M. Fluoroquinolones or macrolides alone versus combined with beta-lactams for adults with community-acquired pneumonia: systematic review and meta-analysis. Int J Antimicrob Agents 2015;46(3):242–8.
115. Liu C, Bayer A, Cosgrove SE, et al. Clinical practice guidelines by the infectious diseases society of America for the treatment of methicillin-resistant Staphylococcus aureus infections in adults and children: executive summary. Clin Infect Dis 2011;52(3):285–92.
116. Siemieniuk RA, Meade MO, Alonso-Coello P, et al. Corticosteroid therapy for patients hospitalized with community-acquired pneumonia: a systematic review and meta-analysis. Ann Intern Med 2015;163(7):519–28.
117. Wan YD, Sun TW, Liu ZQ, et al. Efficacy and safety of corticosteroids for community-acquired pneumonia: a systematic review and meta-analysis. Chest 2016;149(1):209–19.
118. Nie W, Zhang Y, Cheng J, et al. Corticosteroids in the treatment of community-acquired pneumonia in adults: a meta-analysis. PLoS One 2012;7(10):e47926.
119. Prina E, Ceccato A, Torres A. New aspects in the management of pneumonia. Crit Care 2016;20(1):267.
120. Lang TR, Cook J, Rio E, et al. What tendon pathology is seen on imaging in people who have taken fluoroquinolones? A systematic review. Fundam Clin Pharmacol 2017;31(1):4–16.
121. Welte T, Torres A, Nathwani D. Clinical and economic burden of community-acquired pneumonia among adults in Europe. Thorax 2012;67(1):71–9.
122. Ma HM, Tang WH, Woo J. Predictors of in-hospital mortality of older patients admitted for community-acquired pneumonia. Age Ageing 2011;40(6):736–41.
123. Ma HM, Yu RH, Woo J. Recurrent hospitalisation with pneumonia is associated with higher 1-year mortality in frail older people. Intern Med J 2013;43(11):1210–5.
124. Johnstone J, Eurich DT, Majumdar SR, et al. Long-term morbidity and mortality after hospitalization with community-acquired pneumonia: a population-based cohort study. Medicine (Baltimore) 2008;87(6):329–34.
125. Mortensen EM, Kapoor WN, Chang CC, et al. Assessment of mortality after long-term follow-up of patients with community-acquired pneumonia. Clin Infect Dis 2003;37(12):1617–24.
126. Marrie TJ, Huang JQ. Low-risk patients admitted with community-acquired pneumonia. Am J Med 2005;118(12):1357–63.
127. Corrales-Medina VF, Suh KN, Rose G, et al. Cardiac complications in patients with community-acquired pneumonia: a systematic review and meta-analysis of observational studies. PLoS Med 2011;8(6):e1001048.
128. Health, United States, 2011. Available at: https://www.cdc.gov/nchs/data/hus/hus11.pdf. Accessed August 12, 2017.
129. Prescott HC, Sjoding MW, Iwashyna TJ. Diagnoses of early and late readmissions after hospitalization for pneumonia. A systematic review. Ann Am Thorac Soc 2014;11(7):1091–100.
130. NewsCAP: poor nurse-patient communication is a factor in 30-day hospital readmission rates for pneumonia. Am J Nurs 2016;116(11):16.

131. Wortham JM, Shapiro DJ, Hersh AL, et al. Burden of ambulatory visits and antibiotic prescribing patterns for adults with community-acquired pneumonia in the United States, 1998 through 2009. JAMA Intern Med 2014;174(9):1520–2.

132. Niederman MS, McCombs JS, Unger AN, et al. The cost of treating community-acquired pneumonia. Clin Ther 1998;20(4):820–37.

133. Personne V, Chevalier J, Buffel du Vaure C, et al. CAPECO: cost evaluation of community acquired pneumonia managed in primary care. Vaccine 2016; 34(19):2275–80.

134. Mehr DR, Zweig SC, Kruse RL, et al. Mortality from lower respiratory infection in nursing home residents. A pilot prospective community-based study. J Fam Pract 1998;47(4):298–304.

135. Muder RR, Brennen C, Swenson DL, et al. Pneumonia in a long-term care facility. A prospective study of outcome. Arch Intern Med 1996;156(20):2365–70.

136. Jamshed N, Woods C, Desai S, et al. Pneumonia in the long-term resident. Clin Geriatr Med 2011;27(2):117–33.

137. Kruse RL, Mehr DR, Boles KE, et al. Does hospitalization impact survival after lower respiratory infection in nursing home residents? Med Care 2004;42(9): 860–70.

138. Lim WS, Macfarlane JT. A prospective comparison of nursing home acquired pneumonia with community acquired pneumonia. Eur Respir J 2001;18(2): 362–8.

139. Giannella M, Pinilla B, Capdevila JA, et al. Pneumonia treated in the internal medicine department: focus on healthcare-associated pneumonia. Clin Microbiol Infect 2012;18(8):786–94.

140. Arancibia F, Ruiz M. Risk factors for drug-resistant cap in immunocompetent patients. Curr Infect Dis Rep 2017;19(3):11.

Septic Arthritis and Prosthetic Joint Infections in Older Adults

Rajeshwari Nair, PhD, MBBS[a,b], Marin L. Schweizer, PhD[a,b,*],
Namrata Singh, MD, MSCI[a,b]

KEYWORDS

- Prosthetic joint infection • Septic arthritis • Biofilm • Older adult

KEY POINTS

- Comorbid conditions and frailty render older adults vulnerable to infections of both native and prosthetic joints.
- Joint infections are associated with loss of joint function and mobility as well as high morbidity among older adults.
- Joint infections are difficult to diagnose; a combination of clinical signs, culture results, and other diagnostic tests are required for appropriate identification of these deep-seated infections.
- Optimization of modifiable and nonmodifiable risk factors aid in the prevention or reduction of the burden of joint infections in older adults.

INTRODUCTION

The incidence of infections in both native joints (ie, septic arthritis) and prosthetic joints, is increasing. This increase is linked to the aging of our populations, which leads to a potential reduction in immune responses, more degenerative joint diseases, more hip fractures, and increased use of invasive joint operations.[1] These infections are associated with high morbidity among older patients, including potential loss of joint function and mobility.[2] The aim of this review is to summarize existing information on septic arthritis and prosthetic joint infection (PJI), including the epidemiology,

All the authors have no financial disclosures. M.L. Schweizer and R. Nair are funded through VA Health Services Research and Development Career Development Award (award 11-215 to M.L. Schweizer).

[a] Department of Internal Medicine, University of Iowa Carver College of Medicine, Newton Road, Iowa City, IA 52242, USA; [b] The Center for Comprehensive Access and Delivery Research and Evaluation (CADRE), Iowa City Veterans Affairs Healthcare System, 601 Highway 6 West, Iowa City, IA 52246, USA
* Corresponding author. Iowa City VA Health Care System, 601 Highway 6 West, Mailstop 152, Iowa City, IA 52246.
E-mail address: marin-schweizer@uiowa.edu

Infect Dis Clin N Am 31 (2017) 715–729
http://dx.doi.org/10.1016/j.idc.2017.07.013
0891-5520/17/Published by Elsevier Inc.

id.theclinics.com

pathogenesis, clinical manifestations, diagnosis, management, and prevention of these infections.

SEPTIC ARTHRITIS

The diagnosis of septic arthritis can be particularly challenging in patients with underlying joint disorders that are common in older adults. Mortality from bacterial arthritis in adults ranges from 10% to 25%.[3]

Epidemiology

Burden

The incidence rates of septic arthritis in the developed world range from about 2 to 7 cases per 100,000 person-years and seem to be increasing.[4] Several factors account for this: an aging population, more orthopedic and invasive procedures, and more frequent use of immunosuppressive therapies.[5] Geirsson and colleagues[4] evaluated changes in the rate of septic arthritis among Icelandic adults, finding that between 1990 and 2002, the incidence in adults increased by 0.61 cases per 100,000 population per year. They further reported iatrogenic causes for 42% of septic arthritis cases (77/184) in adults owing to arthrocentesis (33 cases), open joint surgery (26 cases), and arthroscopy (18 cases). A similar study in New Zealand also found an increased rate of septic arthritis disease in older adults, although with a lower rate of iatrogenic (42/248 cases; 16.9%).[6]

Risk factors

Risk factors of septic arthritis, as determined by a large, prospective study of patients with joint diseases over a 3-year period, were age 80 years or greater, diabetes, rheumatoid arthritis, hip or knee prostheses, and skin infection.[7] Immunosuppression is also a risk; a large, prospective, observational study in England indicates that patients with rheumatoid arthritis who are treated with tumor necrosis factor inhibitors are at increased risk for septic arthritis.[8] The most common route for the pathogen to enter a joint is via hematogenous spread. Older adults are particularly susceptible to this route of infection because of primary diseases affecting their joints, like rheumatoid arthritis and crystal arthritides, and because of comorbid conditions that include diabetes, skin infections, and cancer. Other routes include direct inoculation such as through trauma, or rarely, iatrogenic, such as therapeutic intraarticular corticosteroid injection.[5,9]

Clinical Manifestations

The most typical presentation is a few days of redness, warmth, pain, and swelling with decreased range of motion of the involved joint.[10] Suspicion for septic arthritis needs to be maintained even if the patient lacks symptoms of systemic infection like fever. It has been reported that only about 30% to 40% of patients with septic arthritis have a temperature of greater than 39°C.[11]

Typically, septic arthritis is monoarticular with predominant involvement of large joints like the knees, but the possibility of polyarticular involvement needs to be considered, especially in adults with underlying joint diseases like rheumatoid arthritis (**Box 1**). Dubost and colleagues[12] reported 25 cases of polyarticular septic arthritis over a 13-year period and cautioned that "septic polyarthritis should be considered even when the clinical picture is not florid—when patients have low fever and normal white blood cell counts." Polyarticular septic arthritis has been thought to represent an average of about 15% of the septic arthritis cases in the literature.[12] Atypical joint

> **Box 1**
> **Differential diagnoses of acute monoarticular arthritis**
>
> 1. Septic arthritis
>
> 2. Crystalline arthritis like gout, pseudogout
>
> 3. Lyme disease
>
> 4. Foreign body synovitis
>
> 5. Hemarthrosis
>
> 6. Avascular necrosis
>
> 7. Monoarticular presentation or flare of a systemic rheumatic disease like rheumatoid arthritis

involvement, like of the sacroiliac or sternoclavicular joints, is sometimes seen in intravenous drug abusers.[13]

Pathogenesis

Among adults, *Staphylococcus aureus* is the most common cause of septic arthritis, followed by other gram-positive bacteria (**Fig. 1**).[14–16] In a study spanning 2 decades, *Staphylococci* accounted for 55% of septic arthritis among non–intravenous drug users.[17] Similar findings were reported from another study where 65% of septic arthritis cases were caused by *Staphylococci*.[14] Although less of a concern in Europe,[14] in the United States and other parts of the world, methicillin-resistant *S aureus* is a notable cause of septic arthritis, including among older adults.[18–21]

Gram-negative bacteria, especially enteric *Escherichia coli*, cause 23% to 30% of septic arthritis cases in the elderly.[15,16] Although specific risk factors for developing

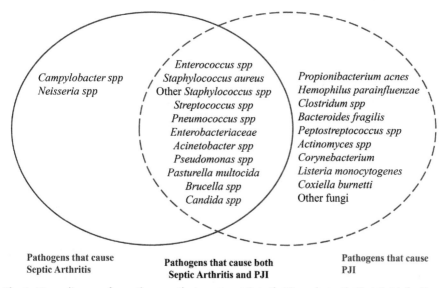

Fig. 1. Venn diagram for pathogens that cause septic arthritis and prosthetic joint infections (PJIs).

septic arthritis owing to gram-negative rods are not clear, we speculate that this is due to hematogenous spread to the joint from bacteremia after urosepsis. This higher incidence is likely due to comorbidities such as urinary tract infections, and chronic joint diseases such as osteoarthritis and rheumatoid arthritis in elderly patients. Gonococcal septic arthritis is exceedingly rare in older adults.

Diagnosis

The definitive diagnosis of septic arthritis is achieved by the detection of a causal pathogen in the synovial fluid of the affected joint. This also requires an integrative approach of thorough clinical history, examination, and laboratory investigations. Efforts should be directed to avoid delays in the diagnosis of septic arthritis, especially in high-risk groups like elderly patients with other comorbidities, immunosuppression, and those with polyarticular infections.

Removing synovial fluid from the affected joint, which should be performed using aseptic technique, is both a therapeutic and diagnostic procedure. Although there is not a single laboratory test with sufficient sensitivity, specificity, and predictive value that can be used alone to diagnose septic arthritis, laboratory studies of synovial fluid, cell count, gram stain, and cultures remain the gold standard.[9] Synovial fluid sampling should be obtained when possible before the start of antibiotics to improve the diagnostic yield. Synovial fluid cultures are positive in more than 60% of nongonococcal arthritis cases, whereas the gram stain is positive in only 50% of the cases.[22] Synovial white blood cell counts of greater than 50,000 per mm^3 should be considered septic until proven otherwise. Crystalline arthritis can also present synovial cell counts in this high range and the presence of crystals in an inflamed joint does not rule out septic arthritis.[23] In some reports, up to 5% of patients with proven crystalline arthritis had concomitant septic arthritis.[24] Blood cultures obtained and sent before starting antimicrobial treatment may help with establishing the severity of disease and guide antibiotic treatment.

Additional laboratory tests include peripheral white blood cell counts as well as erythrocyte sedimentation rate (ESR) and C-reactive protein (CRP), both markers of inflammation. With septic arthritis, the levels of the markers should be elevated but normal values cannot exclude the diagnosis of septic arthritis.[10,25] If elevated, these markers can be followed during treatment to monitor response. Another consideration with white blood cell counts, ESR, and CRP is that these can be elevated in patients presenting with a flare of gout or another inflammatory process, and cannot distinguish septic from nonseptic causes of inflamed joints. Serum procalcitonin has recently emerged as a potential biomarker to distinguish bacterial infections from other causes of inflammatory processes and was found to be highly sensitive and specific marker for septic arthritis.[26,27] Assessment of renal function may help to guide the selection of antibiotics, including appropriate dosing; some antibiotics (eg, gentamicin) should be avoided in patients with low creatinine clearance.

Although plain radiography is the imaging technique obtained initially, they usually seem to be normal. As the infection progresses, osteopenia followed by joint space narrowing develops. Ultrasound examination is a useful modality in detecting small joint effusions as well as for evaluation of inaccessible joints like the hips. It also can guide arthrocentesis in difficult to access joints.[28] MRI is a better imaging modality than radiographs or computed tomography for the differentiation between bone and soft tissue infections. However, no one imaging modality or sign is pathognomonic for septic arthritis and a comprehensive history, examination, and joint aspiration are necessary for a final diagnosis.[29]

Management

If not promptly recognized and treated, septic arthritis can lead to loss of joint function and significant morbidity. The key to management of septic arthritis is prompt recognition, joint aspiration, antibiotics, and supportive care. The importance of removing infected fluid from affected joints, which may sometimes require multiple procedures, cannot be overstated. No guidelines exist for choosing the initial drainage method and should be decided based on the clinical situation of the patient. Initial drainage is usually attempted by needle aspiration, although surgical drainage can be attempted as well; both techniques achieve similar results.[30] Daily arthrocentesis should be done until the effusion resolves and the cultures turn negative.[31] Decreasing joint swelling and synovial fluid counts indicate response to treatment. If the effusion is persistent (after 7 days) even after performing serial joint taps, it is an indication for surgical drainage of the joint, either arthroscopically or by an arthrotomy.[9] The indications for arthrotomy include the need for urgent decompression (either owing to neuropathy or compromise of blood supply), joints like the hip that are inaccessible by less invasive methods, a previously damaged joint from an existing articular disease, failure of conservative treatment, and osteomyelitis complicating septic arthritis.[32]

Systemic antibiotic therapy is the other mainstay of treatment for septic arthritis. A large metaanalysis exploring the clinical efficacy of individual antibiotic agents in adults did not find an advantage of one regimen over the other for native joint infections.[33] The empiric antibiotic regimen should be based on local sensitivity patterns, patient risk factors, and then modified as directed by the synovial fluid gram stain and cultures. Because gram-positive cocci are the most common causative pathogens, initial antibiotic regimens should include coverage for these organisms. In patients with other risk factors such as immunosuppression and those with bacteremia from urinary or gastrointestinal source, coverage should also be directed to gram-negative pathogens like *E coli*. The usual treatment course for nongonococcal arthritis such as that caused by some *Streptococci spp.* or gram-negative cocci is 2 weeks, with 3 weeks for *Staphylococcal spp.* and 4 weeks for *Streptococcus pneumoniae* and Gram-negative bacilli.[11]

Prevention

Septic arthritis prevention is mainly composed of timely treatment of other infections such as skin infections and bloodstream infections. Those infections can lead to hematogenous spread of bacteria that seeds the joint, thus causing septic arthritis. Prevention of these infections includes common infection control measures such as source control of catheters and devices.[5] Additionally, because some septic arthritis infections have been caused by intraarticular corticosteroid injections, safe injection practices must be followed at all times.[5]

PROSTHETIC JOINT INFECTIONS

PJI are among the most challenging complications after a total joint arthroplasty. It is projected that by 2030 more than 4 million joint arthroplasties will be done annually.[34] As people live longer, the numbers of individuals who receive a prosthetic joint increases and, therefore, so does the number of people who are at risk for PJI. Although PJI is diagnosed in both young and old adults, most studies address patients are greater than 65 years of age.[35] Accordingly, subsequent sections do not specifically emphasize age as the mean age for the studies cited ranges from 65 to 80 years.

Epidemiology

Burden

The first 2 years after primary arthroplasty represent the greatest risk period, with up to 70% of PJI occur during this period.[36] In the United States, studies conducted using the Nationwide Inpatient Sample estimated an annual incidence rate of PJI of 2% for hip and knee arthroplasties and 1% after shoulder arthroplasties.[37] The Rochester Epidemiology Project, a population-based study that covered a 40-year time span, reported a standardized incidence rate of 1.5 infections per 1000 person–joint-years for hip or knee arthroplasty, with a cumulative incidence of infection of 0.5%, 0.8%, and 1.4% after 1, 5, and 10 years of follow-up, respectively.[38] A systematic review estimated that 3.3% of patients undergoing elbow arthroplasties develop a PJI.[39]

The overall hospital costs of PJI was noted to be $566 million in 2009, $900 million in 2012, and is projected to exceed $1.6 billion by 2020 in the United States alone, not accounting for other direct and indirect costs.[37] These costs depend on the strategy used to treat PJI patients. Revision surgeries such as debridement, 1-stage, and 2-stage exchange arthroplasty to treat PJI are observed to be 3, 3.4, and 6 times higher in cost, respectively, than the cost of a primary arthroplasty.[40] These costs quickly add up owing to multiple surgeries in a single patient, administration of antimicrobials, nursing home stays, and costs incurred by immobility of patients who are treated with a 2-stage exchange arthroplasty.

Risk factors

Although advanced age alone is a risk factor for PJI, several other patient-specific characteristics, including the severity of underlying illness at the time of admission for joint surgery, increase the risk of PJI (**Box 2**).[41–43] Scoring systems such as the National Nosocomial Infections Surveillance System surgical score and the Mayo PJI score aggregate the number of risk factors and can aid in identification of patients with an increased risk of PJI.[43,44] Factors related to the surgical procedure itself including longer procedure time and postoperative wound drainage also seem to increase PJI, although this association is confounded by comorbidities, choice of treatment option, and longer durations of hospital stay (**Box 3**).[43] Finally, although metal-on-metal bearing surface primary arthroplasty and use of megaprostheses increases the risk of PJI, efforts to mitigate prosthesis-related risk factors such as antibiotic-impregnated cement and the use of metal alloy to modify the prosthesis surface reduce the risk for PJI.[45]

Clinical Manifestations

Signs and symptoms of PJI depend on host factors such as immune response, the joint involved, soft tissue surrounding the joint, and virulence of the infecting organism. There is no evidence of differences in clinical manifestations owing to age, frailty, or loss of function. The most frequently reported signs and symptoms include pain, effusion or swelling in the joint, erythema or warmth around the joint, and fever, chills, drainage, or presence of a sinus tract communicating with the prosthesis.[46] PJI patients with hematogenous acquisition of S aureus typically present with fever and chills compared with patients with perioperative acquisition of S aureus, in whom open wound, sinus tract, or abscess are more common presenting signs.

Pathogenesis

Microorganisms such as S aureus, S epidermidis, and Pseudomonas aeruginosa that typically cause PJI form biofilms on orthopedic implants.[47] S aureus and coagulase-negative staphylococci and are the most common pathogens responsible for PJI.[48]

Box 2
Patient-specific risk factors for infection after arthroplasty

Modifiable risk factors

Obesity
   Severely obese (BMI $\geq$35 kg/m^2) or morbidly obese (BMI >40 kg/m^2)

Malnutrition
   BMI less than 17, serum albumin less than 35 g/L, lymphocytes less than 1500/mm^3

Diabetes

Human immunodeficiency virus infection
   CD4 lymphocytes below 400/mm^3 or less than 20%, viral load greater than 50 copies/mL

Rheumatoid arthritis and treatment

Anticoagulants

Poor source control
   Skin, urinary tract, digestive, respiratory, oral or dental infection

Smoking

Alcoholism

Intravenous drugs

Socioeconomic status
   Associated with malnutrition, smoking, other comorbidities

Poor hygiene

Nonmodifiable risk factors

Age

Gender

Genetic predisposition
   Genes for proteins involved in bone resorption
   Genetic polymorphism of immune response

History of surgery at same site including revision arthroplasty

History of infection at surgical site

Bacterial colonization
   Urinary tract, nares

Immunosuppression owing to chronic diseases
   Chronic renal disease, hemodialysis, or renal transplantation
   Cancer
   Stem cell transplantation
   Cirrhosis

Abbreviation: BMI, body mass index.
   Data from Refs.[45,63–65]

S aureus is the causative organism in 20% to 25% of all PJI.[49] Coagulase-negative *staphylococci*, although sometimes a pathogen, is also a frequent contaminant, which can make interpreting cultures positive for this organism difficult. Additionally, *Propionibacterium acnes*, a low-virulence anaerobic Gram-positive bacillus, may be both a contaminant or a cause of PJI, particularly in shoulders.[35] In addition, 7% to 15% of PJI could be culture negative despite clinical evidence of infection such as purulence, sinus tract, or acute inflammation on histology.[50] Prior antimicrobial therapy is one of the most important risk factors for culture-negative PJI. Other factors include inability

---

Box 3
Surgical considerations for prosthetic joint infections

Perioperative risk factors

- Duration of surgery
- Suboptimal antimicrobial prophylaxis
- Uncontrolled blood sugar
- Blood transfusion

Postoperative complications

- Wound dehiscence
- Superficial surgical site infection
- Wound drainage
- Hematoma

Data from Refs.[63,64,66]

---

to detect a pathogen based on available microbiological diagnostic methods or, in some cases, misclassification as infection.[35]

Diagnosis

As with septic arthritis, the diagnosis of PJI is frequently based on a combination of clinical findings, laboratory tests, microbiological results, radiographic results, intraoperative evaluation by the surgeon, and histologic evaluation of tissue. The Infectious Diseases Society of America guidelines, widely accepted in the United States, use the following criteria as definitive evidence of PJI: the presence of a sinus tract, purulence surrounding the prosthesis without another known etiology, and 2 or more sterile cultures with the identical microorganism.[51] In addition, growth of a virulent organism from a single culture or the findings of acute inflammation by periprosthetic tissue histology are also highly supportive of a diagnosis of PJI. Finally, for cases that do not meet these criteria, the Infectious Diseases Society of America guidelines specifically state that clinical judgment is important to determining if patients have a PJI.

Identification of the organism causing the PJI facilitates pathogen-directed antimicrobial therapy. Gram stain, cultures, and cell counts on synovial fluid may be obtained as an aspirate or during surgery (**Table 1**). Intraoperative cultures, with the

---

Table 1
Threshold value for cell counts of laboratory tests used in diagnosis of prosthetic joint infections

Peripheral Blood (Hip and Knee)	Synovial Fluid Analysis (Neutrophil Percentage)
• WBC: 11,000 × 10⁹ cells/liter	• Knee: 1100 cells/μL (64%)
• CRP: 10 mg/L	27,800 cells/μL (89%) if <6 wk after implantation
• ESR: 30 mm/h	• Hip: 4200 cells/μL (80%)
• IL-6: 10 pg/mL	
• Procalcitonin: 0.3 ng/mL	

Abbreviations: CRP, C-reactive protein; ESR, erythrocyte sedimentation rate; IL-6, interleukin-6; WBC, white blood cell count.
Data from Tande AJ, Patel R. Prosthetic joint infection. Clin Microbiol Rev 2014;27(2):302–45.

Infectious Diseases Society of America guidelines recommendation of at least 6 samples obtained from affected tissue, may also support a specific microbiological diagnosis, although these tend to be less sensitive in general. Testing of removed prosthetic components by ultrasonication and polymerase chain reaction assays provides rapid turnaround time and greater sensitivity compared with conventional culture.[35] As with septic arthritis, additional laboratory studies, including white blood cell counts, ESR, and CRP from peripheral blood samples may help to clarify the diagnosis of PJI when clinical and microbiological criteria are unclear (see **Table 1**). The combination of an elevated ESR and CRP (or normal values for both) offers reasonable positive and negative predictive values.[51] Radiographic studies are less helpful for diagnosing PJI owing to challenges with interpreting the images owing to distortion and lack of specific findings.[51]

Management

The long-term goals of PJI treatment are to eradicate the infection, reduce pain, and restore the functional capacity of the infected joint.[35] Revision surgery and antibiotics represent definitive therapy for eradication of infection from a prosthetic joint (**Fig. 2**). Surgery also leads to better absorption of antimicrobial therapy, which can help to eliminate residual bacteria.[51] Antibiotic treatment for PJI should be selected based on the microorganism isolated on culture and corresponding antimicrobial susceptibility.[51] Patients are subject to arthrodesis or amputation in cases where the limb and prosthesis cannot be salvaged or if the older patient is too frail to have a 2-stage exchange that involves multiple surgical admissions.[51] These terminal procedures permanently alter the quality of life owing to limb shortening and a decreased range of motion at the joint or limb loss, and are typically considered life-saving options.

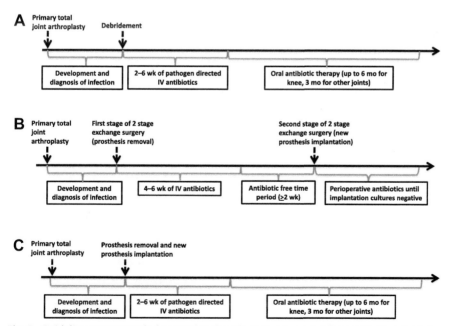

Fig. 2. Guideline recommended surgical and medical management for prosthetic joint infections. (*A*) Debridement. (*B*) Two-stage exchange. (*C*) One-stage exchange. IV, intravenous.

Appropriate choice of surgical procedure and antibiotics based on susceptibility are crucial for the success of PJI treatment. Selection of a procedure depends on patient comorbidities, time to PJI from primary arthroplasty, virulence and susceptibility of the isolated pathogen, and the condition of the infected site (**Fig. 3**). Additionally, selection of antibiotic therapy and duration of antibiotic administration depends on the type of surgery and susceptibility of the pathogen. Both treatment modalities may vary depending on patient and physician preferences. Regardless of the treatment option, patients should be monitored at regular intervals for clinical signs of infection and trends in levels of biomarkers such as ESR and CRP compared with baseline levels, which potentially indicate infection resolution.

Prevention and Suppression

It is critical to identify potential risk factors in patients undergoing elective arthroplasty to reduce the risk of PJI. Factors such as better glycemic control, cessation of smoking, reduction of alcohol consumption, and cessation of intravenous drug abuse are known to be effective in the prevention of PJI.[52] A large, pragmatic, quasiexperimental study conducted in the United States showed that screening patients for presence of *S aureus*, decolonization in the preoperative period, and use of prophylactic antibiotics depending on methicillin susceptibility status of the colonizing *S aureus* strain, reduced the incidence of PJI in patients undergoing hip and knee arthroplasty.[53] Optimization of nonmodifiable factors such as renal, hepatic, or immune system insufficiency, nutritional status, and metabolic status of obese patients favor better surgical outcomes.[52] In addition, adherence to surgical safety checklists and adequate maintenance of the operating room environment are intraoperative measures that reduce the incidence of PJI.[52,54]

Prolonged suppressive antibiotic therapy (PSAT) is considered in conjunction or as an alternative to surgery (**Box 4**). PSAT is the use of oral antibiotics for durations longer than those recommended for curative treatment, although this definition varies in the published evidence.[55–57] Studies have identified PSAT to be an effective option among elderly patients over 80 years of age with a PJI and these studies observed a survival rate of about 60% with a 2-year follow-up.[58,59] Nevertheless, existing evidence on the clinical effectiveness of PSAT is weak and is based on underpowered studies.[51] There is lack of valid evidence on the patient population who may benefit with PSAT, patients in whom PSAT should be contraindicated or be considered as antibiotic overuse, duration of PSAT, and effectiveness of antibiotics for use in PSAT. The effectiveness of these antibiotics is determined by weighing favorable

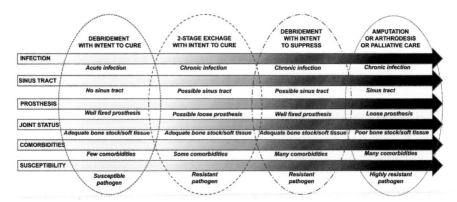

Fig. 3. Patient- and pathogen-specific characteristics for selection of a surgical procedure.

> **Box 4**
> **Patient who may benefit from prolonged suppressive antibiotic therapy**
>
> - Refuse surgery or surgery is contraindicated
> - Are immunosuppressed
> - The infection is due to a virulent, biofilm forming pathogen such as *Staphylococcus aureus*
> - Are managed with less invasive surgical options such as debridement or 1-stage exchange arthroplasty

clinical outcomes such as microbiological cure, reduced readmissions, or improved functional mobility against adverse drug events such as drug reactions or *Clostridium difficile* infection.[51] The current strategy to monitor for adverse effects while on PSAT is to perform complete blood count, check liver function, and measure of serum creatinine every 2 weeks for 1 month, monthly for 2 months, followed by annual measurements.[60] However, there is no evidence or consensus for stopping PSAT among patients with PJI.

In addition to the heterogeneity in patient population treated with PSAT, there is also wide variation in the antibiotics, dose, and duration for administration of PSAT by health care providers. The decision to prescribe antibiotics is not only influenced by therapeutic goals, but also factors such as an organization's prescribing culture and the specialty of the healthcare provider.[61] Orthopedic surgeons are at high risk for malpractice suits and were observed to prescribe more medications compared with clinicians from other specialties.[62] In addition, pressure from consumers (patients, relatives, and caregivers) is also observed to influence the decision to prescribe PSAT.[61]

SUMMARY

- Joint infections are associated with increases in morbidity and mortality, and the incidence of these infections is increasing.[4,34]
- Septic arthritis and PJI have many common risk factors such as older age, presence of comorbidities (eg, prior joint disease, diabetes), immunosuppression, and severe underlying illness.[7,42,63]
- Potentially modifiable risk factors for these infections include uncontrolled blood sugar, drug and alcohol abuse, and other infections such as skin infections and central line–associated bloodstream infections.[5,7,52]
- Joint infections are challenging to diagnose and difficult to treat, especially among older adults owing to nondescript symptoms of infection and varying clinical presentation.
- Treatment of joint infection is difficult both owing to patient frailty and the development of biofilms in the joints. PSAT is considered as an option for patients with septic arthritis and PJI, in whom surgery is contraindicated.
- *S aureus* is the most common cause of septic arthritis and PJI, and thus interventions can be directed at preventing *S aureus* infections.

REFERENCES

1. Kaandorp CJ, Krijnen P, Moens HJ, et al. The outcome of bacterial arthritis: a prospective community-based study. Arthritis Rheum 1997;40(5):884–92.
2. Coakley G, Mathews C, Field M, et al. BSR & BHPR, BOA, RCGP and BSAC guidelines for management of the hot swollen joint in adults. Rheumatology 2006;45(8):1039–41.

3. Goldenberg DL. Infectious arthritis complicating rheumatoid arthritis and other chronic rheumatic disorders. Arthritis Rheum 1989;32(4):496–502.
4. Geirsson AJ, Statkevicius S, Vikingsson A. Septic arthritis in Iceland 1990-2002: increasing incidence due to iatrogenic infections. Ann Rheum Dis 2008;67(5): 638–43.
5. Mathews CJ, Weston VC, Jones A, et al. Bacterial septic arthritis in adults. Lancet 2010;375(9717):846–55.
6. Kennedy N, Chambers ST, Nolan I, et al. Native joint septic arthritis: epidemiology, clinical features, and microbiological causes in a New Zealand population. J Rheumatol 2015;42(12):2392–7.
7. Kaandorp CJ, Van Schaardenburg D, Krijnen P, et al. Risk factors for septic arthritis in patients with joint disease. A prospective study. Arthritis Rheum 1995;38(12):1819–25.
8. Galloway JB, Hyrich KL, Mercer LK, et al. Risk of septic arthritis in patients with rheumatoid arthritis and the effect of anti-TNF therapy: results from the British Society for Rheumatology Biologics Register. Ann Rheum Dis 2011;70(10):1810–4.
9. Garcia-Arias M, Balsa A, Mola EM. Septic arthritis. Best Pract Res Clin Rheumatol 2011;25(3):407–21.
10. Gupta MN, Sturrock RD, Field M. A prospective 2-year study of 75 patients with adult-onset septic arthritis. Rheumatology 2001;40(1):24–30.
11. Smith JW, Chalupa P, Shabaz Hasan M. Infectious arthritis: clinical features, laboratory findings and treatment. Clin Microbiol Infect 2006;12(4):309–14.
12. Dubost JJ, Fis I, Denis P, et al. Polyarticular septic arthritis. Medicine 1993;72(5): 296–310.
13. Vyskocil JJ, McIlroy MA, Brennan TA, et al. Pyogenic infection of the sacroiliac joint. Case reports and review of the literature. Medicine 1991;70(3):188–97.
14. Dubost JJ, Couderc M, Tatar Z, et al. Three-decade trends in the distribution of organisms causing septic arthritis in native joints: single-center study of 374 cases. Joint Bone Spine 2014;81(5):438–40.
15. Joseph ME, Sublett KL, Katz AL. Septic arthritis in the geriatric population. J Okla State Med Assoc 1989;82(12):622–5.
16. McGuire NM, Kauffman CA. Septic arthritis in the elderly. J Am Geriatr Soc 1985; 33(3):170–4.
17. Nolla JM, Lora-Tamayo J, Gomez Vaquero C, et al. Pyogenic arthritis of native joints in non-intravenous drug users: a detailed analysis of 268 cases attended in a tertiary hospital over a 22-year period. Semin Arthritis Rheum 2015;45(1): 94–102.
18. Frazee BW, Fee C, Lambert L. How common is MRSA in adult septic arthritis? Ann Emerg Med 2009;54(5):695–700.
19. Helito CP, Noffs GG, Pecora JR, et al. Epidemiology of septic arthritis of the knee at Hospital das Clinicas, Universidade de Sao Paulo. Braz J Infect Dis 2014; 18(1):28–33.
20. Lim SY, Pannikath D, Nugent K. A retrospective study of septic arthritis in a tertiary hospital in West Texas with high rates of methicillin-resistant Staphylococcus aureus infection. Rheumatol Int 2015;35(7):1251–6.
21. Lin WT, Wu CD, Cheng SC, et al. High prevalence of methicillin-resistant Staphylococcus aureus among patients with septic arthritis caused by Staphylococcus aureus. PLoS One 2015;10(5):e0127150.
22. Goldenberg DL. Septic arthritis. Lancet 1998;351(9097):197–202.
23. Shah K, Spear J, Nathanson LA, et al. Does the presence of crystal arthritis rule out septic arthritis? J Emerg Med 2007;32(1):23–6.

24. Papanicolas LE, Hakendorf P, Gordon DL. Concomitant septic arthritis in crystal monoarthritis. J Rheumatol 2012;39(1):157–60.

25. Li SF, Cassidy C, Chang C, et al. Diagnostic utility of laboratory tests in septic arthritis. Emerg Med J 2007;24(2):75–7.

26. Maharajan K, Patro DK, Menon J, et al. Serum procalcitonin is a sensitive and specific marker in the diagnosis of septic arthritis and acute osteomyelitis. J Orthop Surg Res 2013;8:19.

27. Hugle T, Schuetz P, Mueller B, et al. Serum procalcitonin for discrimination between septic and non-septic arthritis. Clin Exp Rheumatol 2008;26(3):453–6.

28. Minardi JJ, Lander OM. Septic hip arthritis: diagnosis and arthrocentesis using bedside ultrasound. J Emerg Med 2012;43(2):316–8.

29. Graif M, Schweitzer ME, Deely D, et al. The septic versus nonseptic inflamed joint: MRI characteristics. Skeletal Radiol 1999;28(11):616–20.

30. Goldenberg DL, Brandt KD, Cohen AS, et al. Treatment of septic arthritis: comparison of needle aspiration and surgery as initial modes of joint drainage. Arthritis Rheum 1975;18(1):83–90.

31. Ross JJ. Septic arthritis of native joints. Infect Dis Clin North Am 2017;31(2): 203–18.

32. Shirtliff ME, Mader JT. Acute septic arthritis. Clin Microbiol Rev 2002;15(4): 527–44.

33. Stengel D, Bauwens K, Sehouli J, et al. Systematic review and meta-analysis of antibiotic therapy for bone and joint infections. Lancet Infect Dis 2001;1(3): 175–88.

34. Kurtz S, Ong K, Lau E, et al. Projections of primary and revision hip and knee arthroplasty in the United States from 2005 to 2030. J Bone Joint Surg Am 2007; 89(4):780–5.

35. Tande AJ, Patel R. Prosthetic joint infection. Clin Microbiol Rev 2014;27(2): 302–45.

36. Kurtz SM, Ong KL, Lau E, et al. Prosthetic joint infection risk after TKA in the Medicare population. Clin Orthop Relat Res 2010;468(1):52–6.

37. Kurtz SM, Lau E, Watson H, et al. Economic burden of periprosthetic joint infection in the United States. J Arthroplasty 2012;27(8 Suppl):61–5.e1.

38. Tsaras G, Osmon DR, Mabry T, et al. Incidence, secular trends, and outcomes of prosthetic joint infection: a population-based study, Olmsted County, Minnesota, 1969-2007. Infect Control Hosp Epidemiol 2012;33(12):1207–12.

39. Voloshin I, Schippert DW, Kakar S, et al. Complications of total elbow replacement: a systematic review. J Shoulder Elbow Surg 2011;20(1):158–68.

40. Klouche S, Sariali E, Mamoudy P. Total hip arthroplasty revision due to infection: a cost analysis approach. Orthop Traumatol Surg Res 2010;96(2):124–32.

41. Zmistowski B, Alijanipour P. Risk factors for periprosthetic joint infection. In: Springer BD, Parvizi J, editors. Periprosthetic joint infection of the hip and knee. New York: Springer; 2014. p. 15–40.

42. Belmont PJ Jr, Goodman GP, Hamilton W, et al. Morbidity and mortality in the thirty-day period following total hip arthroplasty: risk factors and incidence. J Arthroplasty 2014;29(10):2025–30.

43. Berbari EF, Osmon DR, Lahr B, et al. The Mayo prosthetic joint infection risk score: implication for surgical site infection reporting and risk stratification. Infect Control Hosp Epidemiol 2012;33(8):774–81.

44. Berbari EF, Hanssen AD, Duffy MC, et al. Risk factors for prosthetic joint infection: case-control study. Clin Infect Dis 1998;27(5):1247–54.

45. Diaz-Ledezma C, Parvizi J, Zhou Y, et al. Prosthesis selection. J Arthroplasty 2014;29(2 Suppl):71–6.

46. Sendi P, Banderet F, Graber P, et al. Clinical comparison between exogenous and haematogenous periprosthetic joint infections caused by Staphylococcus aureus. Clin Microbiol Infect 2011;17(7):1098–100.

47. Muszanska AK, Nejadnik MR, Chen Y, et al. Bacterial adhesion forces with substratum surfaces and the susceptibility of biofilms to antibiotics. Antimicrob Agents Chemother 2012;56(9):4961–4.

48. Anguita-Alonso P, Hanssen AD, Patel R. Prosthetic joint infection. Expert Rev Anti Infect Ther 2005;3(5):797–804.

49. Salgado CD, Dash S, Cantey JR, et al. Higher risk of failure of methicillin-resistant Staphylococcus aureus prosthetic joint infections. Clin Orthop Relat Res 2007; 461:48–53.

50. Peel TN, Cheng AC, Buising KL, et al. Microbiological aetiology, epidemiology, and clinical profile of prosthetic joint infections: are current antibiotic prophylaxis guidelines effective? Antimicrob Agents Chemother 2012;56(5):2386–91.

51. Osmon DR, Berbari EF, Berendt AR, et al. Diagnosis and management of prosthetic joint infection: clinical practice guidelines by the Infectious Diseases Society of America. Clin Infect Dis 2013;56(1):e1–25.

52. Alijanipour P, Heller S, Parvizi J. Prevention of periprosthetic joint infection: what are the effective strategies? J Knee Surg 2014;27(4):251–8.

53. Schweizer ML, Chiang HY, Septimus E, et al. Association of a bundled intervention with surgical site infections among patients undergoing cardiac, hip, or knee surgery. JAMA 2015;313(21):2162–71.

54. Shahi A, Parvizi J. Prevention of periprosthetic joint infection. Arch Bone Jt Surg 2015;3(2):72–81.

55. Drancourt M, Stein A, Argenson JN, et al. Oral rifampin plus ofloxacin for treatment of Staphylococcus-infected orthopedic implants. Antimicrob Agents Chemother 1993;37(6):1214–8.

56. Goulet JA, Pellicci PM, Brause BD, et al. Prolonged suppression of infection in total hip arthroplasty. J Arthroplasty 1988;3(2):109–16.

57. Widmer AF, Gaechter A, Ochsner PE, et al. Antimicrobial treatment of orthopedic implant-related infections with rifampin combinations. Clin Infect Dis 1992;14(6): 1251–3.

58. Prendki V, Ferry T, Sergent P, et al. Prolonged suppressive antibiotic therapy for prosthetic joint infection in the elderly: a national multicentre cohort study. Eur J Clin Microbiol Infect Dis 2017;36(9):1577–85.

59. Prendki V, Zeller V, Passeron D, et al. Outcome of patients over 80 years of age on prolonged suppressive antibiotic therapy for at least 6 months for prosthetic joint infection. Int J Infect Dis 2014;29:184–9.

60. Tande AJ, Gomez-Urena EO, Berbari EF, et al. Management of prosthetic joint infection. Infect Dis Clin North Am 2017;31(2):237–52.

61. Charani E, Castro-Sanchez E, Sevdalis N, et al. Understanding the determinants of antimicrobial prescribing within hospitals: the role of "prescribing etiquette". Clin Infect Dis 2013;57(2):188–96.

62. Studdert DM, Mello MM, Sage WM, et al. Defensive medicine among high-risk specialist physicians in a volatile malpractice environment. JAMA 2005; 293(21):2609–17.

63. Peel TN, Dowsey MM, Daffy JR, et al. Risk factors for prosthetic hip and knee infections according to arthroplasty site. J Hosp Infect 2011;79(2):129–33.

64. Zhu Y, Zhang F, Chen W, et al. Risk factors for periprosthetic joint infection after total joint arthroplasty: a systematic review and meta-analysis. J Hosp Infect 2015;89(2):82–9.
65. Marmor S, Kerroumi Y. Patient-specific risk factors for infection in arthroplasty procedure. Orthop Traumatol Surg Res 2016;102(1 Suppl):S113–9.
66. Martin CT, Pugely AJ, Gao Y, et al. Incidence and risk factors for early wound complications after spinal arthrodesis in children: analysis of 30-day follow-up data from the ACS-NSQIP. Spine (Phila Pa 1976) 2014;39(18):1463–70.

Sepsis in Older Adults

Theresa A. Rowe, DO, MS*, June M. McKoy, MD, MPH, JD, MBA

KEYWORDS

- Older adults • Sepsis • Outcomes • Infections

KEY POINTS

- Sepsis disproportionally affects older adults.
- Advanced age has been associated with worse outcomes.
- Older adults with infection can present atypically, making a prompt diagnosis of sepsis challenging.
- Special considerations must be given to selection and dosing of antimicrobials in older adults because of alterations in pharmacokinetics and pharmacodynamics that occur as a result of physiologic changes associated with aging.
- Goals of care should be discussed in all older adults with suspected sepsis.

INTRODUCTION

Sepsis is defined as life-threatening organ dysfunction caused by a host response to infection and represents a spectrum of disease severity ranging from bacteremia to septic shock. Septic shock is a subset of sepsis in which there is circulatory and metabolic dysfunction.[1] Sepsis is a significant burden on our society and disproportionally affects older adults.[2,3] More than 60% of sepsis diagnoses are made in adults aged ≥65 years.[4] The high rate of sepsis among the older population has important implications for our health care system, especially given that the incidence of sepsis is expected to increase with the aging of our population.[5]

EPIDEMIOLOGY

The overall rate of sepsis is increasing.[4,5] Although there are several factors contributing to the increase, the aging of our population plays a significant role. Since 2004, the population of older adults aged ≥65 years living in the United States has

Disclosure Statement: The authors have no disclosures to report.
General Internal Medicine and Geriatrics, Northwestern University Feinberg School of Medicine, 750 North Lakeshore Drive, 10th Floor, Chicago, IL 60611, USA
* Corresponding author.
E-mail address: theresa.rowe@northwestern.edu

Infect Dis Clin N Am 31 (2017) 731–742
http://dx.doi.org/10.1016/j.idc.2017.07.010   **id.theclinics.com**
0891-5520/17/© 2017 Elsevier Inc. All rights reserved.

increased 28% to more than 46 million in 2014 and is projected to more than double to 98 million in 2060.[6]

Using data from the National Inpatient Sample database, Kumar and colleagues[7] estimated that the frequency of hospitalizations of patients with sepsis in the United States increased from 143 per 100,000 persons in the year 2000 to 323 per 100,000 persons in the year 2008, an increase of almost 17% annually. The largest absolute increase was seen in adults aged ≥65 years. Using the same database, Stoller and colleagues[8] later found the incidence of sepsis to have increased from 346 per 100,000 persons in 2008 to 436 per 100,000 persons in 2012. The mean age of patients in the cohort was 69 years in 2008 and 68 years in 2012.[7,8] In an observational study using hospital discharge data, Martin and colleagues[3] determined that incident rates of sepsis in older adults aged ≥65 years increased 20.4% faster than in those aged less than 65 years (mean increase 11.5% vs 9.5% per year, P<.001).

Sepsis also appears to be the most common reason older adults are admitted to an intensive care unit (ICU). In a prospective cohort study of older adults with a mean age of 75 years, approximately 64% of older adults admitted to an ICU met the definition of sepsis.[9]

SUSCEPTIBILITY TO INFECTION

There are several reasons older adults are more likely to develop infections. It is well established that immune function decreases with age, also known as immunosenescence, which puts older adults at increased risk both of developing an infection and for developing an infection with a more severe and protracted course.[10,11] Aging appears to reduce the body's immune response to infection through multiple complex pathways, such as decreased cytokine production and altered expression and function of toll-like receptors. There are also changes in adaptive immunity because of thymic involution that depresses T-cell function. In addition, B cells in older adults often produce antibodies with lower affinity that reduces immunogenicity and thus the protective effects of vaccinations.[10] Poor skin integrity from age-associated changes (eg, thinning and drying) increases the risk of developing skin and soft tissue infections, and swallowing difficulty, immobility, and inadequate oral care have been associated with higher rates of pneumonia.[12–14] Postmenopausal women are more likely to develop urinary tract infections (UTI) because of declining estrogen levels that alter the vaginal flora and promote the colonization of the vagina with uropathogens.[15,16] For older men, prostatic hypertrophy can lead to urinary retention and stasis, predisposing this cohort to UTIs.[17]

Common risk factors in older adults that are associated specifically with sepsis include institutionalization (eg, hospitals, postacute care facilities), instrumentation (eg, chronic indwelling urinary catheters), frailty, malnutrition, and cognitive impairment.[18] In a population-based study of older adults aged ≥65 years, a diagnosis of dementia was associated with a 50% higher risk of severe sepsis (odds ratio [OR] 1.50, 95% confidence interval [CI] 1.32–1.69), after controlling for multiple factors, including age, sex, and other comorbidities.[18] Residing in a long-term care facility has also been shown to increase the risk of developing severe sepsis. In a retrospective study of emergency department visits, nursing home residents were 7 times more likely to be diagnosed with severe sepsis compared with non–nursing home residents (14% vs 1.9%) and to have higher rates of ICU admissions (40% vs 21%).[19]

Many common comorbid diseases in older adults increase the risk of infection and subsequent sepsis, including congestive heart failure, chronic obstructive pulmonary disease (COPD), malignancies, diabetes mellitus, and chronic liver failure.[20] Longstanding diabetes mellitus can result in delayed phagocytosis with decreased clearance of yeast and bacteria by neutrophils,[21] and chronic liver failure causes impairment of complement factor formation and proliferation of cellular immunity.[22] Physiologic changes associated with COPD, including impaired mucociliary clearance, alveolar macrophage dysfunction, and suppressed cough mechanism significantly increase the risk for lower respiratory tract infections in older individuals.[23] Frailty, a common clinical syndrome in older adults, is associated with a decline in activities of daily living (ADLs) causing a cascade of medical problems, including an increase in traumatic falls with injuries that often lead to hospitalization, thus exposing older adults to nosocomial infections.[24]

DIAGNOSTIC CHALLENGES

Older adults with infection often present atypically, making prompt diagnosis and treatment initiation challenging. Fever, the most recognized clinical feature of infection and the most common sign associated with sepsis, is absent in approximately 30% to 50% of older adults with infection. A retrospective cohort study of patients seen in an emergency department found that more than 50% of adults aged $\geq$65 with bacteremia did not present with a fever, defined as a temperature greater than 100.4°F (>38°C). In addition to bacteremia, older adults often have an absent or diminished febrile response to other infections, such as pneumonia, endocarditis, and meningitis.[25–27]

Several studies have shown that older adults often have a basal body temperature lower than the standard normal body temperature of younger adults.[28–30] One study found the average baseline temperature of 50 hospitalized older adults aged $\geq$65 years without infection to be 97.9°F (36.6°C) measured orally, substantially lower than 98.6°F (37°C), the traditionally accepted normal body temperature of younger adults.[31] In 2008, The Infectious Disease Society of America proposed a new definition for fever in older adults. Specifically intended for residents of long-term care facilities, it has also been used in other clinical settings and is defined as follows:

- A single oral temperature greater than 100°F (>37.8°C); or
- Repeated oral temperatures greater than 99°F (>37.2°C); or
- Repeated rectal temperatures greater than 99.5 °F (>37.5°C); or
- Increase in temperature of greater than 2°F (>1.1°C) over baseline temperature.[32]

However, the definition of fever often used to determine a systemic inflammatory response to infection is >38.3°C (100.9°F). Thus, an older adult may not meet the "fever" threshold in many clinical settings.[33] That being said, assessing temperature in older individuals can still provide important clinical information.[34] One strategy in older adult patients is to assess the change in temperature from the individual patient's baseline rather than the absolute temperature value.[22]

Other challenges associated with diagnosing infections in older adults are atypical syndrome-specific signs and symptoms, which may require a higher clinical index of suspicion for infection.[14] For example, pneumonia in older adults can present as confusion, falls, and a decrease in functional status. Although typical localizing symptoms, such as increased sputum production and cough might be absent, an increased respiratory rate and oxygen requirements, detectable via pulse oximetry, may suggest pneumonia.[32,35] Recognizing dysuria, a typical feature of UTI, may be challenging in older adults because other conditions, such as prostate enlargement and genital prolapse, may cause similar sensations.[36] In addition, older adults who are nonverbal may not be able to express feelings of discomfort; their caregivers may have to rely on other changes to recognize symptoms suggestive of a possible infection. Furthermore, differentiating infection from other noninfectious causes, such as congestive heart failure and urinary incontinence, can cause diagnostic uncertainty.

Obtaining accurate clinical information and diagnostic studies can be difficult in subgroups of older individuals. Interpreting biomarkers of sepsis in older adults is challenging because other comorbid conditions can also lead to abnormal findings. For example, lactic acid level is an important marker for sepsis diagnosis and surveillance response to treatment[37]; as its level increases, so does the mortality risk from sepsis. However, dehydration and anemia, common in older individuals, can also result in increased lactic acid levels (low red cell count and contracted volume), making it difficult at times to interpret values clinically. Collecting a urine sample that is not contaminated with skin bacteria can be challenging in a cognitively impaired individual in the acute care hospital or nearly impossible in an agitated or incontinent patient in a nursing home setting. Physical disabilities, such as kyphosis, osteoporosis, and immobility, can also make it difficult to obtain good diagnostic chest radiographs to assess for pulmonary infiltrates suggestive of a lower respiratory tract infection.

CAUSE

The most common infectious sources of sepsis in older adults are respiratory tract infections and genitourinary tract infections.[3,9] Less common causes include skin and soft tissue infections and gastrointestinal infections, with the latter being associated with the highest mortality in older adults.[38]

Older adults are more likely than younger adults to develop infections from gram-negative organisms. Martin and colleagues[3] reported that older adults aged ≥65 years were 1.31 times more likely to have a gram-negative infection compared with adults under the age of 65 (95% CI, 1.27–1.35). The most common organism identified by urine culture in patients who developed sepsis from a urinary source is *Escherichia coli* (50%).[9] Although *E coli* is the predominant cause of UTI in both younger and older adults, older adults are at increased risk for infection from other gram-negative bacteria, such as *Proteus* spp, *Klebsiella* spp, and *Pseudomonas* spp.[39]

Common gram-positive organisms in older adults with bloodstream infections include *Staphylococcus aureus*, *Enterococci* spp, and *Streptococci* spp.[40] In a cohort of older adults aged ≥60 with sepsis due to pneumonia, 16.9% had a positive culture for methicillin-sensitive *S aureus* and 12.3% had a positive culture for methicillin-resistant *S aureus* (MRSA).[9]

MANAGEMENT

The overall management of sepsis in older adults follows the same guidelines as in younger adults and is outlined in the "Surviving Sepsis Campaign, International Guidelines for Initial Management of Sepsis and Septic Shock: 2016," summarized in **Table 1**.[1] Although the underlying principles are the same, there are a few unique considerations when managing older adults.

Antimicrobial Selection and Dosage

Early administration of *effective* antibiotic therapy is essential, because poor outcomes are associated with inadequate therapy across all ages.[41,42] Older adults are at higher risk compared with younger adults for having an infection from a multidrug-resistant organism (MDRO)[43] for multiple reasons, including the following:

Table 1
Selected initial management strategies for sepsis and septic shock

• Patients with hypoperfusion should receive at least 30 mL/kg of intravenous crystalloid within 3 h	Strong recommendation, low quality of evidence
• Patients should be frequently reassessed	Best practice statement
• Norepinephrine is the first choice for patients who need vasopressors	Strong recommendation, moderate quality of evidence
• For patients who require vasopressors, the target mean arterial pressure should be 65 mm Hg	Strong recommendation, moderate quality of evidence
• Broad-spectrum intravenous antibiotics should be started within 1 h of sepsis recognition	Strong recommendation, moderate quality of evidence

- Foreign bodies (eg, urinary catheter, vascular access devices)
- Recent hospitalizations (especially within 90 days)
- Recent exposure to antibiotics
- Residing in a long-term care facility
- Comorbid conditions (eg, COPD, renal failure, diabetes mellitus)
- Prior colonization with an MDRO

In a case-control study of patients 65 years of age and older admitted to a tertiary care hospital with gram-negative bloodstream infections, 8% of these infections were caused by MDROs; initial antibiotic therapy was *ineffective* for more than half (63%) of these patients.[44] In addition, in a prospective cohort study of adults with bacteremia, MRSA was more prevalent in those aged greater than 65 compared with adults aged ≤60 (OR, 1.66, 95% CI 1.06–2.59).[45] Thus, clinicians must be cognizant of the pathogens that can lead to sepsis in the older population when choosing empiric antibiotic therapy and simultaneously of the risk of developing antibiotic resistance.

The Surviving Sepsis Campaign Guidelines strongly recommend initiation of intravenous antimicrobials within 1 hour for both sepsis and septic shock (moderate quality of evidence) (**Table 2**).[1] The specific antibiotic regimen should always be modified based

Table 2
Selected infection management strategies for sepsis and septic shock

• Empiric[a] broad-spectrum[b] therapy	Strong recommendation, moderate quality of evidence
• Regular assessment for narrowing antimicrobial coverage	Best practice statement
• Dosing of antimicrobials should be optimized based on pharmacokinetic/pharmacodynamics principles and specific drug properties	Best practice statement
• Obtain anatomic source control as quickly as practical after diagnosis	Best practice statement

[a] Initial therapy started without a definite pathogen or source.
[b] Use of one or more antimicrobials to ensure coverage of a wide range of pathogens.

on the suspected site of infection, local antibiotic susceptibility patterns, and a patient's own microbiologic history (if available). Modification and deescalation of antibiotics once a source is identified and culture data are made available is *crucial* to adhering to antibiotic stewardship principles. Judicious use of antibiotics can help minimize risks of antibiotic resistance and other commonly associated negative consequences (eg, *Clostridium difficile* infection, adverse drug reactions).[22]

An understanding of the physiologic changes that occur with aging and their impact on pharmacokinetics and pharmacodynamics is critical when selecting antibiotics for older patients with sepsis.[46] Drug-receptor interactions (agonist/antagonist), post–receptor drug effects (signaling and receptor regulation), and drug-drug interactions are all important concepts when dosing antibiotics in the aging population.[47] Clinically, pharmacodynamics can be thought of with respect to toxicity and clinical response. Age is a well-documented risk factor for the development of both liver and kidney toxicities and should be taken into consideration when dosing antibiotics. Decreased systemic perfusion due to age-related atherosclerosis and increased peripheral vascular resistance is further magnified during sepsis.[48] Physiologic changes that occur with aging can affect all stages of pharmacokinetics.[49] With respect to absorption of drugs, slowed gastric emptying, increased gastric pH, and a decrease in small bowel surface area can all affect absorption rates of antibiotics.[49] Furthermore, body fat and total body water decrease with aging, resulting in an increase in the volume for drug distribution within the tissues. A decrease in serum albumin, especially during critical illness, can increase serum levels of drugs that bind to albumin within the body.[49,50] A decrease in the activity of the cytochrome P450 system can also contribute to slower rates of metabolism of medications that are primarily metabolized within the liver.[51] Finally, decreased glomerular filtration rate (GFR) is extremely prevalent in the aging population. Antibiotics, such as vancomycin, tobramycin, and meropenem, require renal dosage adjustment to prevent toxicity.[52] It is critically important that clinicians remember that even though measured levels of creatinine may technically remain within normal range, creatinine clearance is decreased because of a decrease in lean muscle mass in older individuals.[53]

Sedation and Delirium

Older critically ill adults with sepsis are at higher risk for developing delirium than younger adults because of underlying cognitive changes. Delirium has been associated with increased mortality in this population.[54] In a prospective study of older adults aged greater than 60 admitted to an ICU, the number of days someone experienced ICU delirium correlated with an increased risk of death the year following that admission (HR, 1.10; 95% CI, 1.02–1.18).[55] The 2016 Surviving Sepsis Guidelines recommend as a best practice statement that "continuous or intermittent sedation be minimized in mechanically ventilated sepsis patients, targeting specific titration endpoints" to reduce duration of mechanical ventilation and support earlier mobilization.[1] Nonpharmacologic approaches to the management of pain, agitation, and delirium should be explored and use of benzodiazepines should be minimized.[56,57]

OUTCOMES
Mortality

Although advances in diagnosis and management of sepsis have led to significant improvements in outcomes across all ages, overall mortality in older adults remains high. In-hospital mortalities reported in patients aged $\geq$65 are around 30% to 60% and approach 40% to 80% in those aged 80 years and older.[2,4,58] Several studies have found age to be an independent risk factor for mortality,[3,58] although others suggest that factors such as comorbid conditions play a more important role.[4,59,60] In a retrospective study evaluating outcomes of adults admitted with severe sepsis to 171 ICUs in Australia and New Zealand, the mortality in patients without comorbidities was 14% compared with 26.4% in patients with comorbidities. In this same cohort, adults aged ≤44 had a mortality of 7.3% compared with 30.4% in adults aged ≥85 years.[4]

The Sequential (Sepsis-related) Organ Failure Assessment (SOFA) and the quick-SOFA (qSOFA) are newly developed tools used to predict mortality in patients suspected of having sepsis.[61] The qSOFA contains the following 3 components:

- Respiratory rate ≥22 breaths per minute
- Altered mentation
- Systolic blood pressure ≤100 mm Hg

Both the SOFA and qSOFA have been shown to be superior to the systemic inflammatory response syndrome criteria in identifying patients likely to have a prolonged ICU stay or die in the hospital.[1,62,63] Although the SOFA and qSOFA have not been exclusively studied in older adults, they do not rely on fever as a clinical criterion. Further studies are needed relative to the specific applicability of these 2 tools to older adults with suspected sepsis.

Functional Status and Cognitive Impairment

In older adults who survive hospitalization, sepsis has been associated with a variety of other negative consequences, including decreased quality of life and new functional and cognitive impairment.[64,65] A study by Iwashyna and colleagues[65] identified significant changes in cognition and functional status in a cohort of older adults, with a mean age of 78, who survived sepsis. In this cohort, the percentage of patients eventually surviving sepsis with moderate to severe cognitive impairment increased from 6.1% (95% CI, 4.2%–8.0%) before sepsis hospitalization to 16.7% (95% CI, 13.8%–19.7%) after hospitalization. Severe sepsis was found to be associated with a 3-fold higher rate of progression to moderate to severe cognitive impairment (OR 3.34, 95% CI 1.53–7.25). These patients also had a decrease in ADLs and instrumental activities of daily living (IADLs), defined as mean of 1.57 (95% CI, 0.99–2.15, $P<.001$) new functional limitations in ADLs and/or IADLs in patients with no limitations before hospitalization, and a mean of 1.5 (95% CI, 0.87–2.12, $P<.001$) new functional limitations in patients with mild to moderate limitations before hospitalization.

Postacute Care

A significant percentage of older adults with sepsis who survive hospitalization are discharged to a postacute care facility. Martin and colleagues[3] found that older patients aged ≥65 years were less likely to return home compared with younger adults aged less than 65 years (54% vs 76%, $P<.001$) and that admission to a long-term care facility was greater in the older age group (37% vs 15%, $P<.001$). Admission to a postacute care facility after hospitalization for sepsis appears to have remained relatively stable over the past several years, representing approximately 44.9% of hospital discharges in 2008 and 42.6% of hospital discharges in 2012.[8]

GOALS OF CARE

Although there has been improvement in mortalities of sepsis over the past decade, older adults are at risk for a variety of other unwanted outcomes. As discussed earlier, older adults surviving a sepsis hospitalization often suffer decreased quality of life, have increased functional impairments, are less likely to return home, are more likely to be rehospitalized, and have increased reliance on caregivers.[65,66] Goals of care should be discussed with older adults with suspected sepsis when possible and patients' preferences honored. An observational cohort study in adult patients admitted to a general medical service over a 2-year period found that 75% of patients in that study reported preferring to die at home, yet most (66%) died in an institutional setting.[67] It is therefore important to engage in conversations about realistic chances of survival and to identify and discuss each patient's potential functional status and quality of life should they survive hospitalization. Rather than offering antibiotics and other aggressive care in patients not expected to survive sepsis, palliative care services may alleviate pain and suffering and allow for a more peaceful death.[68,69] The Surviving Sepsis Campaign Guidelines provide recommendations for setting goals of care in patient with sepsis[1]:

- Discuss goals of care and prognosis with patients and families (best practice statement).
- Incorporate goals of care into treatment and end-of-life care planning, using palliative care principles where appropriate (strong recommendation, moderate quality of evidence).
- Addressed goals of care as early as feasible, but no later than within 72 hours of ICU admission (weak recommendation, low quality of evidence).

Cost Burden of Sepsis in the Elderly

According to the Agency for Healthcare Research and Quality, the annual cost of sepsis management in 2011 was $20 billion with more than 50% of this cost attributed to the care of individuals over the age of 65 years.[70] Sepsis is regarded as the most expensive condition treated in hospitals in the United States. Furthermore, readmission as a result of sepsis is not only more likely, but also at least 2 to 3 times more costly than readmission for other medical conditions, including COPD, pneumonia, and heart failure.[71]

SUMMARY

Identifying, diagnosing, and treating sepsis in older individuals remain a major challenge for clinicians. Physiologic aging changes and the presence of multiple comorbid conditions can be a barrier to early diagnosis and treatment. Reliance on temperature must be done in context, given that temperature response is often blunted and delayed in older adults. Although rates for surviving sepsis in older adults have improved, overall mortality remains high and older adults surviving sepsis often suffer from significant functional impairment. Further research to determine optimal diagnostic and treatment approaches to sepsis specifically in the older adult population is needed.

REFERENCES

1. Rhodes A, Evans LE, Alhazzani W, et al. Surviving sepsis campaign: international guidelines for management of sepsis and septic shock: 2016. Intensive Care Med 2017;43(3):304–77.
2. Angus DC, Linde-Zwirble WT, Lidicker J, et al. Epidemiology of severe sepsis in the United States: analysis of incidence, outcome, and associated costs of care. Crit Care Med 2001;29(7):1303–10.

3. Martin GS, Mannino DM, Moss M. The effect of age on the development and outcome of adult sepsis. Crit Care Med 2006;34(1):15–21.
4. Kaukonen KM, Bailey M, Suzuki S, et al. Mortality related to severe sepsis and septic shock among critically ill patients in Australia and New Zealand, 2000-2012. JAMA 2014;311(13):1308–16.
5. Lagu T, Rothberg MB, Shieh MS, et al. Hospitalizations, costs, and outcomes of severe sepsis in the United States 2003 to 2007. Crit Care Med 2012;40(3):754–61.
6. Aging Ao. Profile of Older Americans. 2015. Available at: https://aoa.acl.gov/Aging_Statistics/Profile/2015/docs/2015-Profile.pdf. Accessed February 18, 2017.
7. Kumar G, Kumar N, Taneja A, et al. Nationwide trends of severe sepsis in the 21st century (2000-2007). Chest 2011;140(5):1223–31.
8. Stoller J, Halpin L, Weis M, et al. Epidemiology of severe sepsis: 2008-2012. J Crit Care 2016;31(1):58–62.
9. Rowe T, Araujo KL, Van Ness PH, et al. Outcomes of older adults with sepsis at admission to an intensive care unit. Open Forum Infect Dis 2016;3(1):ofw010.
10. Castle SC, Uyemura K, Fulop T, et al. Host resistance and immune responses in advanced age. Clin Geriatr Med 2007;23(3):463–79, v.
11. Norman DC. Clinical features of infection in older adults. Clin Geriatr Med 2016;32(3):433–41.
12. Quagliarello V, Ginter S, Han L, et al. Modifiable risk factors for nursing home-acquired pneumonia. Clin Infect Dis 2005;40(1):1–6.
13. Juthani-Mehta M, De Rekeneire N, Allore H, et al. Modifiable risk factors for pneumonia requiring hospitalization of community-dwelling older adults: the Health, Aging, and Body Composition Study. J Am Geriatr Soc 2013;61(7):1111–8.
14. van Duin D. Diagnostic challenges and opportunities in older adults with infectious diseases. Clin Infect Dis 2012;54(7):973–8.
15. Raz R, Gennesin Y, Wasser J, et al. Recurrent urinary tract infections in postmenopausal women. Clin Infect Dis 2000;30(1):152–6.
16. Jackson SL, Boyko EJ, Fihn SD, et al. Predictors of urinary tract infection after menopause: a prospective study - Reply. Am J Med 2005;118(8):931.
17. Rowe TA, Juthani-Mehta M. Diagnosis and management of urinary tract infection in older adults. Infect Dis Clin North Am 2014;28(1):75–89.
18. Shen HN, Lu CL, Li CY. Dementia increases the risks of acute organ dysfunction, severe sepsis and mortality in hospitalized older patients: a national population-based study. PLoS One 2012;7(8):e42751.
19. Ginde AA, Moss M, Shapiro NI, et al. Impact of older age and nursing home residence on clinical outcomes of US emergency department visits for severe sepsis. J Crit Care 2013;28(5):606–11.
20. Esper AM, Moss M, Lewis CA, et al. The role of infection and comorbidity: factors that influence disparities in sepsis. Crit Care Med 2006;34(10):2576–82.
21. Zykova SN, Jenssen TG, Berdal M, et al. Altered cytokine and nitric oxide secretion in vitro by macrophages from diabetic type II-like db/db mice. Diabetes 2000;49(9):1451–8.
22. Bellmann-Weiler R, Weiss G. Pitfalls in the diagnosis and therapy of infections in elderly patients–a mini-review. Gerontology 2009;55(3):241–9.
23. Reilly JJ Jr, Silverman EK, Shapiro SD. Chapter 260. Chronic Obstructive Pulmonary Disease. In: Longo DL, Fauci AS, Kasper DL, et al, editors. Harrison's Principles of Internal Medicine. 18th edition. New York: McGraw-Hill; 2012. Available at: http://accessmedicine.mhmedical.com/content.aspx?bookid=331&sectionid=40727043. Accessed August 08, 2017.

24. Fried LP, Tangen CM, Walston J, et al. Frailty in older adults: evidence for a phenotype. J Gerontol A Biol Sci Med Sci 2001;56(3):M146–56.
25. Ewig S, Klapdor B, Pletz MW, et al. Nursing-home-acquired pneumonia in Germany: an 8-year prospective multicentre study. Thorax 2012;67(2):132–8.
26. Dhawan VK. Infective endocarditis in elderly patients. Clin Infect Dis 2002;34(6): 806–12.
27. Norman DC. Fever in the elderly. Clin Infect Dis 2000;31(1):148–51.
28. Castle SC, Norman DC, Yeh M, et al. Fever response in elderly nursing home residents: are the older truly colder? J Am Geriatr Soc 1991;39(9):853–7.
29. Castle SC, Yeh M, Toledo S, et al. Lowering the temperature criterion improves detection of infections in nursing home residents. Aging Immunol Infect Dis 1993;4:67–76.
30. Yoshikawa TT, Norman DC. Approach to fever and infection in the nursing home. J Am Geriatr Soc 1996;44(1):74–82.
31. Darowski A, Najim Z, Weinberg J, et al. The febrile response to mild infections in elderly hospital inpatients. Age Ageing 1991;20(3):193–8.
32. High KP, Bradley SF, Gravenstein S, et al. Clinical practice guideline for the evaluation of fever and infection in older adult residents of long-term care facilities: 2008 update by the Infectious Diseases Society of America. Clin Infect Dis 2009;48(2):149–71.
33. Kaukonen KM, Bailey M, Bellomo R. Systemic inflammatory response syndrome criteria for severe sepsis. N Engl J Med 2015;373(9):881.
34. Chester JG, Rudolph JL. Vital signs in older patients: age-related changes. J Am Med Directors Assoc 2011;12(5):337–43.
35. Talbot HK, Falsey AR. The diagnosis of viral respiratory disease in older adults. Clin Infect Dis 2010;50(5):747–51.
36. Juthani-Mehta M, Quagliarello V, Perrelli E, et al. Clinical features to identify urinary tract infection in nursing home residents: a cohort study. J Am Geriatr Soc 2009;57(6):963–70.
37. Walker CA, Griffith DM, Gray AJ, et al. Early lactate clearance in septic patients with elevated lactate levels admitted from the emergency department to intensive care: time to aim higher? J Crit Care 2013;28(5):832–7.
38. Leligdowicz A, Dodek PM, Norena M, et al. Association between source of infection and hospital mortality in patients who have septic shock. Am J Respir Crit Care Med 2014;189(10):1204–13.
39. Das R, Towle V, Van Ness PH, et al. Adverse outcomes in nursing home residents with increased episodes of observed bacteriuria. Infect Control Hosp Epidemiol 2011;32(1):84–6.
40. Blot S, Cankurtaran M, Petrovic M, et al. Epidemiology and outcome of nosocomial bloodstream infection in elderly critically ill patients: a comparison between middle-aged, old, and very old patients. Crit Care Med 2009;37(5):1634–41.
41. Kreger BE, Craven DE, Carling PC, et al. Gram-negative bacteremia. III. Reassessment of etiology, epidemiology and ecology in 612 patients. Am J Med 1980;68(3):332–43.
42. Harbarth S, Garbino J, Pugin J, et al. Inappropriate initial antimicrobial therapy and its effect on survival in a clinical trial of immunomodulating therapy for severe sepsis. Am J Med 2003;115(7):529–35.
43. Kirby JT, Fritsche TR, Jones RN. Influence of patient age on the frequency of occurrence and antimicrobial resistance patterns of isolates from hematology/ oncology patients: report from the Chemotherapy Alliance for Neutropenics

and the Control of Emerging Resistance Program (North America). Diagn Microbiol Infect Dis 2006;56(1):75–82.

44. Pop-Vicas A, Tacconelli E, Gravenstein S, et al. Influx of multidrug-resistant, gram-negative bacteria in the hospital setting and the role of elderly patients with bacterial bloodstream infection. Infect Control Hosp Epidemiol 2009;30(4): 325–31.

45. McClelland RS, Fowler VG Jr, Sanders LL, et al. Staphylococcus aureus bacteremia among elderly vs younger adult patients: comparison of clinical features and mortality. Arch Intern Med 1999;159(11):1244–7.

46. Herring AR, Williamson JC. Principles of antimicrobial use in older adults. Clin Geriatr Med 2007;23(3):481–97, v.

47. Clifford KM, Dy-Boarman EA, Haase KK, et al. Challenges with diagnosing and managing sepsis in older adults. Expert Rev Anti Infect Ther 2016;14(2):231–41.

48. Podnos YD, Jimenez JC, Wilson SE. Intra-abdominal sepsis in elderly persons. Clin Infect Dis 2002;35(1):62–8.

49. Weber S, Mawdsley E, Kaye D. Antibacterial agents in the elderly. Infect Dis Clin North Am 2009;23(4):881–98, viii.

50. Noreddin AM, El-Khatib W, Haynes V. Optimal dosing design for antibiotic therapy in the elderly: a pharmacokinetic and pharmacodynamic perspective. Recent Pat Antiinfect Drug Discov 2008;3(1):45–52.

51. Gregg CR. Drug interactions and anti-infective therapies. Am J Med 1999;106(2): 227–37.

52. Trotman RL, Williamson JC, Shoemaker DM, et al. Antibiotic dosing in critically ill adult patients receiving continuous renal replacement therapy. Clin Infect Dis 2005;41(8):1159–66.

53. Dowling TC, Wang ES, Ferrucci L, et al. Glomerular filtration rate equations overestimate creatinine clearance in older individuals enrolled in the Baltimore Longitudinal Study on Aging: impact on renal drug dosing. Pharmacotherapy 2013; 33(9):912–21.

54. Pisani MA, Murphy TE, Van Ness PH, et al. Characteristics associated with delirium in older patients in a medical intensive care unit. Arch Intern Med 2007;167(15):1629–34.

55. Pisani MA, Kong SY, Kasl SV, et al. Days of delirium are associated with 1-year mortality in an older intensive care unit population. Am J Respir Crit Care Med 2009;180(11):1092–7.

56. Pisani MA, Murphy TE, Araujo KL, et al. Factors associated with persistent delirium after intensive care unit admission in an older medical patient population. J Crit Care 2010;25(3):540.e1-7.

57. Barr J, Fraser GL, Puntillo K, et al. Clinical practice guidelines for the management of pain, agitation, and delirium in adult patients in the intensive care unit. Crit Care Med 2013;41(1):263–306.

58. Nasa P, Juneja D, Singh O, et al. Severe sepsis and its impact on outcome in elderly and very elderly patients admitted in intensive care unit. J Intensive Care Med 2012;27(3):179–83.

59. Holder AL, Gupta N, Lulaj E, et al. Predictors of early progression to severe sepsis or shock among emergency department patients with nonsevere sepsis. Int J Emerg Med 2016;9(1):10.

60. Capp R, Horton CL, Takhar SS, et al. Predictors of patients who present to the emergency department with sepsis and progress to septic shock between 4 and 48 hours of emergency department arrival. Crit Care Med 2015;43(5):983–8.

61. Seymour CW, Liu VX, Iwashyna TJ, et al. Assessment of clinical criteria for sepsis: for the Third International Consensus Definitions for Sepsis and Septic Shock (Sepsis-3). JAMA 2016;315(8):762–74.

62. Raith EP, Udy AA, Bailey M, et al. Prognostic accuracy of the SOFA score, SIRS criteria, and qSOFA Score for in-hospital mortality among adults with suspected infection admitted to the intensive care unit. JAMA 2017;317(3):290–300.

63. Freund Y, Lemachatti N, Krastinova E, et al. Prognostic accuracy of Sepsis-3 criteria for in-hospital mortality among patients with suspected infection presenting to the emergency department. JAMA 2017;317(3):301–8.

64. Winters BD, Eberlein M, Leung J, et al. Long-term mortality and quality of life in sepsis: a systematic review. Crit Care Med 2010;38(5):1276–83.

65. Iwashyna TJ, Ely EW, Smith DM, et al. Long-term cognitive impairment and functional disability among survivors of severe sepsis. JAMA 2010;304(16):1787–94.

66. Prescott HC, Langa KM, Iwashyna TJ. Readmission diagnoses after hospitalization for severe sepsis and other acute medical conditions. JAMA 2015;313(10): 1055–7.

67. Fischer S, Min SJ, Cervantes L, et al. Where do you want to spend your last days of life? Low concordance between preferred and actual site of death among hospitalized adults. J Hosp Med 2013;8(4):178–83.

68. Juthani-Mehta M. Why infection may be a good way to die. Next Avenue 2015.

69. Juthani-Mehta M, Malani PN, Mitchell SL. Antimicrobials at the end of life: an opportunity to improve palliative care and infection management. JAMA 2015; 314(19):2017–8.

70. Torio C (AHRQ), Moore B (Truven Health Analytics). National inpatient hospital costs: the most expensive conditions by Payer, 2013. HCUP Statistical Brief #204. May 2016. Agency for Healthcare Research and Quality, Rockville, MD. Available at: http://www.hcup-us.ahrq.gov/reports/statbriefs/sb204-Most-Expensive-Hospital-Conditions.pdf. Accessed February 18, 2017.

71. Mayr FB, Talisa VB, Balakumar V, et al. Proportion and cost of unplanned 30-day readmissions after sepsis compared with other medical conditions. JAMA 2017; 317(5):530–1.

Clostridium difficile in Older Adults

Curtis J. Donskey, MD[a,b,*]

KEYWORDS

- Elderly • Long-term care facility • *C difficile* infection • Fecal microbiota transplant

KEY POINTS

- *Clostridium difficile* infection (CDI) disproportionately affects the elderly.
- Many cases of CDI have their onset in long-term care facilities (LTCFs) and many hospital-onset cases are transferred to LTCFs.
- CDI may have significant adverse effects on quality of life in elderly individuals, particularly in cases involving multiple recurrences.
- Fecal microbiota transplantation is a promising approach for management of patients with multiple recurrences.

INTRODUCTION

Clostridium difficile is the most common infectious cause of health care-associated diarrhea in developed countries.[1] The incidence of *C difficile* infection (CDI) increased dramatically in North America and Northern Europe beginning in the early 2000s in association with emergence of an epidemic strain termed 027/BI/NAP1. Control of outbreaks often required years of effort and sequential implementation of multiple control measures, including antimicrobial stewardship.[2] Many health care facilities continue to struggle with high endemic rates of CDI. Current estimates from the Centers for Disease Control and Prevention suggest that CDI now causes more health care–associated infections than any other pathogen. In 2011, it was estimated that there were approximately 500,000 CDI cases in the United States that were associated with 29,000 deaths.[1]

The recent increases in the incidence of CDI have occurred in all age groups, but the elderly have been disproportionately affected and long-term care facilities (LTCFs) have borne a significant proportion of the increasing burden of CDI.[3–10] The elderly may be at

Disclosure Statement: This work was supported by the Department of Veterans Affairs. C.J. Donskey has received research grants from Pfizer, Merck, GOJO, Altapure, and Clorox, and serves on advisory boards for 3M and Synthetic Biologics.
[a] Geriatric Research Education and Clinical Center, Cleveland Veterans Affairs Medical Center, 10701 East Boulevard, Cleveland, OH 44106, USA; [b] Case Western Reserve University School of Medicine, 10,000 Euclid Avenue, Cleveland, OH 44106, USA
* Infectious Diseases Section, Louis Stokes Cleveland Veterans Affairs Medical Center, 10701 East Boulevard, Cleveland, OH 44106.
E-mail address: Curtis.Donskey@va.gov

Infect Dis Clin N Am 31 (2017) 743–756
http://dx.doi.org/10.1016/j.idc.2017.07.003
0891-5520/17/Published by Elsevier Inc.

id.theclinics.com

increased risk for initial CDI cases and recurrences of infection due to intrinsic factors associated with aging, such as waning immunity and altered intestinal microbiota. In addition, increased exposure to health care and antibiotics are major contributors to the risk for CDI in the elderly. This article focuses on current concepts related to the pathogenesis, epidemiology, diagnosis, and management of CDI among the elderly.

PATHOGENESIS

C difficile is acquired through ingestion of spores that are ubiquitous in the environment, including in low-levels in food and water. In health care facilities, the hands of health care workers and contaminated environmental surfaces are common sources (**Fig. 1**).[11] After ingestion, spores pass through the stomach and germinate in the small intestine in response to germinants, including bile salts.[12] Gastric acid provides an important host defense by killing ingested pathogens; however, the role of gastric acid as a defense against *C difficile* is controversial. Gastric acid does not kill *C difficile* spores and although some studies have demonstrated an association between medications that inhibit stomach acid and CDI, others have not.[12]

In the colon, vegetative *C difficile* establishes colonization with production of toxin if the indigenous microbiota that provide colonization resistance are disrupted. The primary cause of altered colonization resistance is antibiotic therapy. After establishment of colonization with toxigenic *C difficile* strains, approximately 10% to 60% of hospitalized patients develop CDI, with the remainder developing asymptomatic colonization (**Fig. 2**).[12] The immune system plays a crucial role in determining whether symptomatic illness occurs. An anamnestic antibody response to toxins protects against initial and recurrent CDI.[13] Other host factors may play a role in determining if symptomatic illness occurs, including innate immune responses. For example, a common polymorphism in the interleukin 8 gene promoter has been associated with initial and recurrent CDI.[14]

Elderly individuals may be at increased risk for CDI in part due to waning of natural defenses with advanced age. Gastric acid production may be reduced in the elderly.[15] In addition, the intestinal microbiota of elderly individuals may be altered in comparison with younger individuals.[16] Borriello and colleagues[17] demonstrated that stool microbiota of elderly individuals was less inhibitory to growth of *C difficile* than that of younger

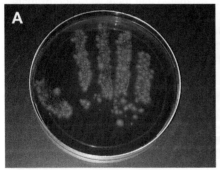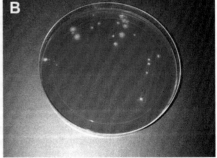

Fig. 1. Typical illustration of acquisition of *C difficile* on sterile gloves after contact with a CDI on the patient's groin (*A*) and the bed rail in the room (*B*). The larger yellow colonies outlining the fingers are *C difficile*. (*Adapted from* Bobulsky GS, Al-Nassir WN, Riggs MM, et al. *Clostridium difficile* skin contamination in patients with *C. difficile*-associated disease. Clin Infect Dis 2008;46(1):448; with permission; and *Courtesy of* Curtis J. Donskey, MD, Cleveland Ohio.)

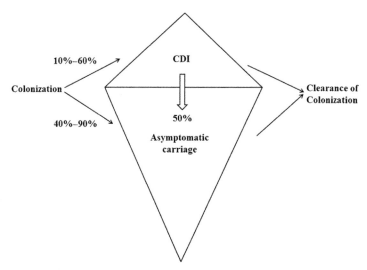

Fig. 2. Outcomes after establishment of colonization by toxigenic *C difficile*. (*Reprinted from* Donskey CJ, Kundrapu S, Deshpande A. Colonization versus carriage of *Clostridium difficile*. Infect Dis Clin North Am 2015;29(1):18; with permission; and *Courtesy of* Curtis J. Donskey, MD, Cleveland Ohio.)

adults. It is plausible that changes associated with aging may contribute to the increased frequency of CDI in the elderly. However, it is likely that loss of natural defense mechanisms among the elderly is primarily iatrogenic: elderly adults are frequently prescribed proton pump inhibitors and antibiotics, often unnecessarily. Given alteration of defenses due to these therapies and increased risk for exposure to spores during hospital and long-term care admissions, it is not surprising that CDI predominantly affects the elderly.

ASYMPTOMATIC CARRIAGE OF TOXIGENIC *CLOSTRIDIUM DIFFICILE*

Asymptomatic carriage of toxigenic *C difficile* is common, particularly in health care settings.[12] Rea and colleagues[18] reported *C difficile* carriage in 2% of elderly subjects in the community versus 10% in the community with outpatient health care exposures and 21% in hospital or LTCF settings. Others have demonstrated that asymptomatic carriage of *C difficile* is common in LTCFs, including on admission.[3–5,10,12] In an outbreak setting, Riggs and colleagues[3] found that 51% of asymptomatic patients on 2 LTCF wards were colonized with toxigenic *C difficile*. Residents with asymptomatic carriage outnumbered those with CDI by a factor of 7 to 1. Antibiotic exposure and recent CDI were risk factors for asymptomatic carriage.

That toxigenic *C difficile* is often carried asymptomatically has important clinical and infection control implications. First, diarrhea due to non-CDI causes is very common in health care facilities.[19] Testing for CDI in an asymptomatic carrier who develops diarrhea due to a non-CDI cause can lead to a diagnosis of CDI and exposure to CDI therapy that is not needed.[20] Second, although current infection control strategies for *C difficile* focus primarily on symptomatic CDI cases, several studies suggest that asymptomatic carriers of toxigenic *C difficile* may be an underappreciated source of transmission.[21–23] For example, using multilocus variable number of tandem repeats analysis (MLVA) genotyping, Curry and colleagues[21] recently demonstrated that incident CDI cases in a tertiary care hospital were as frequently linked to asymptomatic carriers of toxigenic *C difficile* as to CDI cases (29% vs 30%, respectively).

EPIDEMIOLOGY

After the emergence of the NAP1/BI/027 strain in the early 2000s, the incidence of CDI increased dramatically in North America and Northern Europe, and many facilities experienced large outbreaks.[1] The increase in CDI disproportionately involved older adults. In 2009, the incidence of CDI-related hospitals stays for adults 65 to 84 years and 85 years or older was 4-fold and 10-fold greater, respectively, than for adults 45 to 64 years old.[24]

LTCFs have borne a significant proportion of the increasing burden of CDI. In Ohio, mandatory statewide surveillance in 2006 demonstrated that about half of initial CDI cases and three-fourths of recurrent cases had their onset in LTCFs.[9] A more recent national surveillance study estimated that 36% of health care–associated CDI cases in the United States had their onset in LTCFs versus 37% in hospitals.[1] Moreover, many patients diagnosed with CDI in hospitals are discharged to LTCFs.[12] There is evidence that the NAP1/BI/027 strain may be a common cause of infections in LTCF populations. For example, Black and colleagues[25] reported that 67% of patients with CDI discharged to LTCFs were infected with BI/NAP1/027 strains.

Although it is known that CDI is often diagnosed in LTCFs, the source of acquisition of *C difficile* in these cases is not clear. Based on surveillance definitions proposed in 2007, cases of CDI with onset of symptoms more than 48 hours after admission to an LTCF were classified as health care facility (HCF)-onset, HCF-associated cases presumed to be acquired in the LTCF.[26] However, Mylotte[27] postulated that true LTCF-associated CDI is uncommon except in postacute rehabilitation patients, with most cases being acquired in hospitals but having onset of symptoms in the LTCF. He proposed that LTCF-onset CDI cases diagnosed within 1 month of hospital discharge be classified as hospital-associated cases.[27] Subsequently, several studies have reported that many LTCF-associated CDI cases occur within 1 month after hospital discharge.[6–8,10,28,29] For example, the authors found that 85% of LTCF-onset CDI cases in a Department of Veterans Affairs' LTCF had their onset within 1 month after transfer from the hospital (**Fig. 3**).[6]

Studies demonstrating onset of CDI soon after transfer from the hospital provide support for the hypothesis that many cases of LTCF-onset CDI may be acquired during hospital stays. However, studies that include serial cultures and molecular typing are needed to definitively determine the source of acquisition. In such a study, the

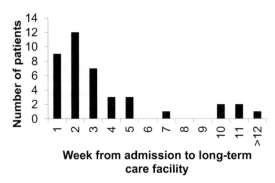

Fig. 3. Timing of onset of CDI in LTCF residents in relation to the time of admission to the LTCF from the hospital. (*Adapted from* Guerrero DM, Nerandzic MM, Jury LA, et al. *Clostridium difficile* infection in a Department of Veterans Affairs long-term care facility. Infect Control Hosp Epidemiol 2011;32(5):513; with permission; and *Courtesy of* Curtis J. Donskey, MD, Cleveland Ohio.)

authors found that LTCF residents frequently acquired colonization with toxigenic *C difficile* after transfer from the hospital, and 3 of 4 initial CDI cases with onset within 1 month of transfer occurred in residents who acquired colonization in the LTCF.[30] These findings suggest that both the hospital and LTCF may be important sources of *C difficile* acquisition.

CLINICAL PRESENTATION

For patients who develop CDI, the typical clinical presentation is diarrhea, ranging in severity from mild to profuse.[31] In most cases, the diarrhea is antibiotic-associated, occurring either during or after completion of antibiotic therapy. Although most cases occur during or within 1 to 2 weeks after completion of antibiotic therapy, increased risk for CDI may persist for up to 90 days after antibiotic exposure.[32] The diarrhea may include presence of mucus in stools and may be associated with abdominal cramping. Fever occurs in a minority of cases. Leukocytosis is a frequent laboratory finding in patients with CDI, and may precede the onset of diarrhea. In patients with antibiotic exposure, a peripheral white blood cell count greater than 20,000/mm^3 with no alternative explanation should raise concern for CDI. A small percentage of patients with CDI never develop diarrhea due to the presence of an ileus. Patients with ileus are at risk for severe complications, including hypotension or shock, toxic megacolon, and intestinal perforation. Factors that reduce bowel motility may increase the risk for ileus (eg, narcotic or antidiarrheal medication exposure, recent intra-abdominal surgery).

Some presentations are not typical of CDI and should lead to consideration of alternative diagnoses. For example, although presence of occult blood is common in stool of CDI cases, frank melena and hematochezia are rare. Vomiting is also uncommon in the absence of ileus. A syndrome with acute onset of vomiting and diarrhea would be more consistent with viral gastroenteritis (eg, norovirus) or staphylococcal food poisoning than with CDI, particularly if multiple patients or LTCF residents and staff members present with similar symptoms. In fact, several pseudo-outbreaks of CDI have been attributed to CDI testing during norovirus outbreaks, with positive CDI results representing detection of asymptomatic carriers of toxigenic *C difficile*.[33] Similarly, a positive test for *C difficile* in a patient with diarrhea after receiving a laxative in the absence of prior antibiotic exposure would suggest asymptomatic carriage rather than CDI.

Although effective treatments are available for CDI, 20% to 30% of patients who respond to initial courses of treatment develop recurrent CDI, usually within 1 to 4 weeks of completing treatment with either vancomycin or metronidazole.[31] The risk of recurrent CDI is even higher in patients who have already had one or more recurrences, and many patients develop repeated episodes that may continue to occur over a period of months or years. Recurrent CDI has a significant impact on health care systems due to need for multiple courses of treatment, increased average length of stay, and increased costs. Recurrent episodes of CDI can also be associated with adverse outcomes. For example, in a recent study conducted in the setting of an outbreak associated with the BI/NAP1/027 strain, 11% of patients with a first recurrence of CDI had serious complications, including shock, toxic megacolon, colectomy, and death.[34]

The presentation of CDI is similar in older and younger adults, but older adults may suffer much greater adverse consequences due to comorbid conditions or debility. In a relatively healthy young adult, having to urgently use the bathroom 8 times per day may be an inconvenience. In an elderly person with decreased mobility, visual impairment, or dementia, having to urgently use the bathroom multiple times per day can be a nearly impossible situation to manage independently. Elderly individuals with multiple medical problems are often in a tenuous state, and CDI can lead to institutionalization. For older adults able to live at home, recurrent CDI often has a significant negative impact on quality of life of patients and their families. Common complaints of patients include loss of independence and inability to travel or enjoy normal activities due to fear of uncontrolled episodes of fecal incontinence or diarrhea.

DIAGNOSIS

The diagnosis of CDI is usually based on a combination of clinical symptoms consistent with the diagnosis and laboratory tests confirming presence of a toxigenic strain or toxin in stool.[31] It is recommended that laboratories should only accept unformed stools (defined by stools taking the shape of the container) for testing unless ileus due to CDI is suspected.[31] In the absence of a positive laboratory test, histopathologic or endoscopic findings may be used to support the diagnosis.

Many laboratories in the United States currently use nucleic acid amplification tests (NAATs) for diagnosis of CDI. Although NAATs have excellent sensitivity, there is increasing concern that asymptomatic carriers of toxigenic C difficile with unformed stool due to other causes (eg, laxatives) are often diagnosed with CDI, resulting in unnecessary treatment and inflation of CDI rates.[20,35] One strategy to address this concern has been to restrict testing to patients with 3 or more unformed stools within 24 hours. Alternatively, a common approach in Europe is to not restrict testing, but to use a 2-step or 3-step testing algorithm in which results of stool toxin testing and clinical assessments are used to guide management for patients with positive initial screening assays for C difficile (ie, a positive toxin assay indicates CDI, whereas a negative toxin assay suggests an asymptomatic carrier who may contribute to transmission as a fecal excretor).[36] Fecal excretors are isolated but not routinely treated or reported as CDI cases. The 2-step or 3-step algorithm approach is supported by recent studies that have demonstrated that patients with evidence of toxigenic C difficile in stool (eg, positive NAAT) but with absence of free toxin based on negative enzyme immunoassay (EIA) for toxin rarely suffer adverse outcomes if they are not treated.[35,36]

Because all CDI testing methods have limitations, it is essential that clinicians and nursing staff understand the advantages and disadvantages of the approach used in their facility. For facilities using NAATs as standalone tests, ongoing education of providers and nursing staff regarding appropriate indications for CDI testing is needed to reduce the risk that asymptomatic carriers will be diagnosed with CDI and treated unnecessarily. In settings in which sensitive screening tests are followed by a relatively sensitive EIA for toxins A and B, it must be appreciated that even relatively sensitive toxin tests miss some patients with CDI. Planche and Wilcox[36] cautioned that the need for CDI treatment in toxin-negative patients is a clinical decision.

Performance of a test of cure after CDI treatment is not recommended.[31] It has been demonstrated that PCR and glutamate dehydrogenase tests often remain positive after resolution of symptoms and approximately 20% of patients may have positive tests at the end of treatment. Moreover, after discontinuation of metronidazole or vancomycin treatment, as many as 56% of patients who remain asymptomatic have positive cultures 1 to 4 weeks after treatment cessation. Resolution of diarrhea is the appropriate criteria for assessing the efficacy of treatment.

Repeat testing during the same episode of diarrhea is a common practice that is also discouraged in current guidelines.[31] Repeat testing increases the possibility of false-positive results and does not substantially increase the yield of true positives. In practice, some laboratories prohibit repeat testing after an initial negative test for 5 or 7 days as a means to avoid inappropriate repeat testing.

In severe CDI cases, computed tomography findings may include colonic mural thickening, pericolonic fat changes, trapping of contrast material between thickened folds (accordion sign), and ascites.[31] Sigmoidoscopy or colonoscopy may also be useful in these cases to evaluate for the presence of pseudomembranous colitis. Finally, perirectal swab specimens could potentially be useful as a diagnostic approach in patients with suspected CDI and ileus. In a study of 139 subjects tested for CDI by polymerase chain reaction (PCR) (Xpert *C difficile*), the sensitivity, specificity, positive predictive value, and negative predictive value of testing perirectal swabs versus stool specimens were 96%, 100%, 100%, and 99%, respectively.[37]

Efforts to assess the timeliness of CDI diagnostic testing and to expedite the diagnosis of CDI may be beneficial. Efficient diagnostic testing for CDI will minimize delays in initiation of isolation and treatment of confirmed cases, while allowing rapid discontinuation of empirical therapy and isolation when testing is negative.[38] However, delays in diagnosis are common in practice. In the authors' Veterans Affairs Medical Center and adjacent LTCF, the average time between placing an order and obtaining a test result from the on-site laboratory was 1.8 days, with the time required for collection of stool specimens contributing to most of the delay.[38] An intervention focused on expediting stool sample collection and testing, and reducing rejection of specimens was effective in significantly reducing the time from test order to diagnosis. Notably, in a prior study conducted by the same institution at a time when the affiliated LTCF was separate from the hospital, the average time from onset of diarrhea to diagnosis of CDI was significantly longer in the LTCF than in the hospital (5 vs 2 days, respectively).[6]

It is likely that delays in diagnostic testing are not unique to the authors' LTCF. For example, Quinn and colleagues[39] found that most Iowa LTCFs did not have a protocol to identify residents with CDI and did not perform diagnostic testing unless a resident had severe diarrhea. Given that many LTCFs use off-site laboratories, improving the timeliness of diagnostic testing may be a particular challenge in this setting.

MANAGEMENT

In addition to specific therapy, general measures for all CDI patients include replacing fluid and electrolyte losses; avoiding antiperistaltic agents; and, whenever possible, stopping the inciting antibiotic. In debilitated older adults, it is necessary to consider the potential for complications such as dehydration if it is not possible to maintain adequate fluid intake or falls if there is difficulty making multiple trips to the bathroom. **Table 1** provides a modified version of treatment regimens recommended by the Society for Healthcare Epidemiology of America (SHEA) and the Infectious Diseases Society of America (IDSA) in 2010.[31] In the guidelines, oral metronidazole was recommended for treatment of initial cases of CDI that are mild or moderate in severity, whereas vancomycin was recommended for severe episodes (defined as those with leukocytosis of 15,000 cells/microliter or higher, or a serum creatinine level$\geq$1.5 times the premorbid level).[31] This recommendation was based on a randomized trial that demonstrated a similar response to treatment with metronidazole and vancomycin for mild CDI but a superior response to treatment with vancomycin for severe CDI.[40] A more recent trial demonstrated that vancomycin was superior to metronidazole for all patients with CDI.[41] If a white blood cell count and creatinine are not available, it is reasonable to base the decision to prescribe metronidazole versus vancomycin on the severity of the symptoms. Due to a significant drug-drug interaction resulting in international normalized ratio (INR) elevation, metronidazole should be avoided in patients receiving warfarin or the INR should be closely monitored.

Table 1
Recommendations for treatment of Clostridium difficile infection

Clinical Definition	Supportive Clinical Data	Recommended Treatment	Other Considerations
Initial episode, mild or moderate	White blood cell count<15,000 cells/μL and serum creatinine<1.5 times the premorbid level	Metronidazole, 500 mg 3 times per day by mouth for 10–14 d (alternative: fidaxomicin 200 mg 2 times per day for 10 d)	Metronidazole is inexpensive and may interact with warfarin to increase INR; Fidaxomicin is expensive in comparison with metronidazole or vancomycin
Initial episode, severe[a]	Leukocytosis with white blood cell count≥15,000 cells/μL and serum creatinine>1.5 times the premorbid level	Vancomycin, 125 mg 4 times per day by mouth for 10–14 d (alternative: fidaxomicin 200 mg 2 times per day for 10 d)	
Initial episode, severe, complicated	Hypotension or shock, ileus, megacolon	Vancomycin, 500 mg 4 times per day by mouth or by nasogastric tube, plus metronidazole, 500 mg every 8 h intravenously; If complete ileus, consider adding rectal instillation of vancomycin	Surgical consult is indicated
First recurrence		Same as for initial episode	
Second recurrence		Vancomycin in a tapered and/or pulsed regimen	
Third recurrence or greater		Consider fecal microbiota transplantation	Fidaxomicin as a taper or chaser regimen successful in a small case series[49]

Abbreviation: INR, international normalized ratio.

[a] The criteria proposed for severe or complicated CDI are based on expert opinion.

Adapted from Cohen SH, Gerding DN, Johnson S, et al. Clinical practice guidelines for Clostridium difficile infection in adults: 2010 update by the Society for Healthcare Epidemiology of America (SHEA) and the Infectious Diseases Society of America (IDSA). Infect Control Hosp Epidemiol 2010;31(5):447; with permission.

Fidaxomicin is a macrocyclic antibiotic approved by the Food and Drug Administration for the treatment of CDI in 2011. Fidaxomicin is an attractive alternative agent for CDI because it demonstrated comparable treatment response with vancomycin and lower rates of recurrence attributed to reduced alteration of the indigenous intestinal microbiota that compete with *C difficile*.[42] However, fidaxomicin has not become widely used because the cost is considerably higher than that of vancomycin, particularly if the inexpensive liquid vancomycin formulation is compounded from the intravenous formulation of vancomycin.

CDI is deemed as severe, complicated if hypotension or shock, ileus, or toxic megacolon is present.[31] These patients have a high risk for mortality and may require surgical intervention. Patients with severe, complicated CDI should ideally be managed in an intensive care unit. The management of such cases is outside the scope of this article.

For patients who develop first recurrences of CDI, treatment with the same agent used for the primary CDI episode is typically recommended.[31] One caveat to this recommendation is that the treatment regimen should again be based on the severity of illness as it is for the primary infection (ie, a patient with an initial recurrence that is severe should receive vancomycin rather than metronidazole). For patients with a second recurrence of CDI, a tapering and/or pulsed vancomycin regimen is recommended.

Given the delays in diagnosis that often occur in outpatients or in LTCFs with off-site laboratories, it is often necessary to consider empirical treatment of CDI in older adults. Current practice guidelines recommend empirical treatment only for patients suspected to have severe CDI.[31] Empirical treatment of patients with suspected recurrence of infection is also reasonable given the high likelihood of infection in the setting of typical symptoms recurring after discontinuation of therapy. If significant delays in testing are anticipated, empirical treatment of frail elderly adults with high clinical suspicion for CDI but mild to moderate symptoms may be reasonable in some settings (eg, an LTCF with a high incidence of CDI). If empirical treatment is considered for suspected mild to moderate CDI, the risks of adverse effects of treatment (eg, adverse drug reactions, promotion of colonization by vancomycin-resistant enterococci) must be balanced against the risks of adverse outcomes due to delays in treatment. Clinicians should also be aware that empirical CDI therapy can convert CDI test results from positive to negative.[43] Thus, if empirical treatment is prescribed it is important to ensure that a stool sample is collected before the start of therapy.

FECAL MICROBIOTA TRANSPLANTATION

Fecal microbiota transplantation (FMT) is an effective therapy for patients with multiple recurrences of CDI.[44] However, the methods of administration used most frequently (ie, colonoscopy, nasoduodenal infusion, and enema) are inconvenient for patients and health care facilities. Thus, recent demonstrations that FMT can be administered via oral capsules and as a frozen preparation have been important advances. Louie and colleagues[45] formulated fresh stool suspensions from related donors into oral capsules, and Youngster and colleagues[46] capsulized frozen suspensions from unrelated donors, both with success rates of 90% or higher with 1 or 2 treatments.

The FMT programs at MetroHealth Medical Center and the Cleveland Veterans Affairs Medical Center recently reported successful use of freeze-dried oral capsules containing fecal microbiota in treatment of patients with recurrent CDI.[47] The capsules provided high concentrations of viable bacteria with a predominance of anaerobes derived from a single healthy stool donor. We administered 20 to 40 capsules with the entire dose taken in the outpatient clinic or with a portion taken home for later consumption. Of 20 recurrent CDI patients treated, 17 (85%) had resolution of diarrhea without recurrence of CDI after 1 FMT procedure and an additional patient resolved after a second FMT by freeze-dried capsules. The mean age of the recipients was 68 years (range, 36–89 years). These findings and other recent reports highlight that it is now possible to offer the benefits of FMT to patients with greater palatability and flexibility in delivery.

Prescription of antibiotics other than those used to treat CDI is a major risk factor for recurrence of CDI after initially successful FMT. Given that a significant proportion of antibiotic therapy is unnecessary, it is important for FMT providers to make efforts to avoid overuse of antibiotics after FMT. In FMT practices at MetroHealth Medical Center and the Cleveland Veterans Affairs Medical Center, FMT recipients are encouraged to contact their FMT providers and/or have their physicians contact the FMT providers for consultation regarding antibiotic prescriptions after the transplant. The authors recently reported our experience with this stewardship intervention.[48] Of 73 FMT recipients, 25 (34%) consulted their FMT physicians, either directly or through their non-FMT providers, regarding a total of 43 antibiotic prescriptions. Of the 43 consultations, 26 (60%) antibiotic courses were deemed unnecessary, 7 (16%) were deemed necessary but an alternative regimen less frequently associated with CDI was recommended, and 10 (23%) were deemed necessary and the regimen was considered appropriate. The recommendations were accepted in 39 of 41 (95%) cases. There were no adverse effects attributable to avoidance of antibiotics. These findings demonstrate that engaging patients in stewardship interventions can be an effective strategy to reduce inappropriate antibiotic use after FMT. FMT patients are an ideal population for such interventions because they are motivated to avoid antibiotics because they fear failure of the transplant and are aware that antibiotics are the most important risk for recurrence. Other CDI patients would also be excellent candidates for such interventions if they are educated that receipt of antibiotics other than those used to treat CDI is a major risk factor for recurrence of CDI.

If fecal transplantation is not available or if medical therapy is preferred, there are options for medical treatment of patients with multiple recurrences. One approach that was effective in a small observational trial was fidaxomicin prescribed as a tapering course over 14 to 33 days or as a chaser after completion of oral vancomycin therapy.[49] Only 2 of 11 (18%) subjects with multiple recurrences of CDI developed recurrence after completion of the fidaxomicin taper or chaser. A second approach for management of patients with multiple recurrences is chronic suppressive therapy (eg, once daily oral vancomycin 125 mg). This approach may be appropriate for patients with relatively short life expectancy or for patients who are not good candidates for fecal transplantation due to frequent requirement for antibiotic therapy that would lead to a high risk for failure of the transplant. Preferably, patients such as these with multiple recurrences would be referred to the infectious diseases service for management.

IMMUNE-BASED APPROACHES TO REDUCE RECURRENCE OF *CLOSTRIDIUM DIFFICILE* INFECTION

Because development of an antibody response to toxins protects against initial and recurrent CDI,[13] there is considerable interest in developing immune-based approaches to prevent initial or recurrent cases of CDI. Passive or active immunization against *C difficile* toxins A and B is protective against toxigenic *C difficile* in animal models.[50] In phase 3 randomized trials, infusion of a single dose of monoclonal antibodies to toxins A and B in combination with standard CDI therapy was effective in significantly lowering the risk of recurrent CDI.[50] In addition, 2 phase 3 trials of vaccines for primary prevention of CDI are currently underway.

SUMMARY

CDI disproportionately affects the elderly, particularly those requiring frequent hospital stays or LTCF admission. Recurrences of CDI are common in older adults and may have significant adverse effects on quality of life. Although intrinsic factors associated with aging contribute to the risk for CDI in the elderly, modifiable factors such as antibiotic therapy also play a major role. Ensuring appropriate diagnostic testing and management is challenging for older adults in the community and in LTCFs. FMT approaches that offer greater palatability and flexibility in delivery are emerging and may provide a promising approach for elderly patients with multiple recurrences.

ACKNOWLEDGMENTS

This work was supported by the Veterans Integrated Service Network 10 Geriatric Research Education and Clinical Center (VISN 10 GRECC) and the Veterans Affairs Merit Review Program (C.J. Donskey).

REFERENCES

1. Lessa FC, Mu Y, Bamberg WM, et al. Burden of *Clostridium difficile* infection in the United States. N Engl J Med 2015;372:825–34.

2. Donskey CJ. Fluoroquinolone restriction to control fluoroquinolone-resistant *Clostridium difficile*. Lancet Infect Dis 2017;17:353–4.

3. Riggs MM, Sethi AK, Zabarsky TF, et al. Asymptomatic carriers are a potential source for transmission of epidemic and nonepidemic *Clostridium difficile* strains among long-term care facility residents. Clin Infect Dis 2007;45:992–8.

4. Simor AE, Bradley SF, Strausbaugh LJ, et al. *Clostridium difficile* in long-term-care facilities for the elderly. Infect Control Hosp Epidemiol 2002;23:696–703.

5. Marciniak C, Chen D, Stein AC, et al. Prevalence of *Clostridium difficile* colonization at admission to rehabilitation. Arch Phys Med Rehabil 2006;87:1086–90.

6. Guerrero DM, Nerandzic MM, Jury LA, et al. *Clostridium difficile* infection in a Department of Veterans Affairs long-term care facility. Infect Control Hosp Epidemiol 2011;32:513–5.

7. Pawar D, Tsay R, Nelson DS, et al. Burden of *Clostridium difficile* infection in long-term care facilities in Monroe County, New York. Infect Control Hosp Epidemiol 2012;33:1107–12.

8. Hunter JC, Mu Y, Dumyati GK, et al. Burden of nursing home-onset *Clostridium difficile* infection in the United States: estimates of incidence and patient outcomes. Open Forum Infect Dis 2016;3:ofv196.

9. Campbell R, Giljahn L, Machesky K, et al. *Clostridium difficile* infection in Ohio hospitals and nursing homes during 2006. Infect Control Hosp Epidemiol 2009;30:526–33.

10. Jinno S, Kundrapu S, Guerrero DM, et al. Potential for transmission of *Clostridium difficile* by asymptomatic acute care patients and long-term care facility residents with prior *C. difficile* infection. Infect Control Hosp Epidemiol 2012;33:638–9.

11. Bobulsky GS, Al-Nassir WN, Riggs MM, et al. *Clostridium difficile* skin contamination in patients with *C. difficile*-associated disease. Clin Infect Dis 2008;46: 447–50.

12. Donskey CJ, Kundrapu S, Deshpande A. Colonization versus carriage of *Clostridium difficile*. Infect Dis Clin North Am 2015;29:13–28.

13. Kyne L, Warny M, Qamar A, et al. Asymptomatic carriage of *Clostridium difficile* and serum levels of IgG antibody against toxin A. N Engl J Med 2000;342:390–7.

14. Jiang ZD, DuPont HL, Garey K, et al. A common polymorphism in the interleukin 8 gene promoter is associated with *Clostridium difficile* diarrhea. Am J Gastroenterol 2006;101:1112–6.

15. Bhutto A, Morley JE. The clinical significance of gastrointestinal changes with aging. Curr Opin Clin Nutr Metab Care 2008;11:651–60.

16. Hopkins MJ, Macfarlane GT. Changes in predominant bacterial populations in human faeces with age and with *Clostridium difficile* infection. J Med Microbiol 2002;51:448–54.

17. Borriello SP, Barclay FE, Welch AR. Evaluation of the predictive capability of an in-vitro model of colonization resistance to *Clostridium difficile* infection. Microb Ecol Health Dis 1988;1:61–4.

18. Rea MC, O'Sullivan O, Shanahan F, et al. *Clostridium difficile* carriage in elderly subjects and associated changes in the intestinal microbiota. J Clin Microbiol 2012;50:867–75.

19. Polage CR, Solnick JV, Cohen SH. Nosocomial diarrhea: evaluation and treatment of causes other than *Clostridium difficile*. Clin Infect Dis 2012;55:982–9.

20. Kundrapu S, Sunkesula V, Tomas M, et al. Response to Prior and Fitzpatrick. Infect Control Hosp Epidemiol 2016;37:362–3.

21. Curry SR, Muto CA, Schlackman JL, et al. Use of multilocus variable number of tandem repeats analysis genotyping to determine the role of asymptomatic carriers in *Clostridium difficile* transmission. Clin Infect Dis 2013;57:1094–102.

22. Longtin Y, Paquet-Bolduc B, Gilca R, et al. Effect of detecting and isolating *C difficile* carriers at hospital admission on the incidence of *C difficile* infections: a quasi-experimental controlled study. JAMA Intern Med 2016;176:796–804.

23. Blixt T, Gradel KO, Homann C, et al. Asymptomatic carriers contribute to nosocomial *Clostridium difficile* infection: a cohort study of 4508 patients. Gastroenterology 2017;152:1031–41.

24. Lucado J, Gould C, Elixhauser A. *Clostridium difficile* infections (CDI) in hospital stays, 2009-Healthcare Cost and Utilization Project (HCUP) Statistical Briefs - Rockville (MD): NCBI Bookshelf; 2012.

25. Black SR, Weaver KN, Jones RC, et al. *Clostridium difficile* outbreak strain BI is highly endemic in Chicago area hospitals. Infect Control Hosp Epidemiol 2011; 32:897–902.

26. McDonald L, Coignard B, Dubberke E, et al. Recommendations for surveillance of *Clostridium difficile*-associated disease. Infect Control Hosp Epidemiol 2007; 28:140–5.

27. Mylotte J. Surveillance for *Clostridium difficile*-associated diarrhea in long-term care facilities: what you get is not what you see. Infect Control Hosp Epidemiol 2008;29:760–3.

28. Kim JH, Toy D, Muder RR. *Clostridium difficile* infection in a long-term care facility: hospital-associated illness compared with long-term care-associated illness. Infect Control Hosp Epidemiol 2011;32:656–60.

29. Mylotte JM, Russell S, Sackett B, et al. Surveillance for *Clostridium difficile* infection in nursing homes. J Am Geriatr Soc 2013;61:122–5.

30. Ponnada S, Guerrero DM, Jury LA, et al. Acquisition of *Clostridium difficile* colonization and infection after transfer from a veterans affairs hospital to an affiliated long-term care facility. Infect Control Hosp Epidemiol 2017;38:1–7.

31. Cohen SH, Gerding DN, Johnson S, et al. Clinical practice guidelines for *Clostridium difficile* infection in adults: 2010 update by the Society for Healthcare Epidemiology of America (SHEA) and the Infectious Diseases Society of America (IDSA). Infect Control Hosp Epidemiol 2010;31:431–55.

32. Hensgens MP, Goorhuis A, Dekkers OM, et al. Time interval of increased risk for *Clostridium difficile* infection after exposure to antibiotics. J Antimicrob Chemother 2012;67:742–8.

33. Koo HL, Ajami NJ, Jiang ZD, et al. A nosocomial outbreak of norovirus infection masquerading as CDI. Clin Infect Dis 2009;48:e75–7.

34. Pepin J, Routhier S, Gagnon S, et al. Management and outcomes of a first recurrence of *Clostridium difficile*-associated disease in Quebec, Canada. Clin Infect Dis 2006;42:758–64.

35. Polage CR, Gyorke CE, Kennedy MA, et al. Overdiagnosis of *Clostridium difficile* infection in the molecular test era. JAMA Intern Med 2015;175:1792–801.

36. Planche T, Wilcox MH. Diagnostic pitfalls in *Clostridium difficile* infection. Infect Dis Clin North Am 2015;29:63–82.

37. Kundrapu S, Sunkesula VC, Jury LA, et al. Utility of perirectal swab specimens for diagnosis of *Clostridium difficile* infection. Clin Infect Dis 2012;55: 1527–30.

38. Kundrapu S, Jury LA, Sitzlar B, et al. Easily modified factors contribute to delays in diagnosis of *Clostridium difficile* infection: a cohort study and intervention. J Clin Microbiol 2013;51:2365–70.

39. Quinn LK, Chen Y, Herwaldt LA. Infection control policies and practices for Iowa long-term care facility residents with *Clostridium difficile* infection. Infect Control Hosp Epidemiol 2007;28:1228–32.

40. Zar FA, Bakkanagari SR, Moorthi KM, et al. A comparison of vancomycin and metronidazole for the treatment of *Clostridium difficile*-associated diarrhea, stratified by disease severity. Clin Infect Dis 2007;45:302–7.

41. Johnson S, Louie TJ, Gerding DN, et al. Vancomycin, metronidazole, or tolevamer for *Clostridium difficile* infection: results from two multinational, randomized, controlled trials. Clin Infect Dis 2014;59:345–54.

42. Louie TJ, Miller MA, Mullane KM, et al. Fidaxomicin versus vancomycin for *Clostridium difficile* infection. N Engl J Med 2011;364:422–31.

43. Sunkesula VC, Kundrapu S, Muganda C, et al. Does empirical *Clostridium difficile* infection (CDI) therapy result in false-negative CDI diagnostic test results? Clin Infect Dis 2013;57:494–500.

44. Van Nood E, Vrieze A, Nieuwdorp M, et al. Duodenal infusion of donor feces for recurrent *Clostridium difficile*. N Engl J Med 2013;368:407–15.

45. Louie TJ, Cannon K, O'Grady H, et al. Fecal microbiome transplantation (FMT) via oral fecal microbial capsules for recurrent *Clostridium difficile* infection (rCDI) [abstract 89]. San Francisco, CA: ID Week; 2013. Available at: https://idsa.confex.com/idsa/2013/webprogram/Paper41627.html. Accessed November 10, 2015.

46. Youngster I, Russell GH, Pindar C, et al. Oral, capsulized, frozen fecal microbiota transplantation for relapsing *Clostridium difficile* infection. JAMA 2014;312: 1772–8.

47. Hecker MT, Obrenovich ME, Cadnum JL, et al. Fecal microbiota transplantation by Freeze-Dried oral capsules for recurrent *Clostridium difficile* Infection. Open Forum Infect Dis 2016;3:ofw091.

48. Hecker MT, Ho E, Donskey CJ. Fear of failure: engaging patients in antimicrobial stewardship after fecal transplantation for recurrent *Clostridium difficile* infection. Infect Control Hosp Epidemiol 2017;38:127–9.

49. Soriano MM, Danziger LH, Gerding DN, et al. Novel fidaxomicin treatment regimens for patients with multiple *Clostridium difficile* infection recurrences that are refractory to standard therapies. Open Forum Infect Dis 2014;1:ofu069.

50. Wilcox MH, Gerding DN, Poxton IR, et al. Bezlotoxumab for prevention of recurrent *Clostridium difficile* infection. N Engl J Med 2017;376:305–17.

Influenza in Older Adults

H. Keipp Talbot, MD, MPH

KEYWORDS

- Influenza • Vaccine • Aging • Antivirals

KEY POINTS

- Influenza viruses circulate yearly and cause significant disease in the elderly.
- Influenza often presents atypically in older adults.
- New influenza vaccines are being developed for older adults to overcome immune senescence.

INTRODUCTION

Influenza viruses cause significant morbidity and mortality in older adults. Prevention and treatment are critical for the reduction of morbidity and mortality in this population, but there are several challenges in the diagnosis, treatment, and prevention of influenza infection and its complications in older adults. This article will describe influenza, its epidemiology, clinical presentation, diagnostic modalities, treatment, and current prevention techniques. Despite the identification of influenza early in the last century, much is still not known about how to protect older adults from influenza infection and its complications. Current treatment and prevention strategies are imperfect, particularly in older frail adults.

VIROLOGY

Influenza is a segmented RNA virus of the orthomyxoviridae family that circulates annually.[1] Influenza A and B are both known to cause disease in people. Because the virus is a segmented RNA virus, it has the capability of making minor (called antigenic drift) or major (called antigenic shift) changes to its genome, causing seasonal or pandemic outbreaks of disease, respectively. Influenza A subtypes are differentiated by the type of hemagglutinin and neuraminidase found on their outer surface (eg, H1N1 and H3N2 subtypes). The hemagglutinin protein is responsible for viral receptor binding and fusion with the host respiratory epithelial cell. This surface protein undergoes frequent genetic mutations that allow for the circulating strain to potentially escape recognition by the host's immune system. The neuraminidase, also a glycoprotein, facilitates the release of daughter virions from infected cells. For unknown

Departments of Medicine and Health Policy, Vanderbilt University Medical Center, A2200 MCN, 1161 21st Avenue South, Nashville, TN 37232, USA
E-mail address: Keipp.talbot@vanderbilt.edu

Infect Dis Clin N Am 31 (2017) 757–766
http://dx.doi.org/10.1016/j.idc.2017.07.005

id.theclinics.com

reasons, seasonal influenza A/H3N2 viruses are associated with higher morbidity and mortality than either seasonal influenza A/H1N1 or influenza B viruses.[2] There are 2 main lineages of influenza B that circulate in the human population, B/Yamagata and B/Victoria. Traditionally 1 of the B lineages has been chosen for inclusion into the yearly vaccine, but most vaccine manufacturers are now including a virus from both B lineages due to poor predictably of the circulating lineage in the coming year. Multiple influenza viruses can circulate in a season (usually December through March), and a patient can be infected by more than 1 virus in a season.[3]

EPIDEMIOLOGY OF INFLUENZA

Because the circulating influenza virus often changes from year to year, the morbidity and the mortality from influenza also fluctuate. In any given year, influenza accounts for 2% to 20% of cardiopulmonary hospitalizations.[4–8] Estimates of hospitalization and death in the United States due to influenza infection range from 1.287 to 2.127 million hospitalizations[9] and 961 to 14,715 deaths,[10] respectively. Many of the deaths are secondary to pneumonia or cardiac complications and are much more common in the older than in the younger populations. Once infected, 67% of elderly become at least temporarily housebound, and 25% become temporarily bedbound.[4] Despite prior exposure to many influenza viruses in the past, the incidence of this morbidity and mortality continues to increase with age likely because of immune senescence and higher number of comorbid conditions present in older adults.

Influenza viruses are among the leading causes of outbreaks in long-term care facilities, with attack rates that span 4% to 94% of residents (mean 33%). Mortality rates in these outbreaks may approach 55%.[11]

CLINICAL PRESENTATION

The classic, textbook presentation of influenza is fever, cough, and general aches (often called an influenza-like illness or ILI) lasting 3 to 7 days.[12] The presentation of older adults with influenza is neither classic, nor simple. Fever may not be prominent even when fever is defined as temperature greater than 99°F, and the presenting complaints may instead consist of exacerbations of underlying health problems like congestive heart failure or chronic obstructive pulmonary disease (COPD).

In one study of veterans with COPD 50 years of age and older, the prominent presentation of influenza was cough, sputum production, and dyspnea.[13] Only 64% of laboratory-confirmed cases of influenza were associated with either documented or subjective fever.[13] In a cohort of vaccinated adults 60 years of age and older, fever was even less common, with only 39% of patients with laboratory-confirmed influenza complaining of fever, while 94% reported coryza.[14] The lack of fever in this cohort, however, could have been due to vaccination of everyone in the cohort.

In the inpatient setting, the most common presentation of influenza is cough (96%), with only 64% of patients reporting being feverish.[15] One hospital-based surveillance study found that only 51% of hospitalized adults with influenza had the classic ILI presentation.[16] Because of this atypical presentation, influenza is often not associated with the reason for hospitalization by many providers.[7] Providers should have a low threshold for testing and treating older adults.

DIAGNOSIS

The diagnosis of influenza is not only important to epidemiologists but also to individual clinicians who care for older individuals. The laboratory method that has been available for clinical use the longest has been culture isolation of influenza, which requires several days until definitive results are available. With recommendations to start antiviral treatment within 48 hours of symptom onset, the delay in culture results makes it less than ideal for rapid therapeutic intervention. Rapid antigen testing is a popular modality to obtain an influenza diagnosis quickly. This works well in children who secrete large amounts of virus. Adults, however, shed much less virus than children and tend to shed for shorter periods of time, thus reducing the utility of rapid antigen tests in this population. A study in hospitalized patients found the sensitivity of the rapid antigen test performed at bedside was only 19% (95% confidence interval [CI], 8.51%–37.9%); and the sensitivity of conventional influenza culture was 34.6% (95% CI, 19.4%–53.8%).

Recently, polymerase chain reaction (PCR), a common diagnostic tool in research settings, has been shown to be more sensitive than culture for the detection of influenza.[17,18] With the introduction of PCR into clinical laboratories, the sensitivity of influenza diagnosis has improved. The sensitivity of PCR in adults 40 years of age and older is greater than 90%.[19] Unfortunately, not all clinical laboratories perform PCR at all, or if they do, some may not perform this test daily. When possible, PCR should be used for diagnosis, as it is the most sensitive method. If PCR not available, results of antigen testing should be remembered to have poor sensitivity.

TREATMENT

Currently 2 classes of antiviral medications active against influenza, the adamantanes and neuraminidase inhibitors, are licensed in the United States. Because of the development of resistance to adamantanes, these agents are no longer used clinically.[20] Neuraminidase inhibitors are currently the only recommended pharmacologic treatment for influenza. They work by blocking the neuraminidase glycoprotein noted earlier.[21] Three neuraminidase inhibitors are currently available in the United States: peramivir, oseltamivir, and zanamivir. Peramivir is the most recently licensed neuraminidase inhibitor and is given intravenously; oseltamivir is given orally, and zanamivir is delivered by inhalation. Both peramivir and oseltamivir need to be dosed based on renal function. Zanamivir should be used cautiously in adults with reactive airway disease, as some patients have developed bronchospasm. Early studies of neuraminidase inhibitors noted relief of symptoms 1 day sooner than with placebo,[22,23] but these early studies were performed in healthy young adults. Meta-analyses were performed on the data to look at high-risk individuals, including those 65 years of age and older.[24] These studies showed that relief of symptoms came 2 days earlier for zanamivir but only 0.5 days earlier for oseltamivir in this high-risk population.[21] Because of low numbers, it was unclear if treatment lowered the incidence of complications involving the lowering respiratory tract or hospitalization rates.

The Emerging Infections Program, which performs surveillance for influenza at hospitals in multiple states, evaluated the impact of antiviral treatment on influenza cases and found antivirals decreased the odds of extended care after hospital discharge and reduced length of stay.[25] Similarly, a cohort study in Canada[26] found that treatment with antivirals reduced mortality caused by influenza infection. Both these studies should be evaluated cautiously, as there were likely differences in the patients who received antiviral treatment (ie, prescription of these agents was at the discretion of the treating physician).

Peramivir underwent phase II trials under emergency use authorization during the 2009 influenza pandemic, as no other intravenous treatments were available. It was then approved for use in the United States by the US Food and Drug Administration in 2014. Phase III studies in Japan have shown peramivir to be noninferior to oseltamivir.[27]

According to recommendations from the US Centers for Disease Control and Prevention, neuraminidase inhibitors should be started within 48 hours of symptom onset for anyone 65 years of age or older. Hence it is recommended to start antivirals empirically until influenza testing results are available. The benefit of neuraminidase inhibitors after 48 hours of symptom onset is controversial.[28,29]

PREVENTION
Vaccination

The current influenza vaccines contain 15 mcg each of hemagglutinin of an A/H3N2, A/H1N1, and a B virus. Because of historically poor predictions of what influenza B lineage would circulate each year, many manufacturers have expanded the vaccine content to include a B virus from both lineages, creating what is known as a quadrivalent inactivated influenza vaccine (IIV4). The vaccine must be reformulated each year because of the changes in strain circulation.

Influenza vaccines were developed prior to World War II to prevent death and pneumonia in military recruits. In 1960 the US Surgeon General recommended the use of influenza vaccine in adults 65 years of age and older.[30] This recommendation was made because of the high burden of morbidity and mortality in older adults. These recommendations were made not based on clinical trials showing clinical efficacy but rather, on extrapolation of data from trials in younger adults. Unfortunately for the same reasons that influenza is associated with more severe disease in older adults, older adults mount inadequate immunologic responses to influenza vaccine and have lower levels of clinical effectiveness. Older adults tend to have lower antibody responses to influenza vaccines.[31] It is debated if this is because of poor immune responses or blunting of responses caused by prior influenza immunizations. Either way, antibody responses to influenza vaccines are lower than responses identified in younger adults. Similarly cell-mediated immune responses are lower.[32] The degree to which these impact clinical effectiveness is not well-known.

Three randomized clinical trials (RCTs)[33–35] have evaluated the efficacy of trivalent inactivated influenza vaccines in older adults. The first of the 3 RCTs used only ILI, and not laboratory-confirmed disease, as an endpoint.[33] Because many illnesses also present with influenza-like symptoms (eg, other respiratory viruses circulating at the same time as influenza), the study was unable to show any vaccine effectiveness. The remaining 2 RCTs used serologic diagnosis of influenza as the efficacy endpoint. In the first of these 2 studies conducted by Govaert and colleagues,[34] vaccine efficacy for serologically confirmed influenza was 56%, but this study was not adequately powered to examine the efficacy of the vaccine in those adults 70 years of age and older and only evaluated a healthy, independently living population. The second randomized study, which enrolled 653 subjects aged over 60 years old in Thailand,[35] also used serologic evidence of infection as the endpoint. Overall, the relative risk reduction in the vaccinated population was 65% (95% CI, 16%–85%), but the study was also inadequately powered either to show a reduction in influenza in adults 70 years of age and older. Hence, no RCTs have been conducted to show influenza vaccine effectiveness in adults 70 years of age and older.

In order to overcome this lack of evidence, new effectiveness studies have been designed to evaluate the prevention of illness in older adults. These studies are observational but prospectively test patients presenting for medical care with an acute respiratory illness for influenza with PCR. To date, these studies show influenza vaccine to be 40% to 60% effective for the prevention of hospitalization in adults 50 years of age and older when circulating and influenza vaccine strains are similar.[5,8,36–41] Data remain lacking in the group 70 years of age and older.

In an attempt to overcome immune senescence that occurs in older adults, new influenza vaccines are being designed to protect this population from influenza. Currently there are 2 licensed influenza vaccines for use specifically in adults 65 years of age and older in the United States, a high dose vaccine and an MF59 adjuvanted vaccine. The first enhanced vaccine licensed for use in the United States was the high-dose influenza vaccine. The amount of hemagglutinin for each influenza strain was quadrupled, increasing the total amount of antigen from 45 mcg to 180 mcg. Early trials showed a significant antibody increase to influenza A (but not influenza B).[42] A large phase IIIb/IV study showed a relative effectiveness of 24% for the high-dose versus the standard-dose influenza vaccine.[43] A study using Medicare data looked at the relative vaccine effectiveness of the high dose compared with the standard dose during the 2012 to 2013 influenza season and found the high-dose vaccine to be 22% more effective.[44] More recently, an adjuvanted influenza vaccine (aIIV) was licensed in the United States. This vaccine uses the traditional amount of hemagglutinin (45 mcg) but adds an adjuvant named MF59. This vaccine has been used for many years in Europe. A small randomized study was conducted for licensure, which showed similar but not superior antibody responses for the adjuvanted vaccine compared with the nonadjuvanted inactivated influenza vaccine.[45] An observational study in Italy compared the effectiveness of the adjuvanted vaccine with a nonadjuvanted vaccine over 3 influenza seasons and found the risk of hospitalization for influenza or pneumonia was 25% lower for aIIV.[46]

Attempts are currently underway to develop a universal vaccine that will work for any circulating influenza virus, so that patients would not necessarily need yearly vaccination nor would experts have to predict which influenza viral strains would need to be included in the following year's vaccine. Until the development of such a vaccine, patients (and health care workers) need yearly vaccination. **Table 1** lists the currently available vaccines licensed in the United States.

Influenza vaccine is usually given early in the fall to allow for the body to make an immune response prior to influenza season. As vaccine is introduced earlier and earlier each year, concerns have arisen about waning immunity, meaning that the protection provided by the vaccine may wane prior to the cessation of influenza circulation. Unfortunately there is little evidence about the true duration of protection, leaving many providers wondering when to give vaccine. Despite concerns about vaccinating too early, it is important not to miss an opportunity to vaccinate all older adults.

Herd Protection

One of the most effective ways to prevent an individual from an infectious agent is to vaccinate the population. Multiple studies[47–50] have shown that vaccinating health care workers in nursing homes provides protection from influenza infection in patients. These studies have compared nursing homes where employees are vaccinated with nursing homes where employees are not vaccinated. The largest of these studies had 22 long-term care facilities. The patient mortality in the facilities without vaccination of employees was 15.3%, while the mortality of patients in facilities that vaccinated employees was 11.2%.[47] This suggests that the introduction of influenza into a facility occurred from the staff, but other sources, such as visitors, cannot be excluded. Hence, vaccination of employees likely blocks at least some introduction of influenza into the facility. One ecologic study has hinted that immunization of

Table 1
Currently licensed influenza vaccine formulations in the United States

	Inactivated Influenza Vaccine – Trivalent (IIV3)	Inactivated Influenza Vaccine – Quadrivalent (IIV4)	Inactivated Influenza Vaccine High-Dose Trivalent (IIV3-HD)	Inactivated Influenza Vaccine – Adjuvanted Trivalent (aIIV3)	Recombinant Influenza HA Vaccine (rIIV3)	Inactivated Influenza Vaccine Cell Culture (ccIIV3)
A/H3N2	x	x	X	x	x	x
A/H1N1	x	x	X	x	x	x
Either B/Victoria or B/Yamagata	x		x	x	x	x
Both B/Victoria & B/Yamagata		x				
Egg Culture	x	x	X	x	No	Seed stock only

younger adults in the community may also protect older adults from influenza infection.[51]

Antiviral Medications

Antiviral medications may be used for treatment and prevention of influenza. Both oseltamivir and zanamivir have been licensed for prophylaxis.

The use of antiviral medications is ideal in the setting of outbreaks in long-term care facilities. An RCT compared the impact of treating individuals with influenza versus treating the infected individuals and giving prophylactic doses to noninfected residents. With the use of prophylactic treatment, there was a reduction in the duration of outbreaks (24 vs 11 days) and a reduction in the attack rate (36% vs 23%).[52]

One study used daily oseltamivir in a blind RCT to prevent outbreaks from occurring in long-term care facilities.[53] This study included 572 volunteers from 31 centers and found a reduction in laboratory-confirmed clinical cases (4.4% vs 0.4%).

If a case of influenza is identified in a long-term care facility, all patients should receive antiviral prophylaxis; vaccination of staff and residents should be completed, and appropriate infection control policies (droplet precautions) should go into effect.

SUMMARY

Influenza causes significant morbidity and mortality in older adults, and prevention with vaccination and antiviral medications is important to reduce the morbidity and mortality of influenza. Future research will need to create an influenza vaccine that not only is effective regardless of the circulating strain but creates a protective response in an aging immune system.

REFERENCES

1. Knipe D, Howley P, editors. Fields virology, vol. 2, 5th edition. Wolters kluwer; 2007.
2. Thompson WW, Shay DK, Weintraub E, et al. Mortality associated with influenza and respiratory syncytial virus in the United States. JAMA 2003;289(2):179–86.
3. Perez-Garcia F, Vasquez V, de Egea V, et al. Influenza A and B co-infection: a case-control study and review of the literature. Eur J Clin Microbiol Infect Dis 2016;35(6):941–6.
4. Falsey AR, Hennessey PA, Formica MA, et al. Respiratory syncytial virus infection in elderly and high-risk adults. N Engl J Med 2005;352(17):1749–59.
5. Talbot HK, Griffin MR, Chen Q, et al. Effectiveness of seasonal vaccine in preventing confirmed influenza-associated hospitalizations in community dwelling older adults. J Infect Dis 2011;203(4):500–8.
6. Talbot HK, Poehling KA, Williams JV, et al. Influenza in older adults: impact of vaccination of school children. Vaccine 2009;27(13):1923–7.
7. Talbot HK, Williams JV, Zhu Y, et al. Failure of routine diagnostic methods to detect influenza in hospitalized older adults. Infect Control Hosp Epidemiol 2010;31(7):683–8.
8. Talbot HK, Zhu Y, Chen Q, et al. Effectiveness of influenza vaccine for preventing laboratory-confirmed influenza hospitalizations in adults, 2011-2012 influenza season. Clin Infect Dis 2013;56(12):1774–7.
9. Thompson WW, Shay DK, Weintraub E, et al. Influenza-associated hospitalizations in the United States. JAMA 2004;292(11):1333–40.

10. Centers for Disease Control and Prevention (CDC). Estimates of deaths associated with seasonal influenza — United States, 1976-2007. MMWR Morb Mortal Wkly Rep 2010;59(33):1057–62.
11. Utsumi M, Makimoto K, Quroshi N, et al. Types of infectious outbreaks and their impact in elderly care facilities: a review of the literature. Age Ageing 2010;39(3):299–305.
12. Cate TR. Clinical manifestations and consequences of influenza. Am J Med 1987;82(6A):15–9.
13. Neuzil KM, O'Connor TZ, Gorse GJ, et al. Recognizing influenza in older patients with chronic obstructive pulmonary disease who have received influenza vaccine. Clin Infect Dis 2003;36(2):169–74.
14. Shahid Z, Kleppinger A, Gentleman B, et al. Clinical and immunologic predictors of influenza illness among vaccinated older adults. Vaccine 2010;28(38):6145–51.
15. Falsey A, Baran A, Walsh E. Should clinical case definitions of influenza in hospitalized older adults include fever? Influenza Other Respir Viruses 2015;9(S1):23–9.
16. Babcock HM, Merz LR, Fraser VJ. Is influenza an influenza-like illness? Clinical presentation of influenza in hospitalized patients. Infect Control Hosp Epidemiol 2006;27(3):266–70.
17. Poehling KA, Edwards KM, Weinberg GA, et al. The underrecognized burden of influenza in young children. N Engl J Med 2006;355(1):31–40.
18. Weinberg GA, Erdman DD, Edwards KM, et al. Superiority of reverse-transcription polymerase chain reaction to conventional viral culture in the diagnosis of acute respiratory tract infections in children. J Infect Dis 2004;189(4):706–10.
19. Steininger C, Kundi M, Aberle SW, et al. Effectiveness of reverse transcription-PCR, virus isolation, and enzyme-linked immunosorbent assay for diagnosis of influenza A virus infection in different age groups. J Clin Microbiol 2002;40(6):2051–6.
20. Fiore AE, Fry A, Shay D, et al. Antiviral agents for the treatment and chemoprophylaxis of influenza — recommendations of the Advisory Committee on Immunization Practices (ACIP). MMWR Recomm Rep 2011;60(1):1–24.
21. Moscona A. Neuraminidase inhibitors for influenza. N Engl J Med 2005;353(13):1363–73.
22. Treanor JJ, Hayden FG, Vrooman PS, et al. Efficacy and safety of the oral neuraminidase inhibitor oseltamivir in treating acute influenza: a randomized controlled trial. US Oral Neuraminidase Study Group. JAMA 2000;283(8):1016–24.
23. Hayden FG, Osterhaus AD, Treanor JJ, et al. Efficacy and safety of the neuraminidase inhibitor zanamivir in the treatment of influenzavirus infections. GG167 Influenza Study Group. N Engl J Med 1997;337(13):874–80.
24. Cooper NJ, Sutton AJ, Abrams KR, et al. Effectiveness of neuraminidase inhibitors in treatment and prevention of influenza A and B: systematic review and meta-analyses of randomised controlled trials. BMJ 2003;326(7401):1235.
25. Chaves SS, Perez A, Miller L, et al. Impact of prompt influenza antiviral treatment on extended care needs after influenza hospitalization among community-dwelling older adults. Clin Infect Dis 2015;61(12):1807–14.
26. McGeer A, Green KA, Plevneshi A, et al. Antiviral therapy and outcomes of influenza requiring hospitalization in Ontario, Canada. Clin Infect Dis 2007;45(12):1568–75.

27. Wester A, Shetty AK. Peramivir injection in the treatment of acute influenza: a review of the literature. Infect Drug Resist 2016;9:201–14.

28. Fry AM, Goswami D, Nahar K, et al. Efficacy of oseltamivir treatment started within 5 days of symptom onset to reduce influenza illness duration and virus shedding in an urban setting in Bangladesh: a randomised placebo-controlled trial. Lancet Infect Dis 2014;14(2):109–18.

29. Spagnuolo PJ, Zhang M, Xu Y, et al. Effects of antiviral treatment on influenza-related complications over four influenza seasons: 2006–2010. Curr Med Res Opin 2016;32(8):1399–407.

30. Langmuir AD, Henderson DA, Serfling RE. The epidemiological basis for the control of influenza. Am J Public Health Nations Health 1964;54:563–71.

31. Goodwin K, Viboud C, Simonsen L. Antibody response to influenza vaccination in the elderly: a quantitative review. Vaccine 2006;24(8):1159–69.

32. Murasko DM, Bernstein ED, Gardner EM, et al. Role of humoral and cell-mediated immunity in protection from influenza disease after immunization of healthy elderly. Exp Gerontol 2002;37(2–3):427–39.

33. Allsup S, Haycox A, Regan M, et al. Is influenza vaccination cost effective for healthy people between ages 65 and 74 years? A randomised controlled trial. Vaccine 2004;23(5):639–45.

34. Govaert TM, Thijs CT, Masurel N, et al. The efficacy of influenza vaccination in elderly individuals. A randomized double-blind placebo-controlled trial. JAMA 1994;272(21):1661–5.

35. Praditsuwan R, Assantachai P, Wasi C, et al. The efficacy and effectiveness of influenza vaccination among Thai elderly persons living in the community. J Med Assoc Thai 2005;88(2):256–64.

36. Sullivan SG, Chilver MB, Higgins G, et al. Influenza vaccine effectiveness in Australia: results from the Australian Sentinel Practices Research Network. Med J Aust 2014;201(2):109–11.

37. Andrews N, McMenamin J, Durnall H, et al. Effectiveness of trivalent seasonal influenza vaccine in preventing laboratory-confirmed influenza in primary care in the United Kingdom: 2012/13 end of season results. Euro Surveill 2014; 19(27):5–13.

38. Dawood FS, Prapasiri P, Areerat P, et al. Effectiveness of the 2010 and 2011 Southern Hemisphere trivalent inactivated influenza vaccines against hospitalization with influenza-associated acute respiratory infection among Thai adults aged ≥ 50 years. Influenza Other Respir Viruses 2014;8(4):463–8.

39. Kwong JC, Campitelli MA, Gubbay JB, et al. Vaccine effectiveness against laboratory-confirmed influenza hospitalizations among elderly adults during the 2010-2011 season. Clin Infect Dis 2013;57(6):820–7.

40. Kissling E, Valenciano M, Falcao J, et al. "I-MOVE" towards monitoring seasonal and pandemic influenza vaccine effectiveness: lessons learnt from a pilot multi-centric case-control study in Europe, 2008-9. Euro Surveill 2009;14(44) [pii: 19388].

41. Chen Q, Griffin MR, Nian H, et al. Influenza vaccine prevents medically attended influenza-associated acute respiratory illness in adults aged ≥50 years. J Infect Dis 2015;211(7):1045–50.

42. Falsey AR, Treanor JJ, Tornieporth N, et al. Randomized, double-blind controlled phase 3 trial comparing the immunogenicity of high-dose and standard-dose influenza vaccine in adults 65 years of age and older. J Infect Dis 2009;200(2):172–80.

43. DiazGranados CA, Dunning AJ, Kimmel M, et al. Efficacy of high-dose versus standard-dose influenza vaccine in older adults. N Engl J Med 2014;371(7): 635–45.

44. Izurieta HS, Thadani N, Shay DK, et al. Comparative effectiveness of high-dose versus standard-dose influenza vaccines in US residents aged 65 years and older from 2012 to 2013 using Medicare data: a retrospective cohort analysis. Lancet Infect Dis 2015;15(3):293–300.

45. Frey SE, Reyes MR, Reynales H, et al. Comparison of the safety and immunogenicity of an MF59(R)-adjuvanted with a non-adjuvanted seasonal influenza vaccine in elderly subjects. Vaccine 2014;32(39):5027–34.

46. Mannino S, Villa M, Apolone G, et al. Effectiveness of adjuvanted influenza vaccination in elderly subjects in northern Italy. Am J Epidemiol 2012;176(6):527–33.

47. Hayward AC, Harling R, Wetten S, et al. Effectiveness of an influenza vaccine programme for care home staff to prevent death, morbidity, and health service use among residents: cluster randomised controlled trial. BMJ 2006;333(7581):1241.

48. Potter J, Stott DJ, Roberts MA, et al. Influenza vaccination of health care workers in long-term-care hospitals reduces the mortality of elderly patients. J Infect Dis 1997;175(1):1–6.

49. Carman WF, Elder AG, Wallace LA, et al. Effects of influenza vaccination of health-care workers on mortality of elderly people in long-term care: a randomised controlled trial. Lancet 2000;355(9198):93–7.

50. Lemaitre M, Meret T, Rothan-Tondeur M, et al. Effect of influenza vaccination of nursing home staff on mortality of residents: a cluster-randomized trial. J Am Geriatr Soc 2009;57(9):1580–6.

51. Taksler GB, Rothberg MB, Cutler DM. Association of influenza vaccination coverage in younger adults with influenza-related illness in the elderly. Clin Infect Dis 2015;61(10):1495–503.

52. Booy R, Lindley RI, Dwyer DE, et al. Treating and preventing influenza in aged care facilities: a cluster randomised controlled trial. PLoS One 2012;7(10): e46509.

53. Peters PH Jr, Gravenstein S, Norwood P, et al. Long-term use of oseltamivir for the prophylaxis of influenza in a vaccinated frail older population. J Am Geriatr Soc 2001;49(8):1025–31.

Respiratory Syncytial Virus and Other Noninfluenza Respiratory Viruses in Older Adults

Fumihiro Kodama, MD[a], David A. Nace, MD, MPH[b], Robin L.P. Jump, MD, PhD[c,d],*

KEYWORDS

- Respiratory syncytial virus • Noninfluenza respiratory virus • Outbreak • Elderly
- Long-term care facility • Multiplex respiratory viral panel

KEY POINTS

- Among older adults, the morbidity and mortality of respiratory syncytial virus infections is similar to that of influenza.
- Several other respiratory viruses (human metapneumovirus, parainfluenza virus, rhinovirus, coronavirus and adenovirus) may cause outbreaks among residents of long-term care facilities.
- Supportive care is the mainstay of medical therapy; effective antivirals or vaccinations do not yet exist for noninfluenza respiratory viruses.
- Rapid diagnostic molecular tests will augment our epidemiologic understanding of noninfluenza respiratory viral outbreaks.
- Infection prevention and control measures for contagious individuals includes hand hygiene, cough etiquette, and use of a mask, gown, and gloves by health care workers.

Disclosure Statement: None (F. Kodama and D.A. Nace). Dr R.L.P. Jump has received research funding from Pfizer (ID 13162823) and the Steris Foundation.

[a] Department of Infectious Diseases, Sapporo City General Hospital, 13 Chome 1-1, Kita 11 Jonishi, Chuo-ku, Sapporo, Hokkaido 060-8604, Japan; [b] Division of Geriatric Medicine, Department of Medicine, University of Pittsburgh, 3471 Fifth Avenue, Kaufmann Building Suite 500, Pittsburgh, PA 15213, USA; [c] Division of Infectious Diseases and HIV Medicine, Department of Medicine, Case Western Reserve University, 11100 Euclid Avenue, Cleveland, OH 44195-5029, USA; [d] Geriatric Research, Education, and Clinical Center (GRECC), Specialty Care Center of Innovation, Louis Stokes Cleveland Veterans Affairs Medical Center, 111C(W), 10701 East Boulevard, Cleveland, OH 44106, USA
* Corresponding author. Geriatric Research Education and Clinical Center, Louis Stokes Cleveland Veterans Affairs Medical Center, 111C (W), 10701 East Boulevard, Cleveland, OH 44106.
E-mail address: robinjump@gmail.com

INTRODUCTION

Respiratory tract infections are a common cause of morbidity and mortality in older adults. In 2014, influenza and pneumonia accounted for 2.3% of deaths among adults 65 years or older in the United States.[1] Older adults, especially those older than 75 years of age, experience the highest rate of influenza-associated mortality rate among all age groups.[2] The availability of rapid diagnostic tests, antiviral medications, and, most notably, the seasonal influenza vaccine mitigate some of influenza's devastating effects.[3] Respiratory viruses other than influenza also cause significant morbidity and mortality among older adults, particularly those who are residents of long-term care facilities (LTCFs).[4,5] These viruses include respiratory syncytial virus (RSV), human metapneumovirus (HMPV), parainfluenza virus, rhinovirus, coronavirus, and adenovirus. In this article, we review viruses, other than influenza, that are common causes of respiratory infections in older adults and discuss relevant diagnostic tests, transmission, and infection prevention and control measures.

Epidemiology

In the United States, the National Respiratory and Enteric Virus Surveillance System, a voluntary laboratory-based system affiliated with the Centers for Disease Control and Prevention (CDC), monitors temporal and geographic patterns associated with the detection of RSV, HMPV, parainfluenza viruses, and respiratory adenoviruses.[6] Data from the National Respiratory and Enteric Virus Surveillance System informs reports from the CDC regarding ongoing trends in detection of respiratory viruses. Although comprehensive, the National Respiratory and Enteric Virus Surveillance System data do not include patient demographics and therefore do not specifically provide information about the epidemiology of respiratory viruses in older adults or LTCFs. Additionally, other than to rule out influenza, for which there is effective antiviral therapy, molecular diagnostic tests are not yet widely used in the evaluation of older adults or LTCF residents with respiratory infections. Accordingly, most of our understanding of the epidemiology of noninfluenza respiratory infections among older adults is informed through research studies and descriptions of outbreaks in LTCFs (**Table 1**).

RESPIRATORY SYNCYTIAL VIRUS

First isolated from chimpanzees in 1956, RSV is a nonsegmented, single-stranded, negative-sense RNA virus within the Paramyxoviridae family (**Table 2**).[7] Most recognized for its effect on children, RSV also causes severe infections among older adults. Similar to influenza, it generally circulates from fall through spring, with a peak in January.[8] A protein on the surface of the virus, dubbed the F protein, causes cell membranes of nearby cells to fuse to form the syncytia for which the virus is named.

Epidemiology

Among older adults, RSV causes morbidity and mortality that rivals that of influenza. Falsey and colleagues[9] described RSV infections among older adults over 4 consecutive winters from 1999 to 2003. Among older adults hospitalized with a respiratory viral infection (n = 1388; age 75 ± 12 years), the authors detected roughly similar proportions of RSV and influenza (142 and 170 cases, respectively). Furthermore, they also found that people with RSV and influenza had similar rates of intensive care stays (15% vs 12%) and mortality (8% vs 7%), respectively. Among this community-dwelling population, for whom the prevalence of vaccination against influenza and *Streptococcus pneumoniae* was greater than 75%, the incidence of RSV was similar to that for nonpandemic influenza.

Table 1
Reports of outbreaks of noninfluenza respiratory viral infection in long-term care facilities

Virus	Reference	Date of Outbreak	Location	Description
RSV	Garvie & Gray,[94] 1980	Data not given	United Kingdom	Seventeen of 40 residents aged 69–90 y developed fever, anorexia and a nonproductive cough. Paired sera from 2 cases showed an increase in RSV complement fixation titers from <20–160. One resident died after severe chest infection.
	Sorvillo et al,[10] 1984	Feb–March, 1979	California	Forty-four of 101 residents (40%) affected; 22 (55%) had pneumonia and 8 (20%) died. Serologic evidence of RSV infection in 13 of 16 patients from whom blood was obtained.
	Caram et al,[12] 2009	Jan–Feb, 2008	North Carolina	Routine surveillance detected an RSV outbreak in a 56-room, 120-bed long-term care facility; 22 of 52 residents (42%) developed symptoms of a respiratory tract infection. RSV was detected by RT-PCR in 7 (32%) of the 22 cases. 1 patient was admitted to the hospital and died.
	Meijer et al,[95] 2013	Winter, 2012–2013	The Netherlands	The Sentinel Nursing Home Surveillance Network in the Netherlands identified an outbreak of RSV-B. Of 10 residents tested for RSV, 4 had RSV-B positive. Two residents had pneumonia and 8 were diagnosed with the common cold. All 10 residents recovered within 2 wk after the onset of symptoms.
	Doi et al,[96] 2014	Winter, 2013–2014	Japan	Twenty-four of 99 residents aged from 68 to 97 y developed respiratory symptoms in winter; 5 cases (20.8%) were diagnosed with pneumonia. RSV was detected from 7 of 10 nasopharyngeal samples by RT-PCR. No other pathogens were isolated.
	Spires et al,[87] 2017	Jan, 2015	Tennessee	During a 16-d outbreak, 30 of 41 (73%) of residents infected. High attack rate among staff. From 14 specimens, 6 positive for RSV-B, 7 for HMPV, 1 for influenza; 15 residents hospitalized, 10 with pneumonia; 5 deaths.

(continued on next page)

Table 1
(continued)

Virus	Reference	Date of Outbreak	Location	Description
HMPV	Honda et al,[97] 2006	Jan, 2005	Japan	Eight inpatients developed respiratory tract illness in a 23-bed ward. HMPV detected using RT-PCR in nasal swabs from all patients. Two developed secondary bacterial pneumonia with *Klebsiella pneumoniae*; all patients recovered.
	Boivin et al,[23] 2007	Jan–Feb, 2006	Quebec, Canada	Ninety-six of 364 residents (27%) presented with respiratory or constitutional symptoms during 6 wk in winter of 2006. Of 13 samples nasopharyngeal samples, real-time multiplex RT-PCR showed HMPV in 6 and RSV in 1 subject. Three of 6 confirmed cases died; a total of 9 people died during the outbreak.
	Louie et al,[48] 2005	June–July, 2003	California	Twenty-six of 148 residents (18%) developed respiratory symptoms. Five of 14 respiratory specimens were positive by PCR for HMPV. Eight residents developed pneumonia, and 2 were hospitalized; no deaths.
	Omura et al,[98] 2011	Sept–Oct, 2009	Japan	Twenty-seven of 99 residents became symptomatic. RT-PCR detected HMPV detected from 9 of 9 throat swabs collected.
	Te Wierik et al,[99] 2012	Jan–March, 2010	The Netherlands	Five of 18 clinical cases tested positive for HMPV by RT-PCR. A 5% attack-rate for laboratory-confirmed cases, 13% for clinical cases. Three deaths; at least 1 believed to be owing to HMPV infection.
	Liao et al,[24] 2012	Spring–Summer, 2011	Oregon	Sixteen of 44 residents met case definition of severe respiratory tract infection. Six of 10 nasopharyngeal swab specimens from case patients were positive for HMPV; 5 diagnosed with pneumonia, 4 hospitalized, and 2 died.
	Ibrahim et al,[25] 2013	Dec, 2011–Feb, 2012	West Virginia and Idaho	Among 57 cases of respiratory illness from 2 facilities (28 of 83 residents in West Virginia, 29 of 80 residents in Idaho), 45 (79%) patients had lower respiratory tract infections. Of these, 25 (56%) had pneumonia, 5 (9%) had upper respiratory tract infection, and 6 patients (11%) died.

	Study	Date	Location	Description
HPIV	Glasgow et al,[36] 1995	May, 1993	Ontario, Canada	Twenty-six (6 definite, 2 probable, and 18 suspected) of total 84 residents had respiratory symptoms. Six of 10 paired sera obtained from ill residents showed a 4-fold or greater increase to HPIV type 3. One resident had pneumonia; 1 was hospitalized. No deaths.
	Faulks et al,[37] 2000	Sept, 1999	Wisconsin	Of 49, 25 residents developed new respiratory symptoms. Of 18 who had chest film, 11 showed new infiltrates. Three residents were hospitalized; 4 died. Four of 10 viral cultures were positive with HPIV type 3.
	Ryan et al,[39] 2017	Jan, 2016	Australia	Eleven residents presented with respiratory symptoms in a 30-bed residential aged care facilities. Nine of 10 nasopharyngeal swabs were positive with HPIV type 3 by PCR; 2 residents were hospitalized. No deaths.
Rhinovirus (HRV)	Wald et al,[49] 1995	Aug–Sept, 1993	Wisconsin	One hundred twenty-eight residents developed a new respiratory illness. Throat and nasopharyngeal virus cultures of 67 ill residents yielded 33 culture-positive with rhinovirus. One resident died owing to respiratory failure.
	Louie et al,[48] 2005	June–July, 2003	California	In a 99-bed facility, 56 residents and 26 staff developed a respiratory illness. Twelve residents died. Seven of 13 respiratory specimens were culture positive for rhinovirus.
	Hicks et al,[47] 2006	July–Aug, 2002 (A); July–Sept, 2003 (B)	Pennsylvania	In nursing home A, 40 of 170 residents (24%) had a respiratory illness; 4 of 10 specimens from symptomatic patients tested positive for rhinovirus. In nursing home B, 77 of 124 residents (62%) had a respiratory illness; 6 of 19 respiratory specimens from symptomatic patients tested positive for rhinovirus. Five of 10 (50%) rhinovirus-positive cases in both facilities showed clinical and radiographic evidence of pneumonia. There were 7 deaths from both facilities.
	Longtin et al,[50] 2010	July, 2009	Ontario, Canada	Thirty-two of 60 (53%) residents and 21 of 100 (21%) staff developed respiratory symptoms. HRV was identified in 5 of 14 nasopharyngeal swabs from symptomatic residents; no other pathogens were detected. Seven deaths occurred during the outbreak (6 owing to pneumonia or respiratory infection and 1 owing to failure to thrive).
	Mubareka et al,[100] 2013	Aug–Oct, 2012	Canada	Of 71 residents screened, 56 were positive for an HRV during an outbreak that lasted 5.5 wk. 3 different rhinovirus genotypes were identified suggesting presence of cocirculation of multiple genotypes during a large outbreak.

(continued on next page)

Table 1
(continued)

Virus	Reference	Date of Outbreak	Location	Description
Human Coronavirus (HCoV)	Birch et al,[58] 2005	Aug-Sept, 2002	Melbourne, Australia	Outbreaks of influenza-like illness occurred in 3 geographically distinct aged-care facilities. HCoV-OC43 RNA was detected in 16 of 27 nasopharyngeal swabs obtained from the 92 symptomatic residents; no other viruses isolated.
	Patrick et al,[59] 2006	Jul-Aug, 2003	British Columbia, Canada	Ninety-five of 142 residents (67%) and 53 of 160 staff members (33%) experienced symptoms of respiratory infection. Eight residents died. Initially misdiagnosed as SARS-CoV owing to antibody cross-reactivity. Subsequently, diagnosis corrected as HCoV-OC43 by RT-PCR.
Adenovirus	Kandel et al,[64] 2010	April-May, 2006	Massachusetts	Twelve of 40 residents had acute respiratory disease (4 confirmed, 8 suspected cases). Three positive cultures for HAdV type 4. Deaths in 3 of 4 confirmed cases and 1 of 4 suspected cases.

Abbreviations: HAdV, human adenovirus; HCoV, human coronaviruses; HMPV, human metapneumovirus; HPIV, human parainfluenza virus; RSV, respiratory syncytial virus; RT-PCR, reverse transcriptase polymerase chain reaction; SARS-CoV, severe acute respiratory syndrome coronavirus.

Table 2
Taxonomy of noninfluenza respiratory viruses

Virus	Family	Genome	Subtypes	Seasonality[a]
Respiratory syncytial virus	Paramyxoviridae	Single-stranded negative sense RNA	A, B	Fall through Spring
Human metapneumovirus	Paramyxoviridae	Single-stranded negative sense RNA	A, B	Winter through Spring
Parainfluenza virus	Paramyxoviridae	Single-stranded negative sense RNA	HPIV-1, HPIV-2, HPIV-3, HPIV-4	Spring through Winter
Rhinovirus	Picornaviridae	Single-stranded positive sense RNA	More than 100 serotypes	Fall through Spring
Coronavirus	Coronaviridae	Single-stranded positive sense RNA	HCoV-229E, HCoV-NL63, HCoV-OC43, HCoV-HKU1, SARS-CoV[b] MERS-CoV[b]	Fall through Spring
Adenovirus	Adenoviridae	Double-stranded DNA	More than 50 serotypes; Major groups A-G	Winter through Spring

Abbreviations: HCoV, human coronaviruses; HPIV, human parainfluenza virus; MERS-CoV, Middle East respiratory syndrome coronavirus; SARS-CoV, severe acute respiratory syndrome coronavirus.
[a] Based on temperate climates.
[b] SARS-CoV and MERS-CoV are outside of the scope of this review.

The rates of RSV infections and death parallel that of influenza among LTCF residents as well. An LTCF in California reported a 6-week outbreak of RSV in 1979 with an attack rate of 40% and a case fatality rate of 20%.[10] Among 381 nursing homes in Tennessee, during 4 consecutive years (1995–1999), RSV contributed to an average of 15 hospitalizations, 76 antibiotic courses, and 17 deaths per 1000 persons each year.[11] In comparison, influenza caused an average of 28 hospitalizations, 147 antibiotic courses, and 15 deaths per 1000 persons each year. In 2008, active surveillance for symptomatic and asymptomatic respiratory viral infections detected an RSV outbreak in a 56-room, 120-bed LTCF in North Carolina.[12] Among 52 residents, 22 (42%) developed respiratory tract infections and, of those, 7 (32%) had an RSV infection confirmed using reverse transcriptase polymerase chain reaction (RT-PCR). One resident required hospitalization and subsequently died. This study in particular is notable for using RT-PCR to support timely and accurate recognition of an RSV outbreak. Although active surveillance for RSV may be useful in early diagnosis and, therefore, in outbreak prevention, the expense and resource use involved may render them impractical for most LTCFs.

Clinical Disease

As with influenza, the spectrum of clinical disease caused by RSV infections is diverse and heterogeneous (**Table 3**). Younger adults may be reinfected every 5 to 7 years, and may manifest symptoms of a mild cold or sinus infection or remain asymptomatic. In older adults, RSV may cause self-limiting upper respiratory tract infections, pharyngitis, rhinosinusitis, pneumonia, respiratory failure, and death. Unfortunately, clinical manifestations do not permit identification of specific viral pathogens, including RSV.[5,13] In a prospective study, Walsh and colleagues[13] assessed the clinical characteristics of older adults living in the community or retirement homes who were admitted to the hospital with an acute respiratory illness. Using culture, RT-PCR, serologic analysis, or a combination of these tests, they identified 132 patients with RSV infection and 144 with influenza A virus. They reported that RSV, compared with influenza A, was more commonly associated with nasal congestion (68% vs 55%; $P = .03$), lower temperature at admission (37.7°C vs 38.1°C; $P = .004$) and wheezing by history (73% vs 53%; $P = .002$) or on physical examination (82% vs 68%; $P = .02$). Although these factors were independent predictors for RSV infection persons, none were sufficiently sensitive or specific to accurately discriminate between illnesses caused by RSV versus influenza.

Among RSV-infected adults, disease severity correlates with increased levels of interleukin-6 (IL-6) and viral shedding. IL-6 is a proinflammatory cytokine associated with physical function decline and chronic disease.[14] A study of RSV-infected adults showed that hospitalized patients, compared with outpatients, had greater nasal IL-6 levels and shed RSV longer (13.1 ± 6.3 days vs 9.8 ± 4.8 days, respectively).[15] Furthermore, hospitalized adults who required mechanical ventilation for RSV-related respiratory failure manifested higher peak RSV viral loads compared with those who did not ($\log_{10}$ 3.7 ± 1.7 PFUs/mL vs $\log_{10}$ 2.4 ± 1.1 PFUs/mL, respectively; $P = .02$).[16] Similarly, among adults hospitalized with PCR-confirmed RSV infections (n = 123; age 78 ± 15 years), increasing concentrations of viral RNA were associated with respiratory insufficiency and risk of complications (adjusted odds ratio 1.40 per increase in $\log_{10}$ copies/mL, 95% CI, 1.03–1.90; $P = .034$).[17] Together, these studies indicate that high RSV viral loads correlate with disease severity.

Age-related immune senescence may increase older adults' risk for developing RSV infection and for subsequent hospital admission. Older adults with lower serum RSV neutralizing antibodies are more likely to become infected with RSV and to require

Table 3
Frequency of clinical manifestation of noninfluenza respiratory viral infections among older adults[a]

	Fever	Headache	Nasal Congestion	Dyspnea	Wheezing	Cough	Sputum	Sore Throat	Myalgia	Fatigue	Hoarseness	Chest Pain
Influenza	+++	++++	+++	+++	++++	++	++++	++	++	+++	+++	++
Respiratory syncytial virus	++	+++	+++	+++	+++	+++	++++	++	++	++	+++	+
Human metapneumovirus	++	++	++	++++	+++	++	++++	++	++	++	+++	++
Parainfluenza virus	−	++	−	++	++	++	++	−	+	−	−	++
Rhinovirus	+	++	++	++	++	++	+++	++	+++	+	+++	++
Coronavirus	++	++	+++	+++	++	−	+++	−	++	++	++	−

[a] Adenovirus is excluded owing to the limited number of reports.

Frequencies are shown with symbols; + = 0%–25%, ++ = 26%–50%, +++ = 51%–75%, ++++ = 76%–100%; − = Frequency unknown owing to insufficient data.

Data from Refs.[4,5,13,26,27,36,44–47,101–106]

hospital admission. A prospective study of adults enrolled in day care programs compared serum anti-RSV antibody titers between an infected subgroup (n = 22) and controls matched for age, exposure, and recent respiratory illness.[18] The mean titers of neutralizing antibodies against RSV were significantly lower in RSV-infected patients compared with controls for both group A (12.4 ± 2.2 vs 14.2 ± 2.2, P = .008, respectively) and group B virus (9.1 ± 2.1, vs 10.3 ± 1.5, P = .01, respectively). A similar study evaluated antibody titers among a prospective cohort of adults with RSV infection (n = 130), 61 of whom were hospitalized for RSV.[19] Multivariate analysis showed an increased risk for hospitalization (odds ratio, 5.89; 95% CI, 1.69–20.57; P = .04) among adults with low serum anti-RSV antibody levels, defined as less than a 1:100 dilution.

After infection, RSV-specific antibodies provide some protection from reinfection, but levels usually decrease within months. A study evaluating 20 adults reported an 8-fold increase in RSV antibody titers after RSV infection. Within 1 year, however, the RSV antibody titers decreased by at least 4-fold in 15 of the adults studied (75%).[20] Because immunity is not complete after preceding infections, reinfection can occur throughout life.[21]

HUMAN METAPNEUMOVIRUS

HMPV, first described in 2001, is a common cause of respiratory infections among all age groups and circulates from winter through spring in temperate climates. Like RSV, HMPV is a member of the Paramyxoviridae family and is divided into genotypes A and B, each of which includes subtypes. Given the variety of genotypes, a seasonal shift of predominant genotype can occur each year, similar to influenza virus.[22]

Epidemiology

A prospective study in Tennessee found similar rates of infection by HMPV and influenza among hospitalized adults.[4] Over 3 consecutive winters, Widmer and colleagues[4] enrolled 508 individuals 50 years and older, more than 90% of whom lived in the community, who were hospitalized with respiratory symptoms or nonlocalizing fever. RT-PCR testing on nasal swabs detected HMPV in 4.5% (23/508) and influenza virus in 6.5% (33/508) of hospitalized individuals. Patients with HMPV, compared with those with laboratory-confirmed influenza, were older (median age, 76.2 vs 60.0), had more cardiovascular disease (78.3% vs 51.5%), and were more likely to have received the influenza vaccination (87.0% vs 51.5%). Notably, they were also less likely to report a fever (51.2% vs 87.9%).

Several reports describe notable morbidity and mortality associated with HMPV outbreaks in LTCF residents. In 2006, 27% of residents (96/364) at an LTCF in Quebec City, Canada, presented with respiratory or constitutional symptoms.[23] Of 13 samples obtained by nasopharyngeal swab or nasopharyngeal aspirate, real-time multiplex RT-PCR detected HMPV in 6 residents. The fatality rate was 50% (3 of 6 patients) among confirmed HMPV cases. In 2011, 36% of residents (16/44) at an LTCF in Oregon met the case definition of severe respiratory tract infection and, of those, 5 had pneumonia, 4 were hospitalized, and 2 died. Six of 10 nasopharyngeal swab specimens collected from the 16 afflicted residents tested positive for HMPV.[24] Similarly, in the winter of 2011 to 2012, 2 skilled nursing facilities in Idaho and Washington also experienced HMPV outbreaks.[25] Among the residents with lower respiratory tract infections, 56% (25/45) had pneumonia, and 11% (6/45) died. For 3 of the HMPV outbreaks described, the outbreak investigation queried about the staff caring for the residents and found that some of them also experienced symptoms of acute respiratory illness.

Clinical Disease

The clinical manifestations of HMPV infection in adults, similar to those in children, are nonspecific upper respiratory symptoms including cough and nasal congestion, although asymptomatic infection is common.[26–28]

Several prospective studies assessed the symptoms manifested by older adults. Older adults developed dyspnea and wheezing more frequently than younger adults,[26] although these symptoms are not specific to HMPV.[4] Compared with influenza, however, fever is reported less frequently (51.2% vs 87.9%).[4] In a prospective study of adults hospitalized for community-acquired pneumonia, Johnstone and colleagues[29] used RT-PCR on nasopharyngeal swabs to detect HMPV in 4% of cases (8/193) during influenza season; concomitant blood, sputum, and assays for other virus and atypical bacterial pathogens were negative. Specific risk factors for HMPV infection for older adults and residents of LTCF are not yet known.

PARAINFLUENZA VIRUS

Human parainfluenza virus (HPIV), a single-stranded negative sense RNA virus, is yet another member of the Paramyxoviridae family. First detected in the 1950s, this virus has 4 major serotypes, HPIV-1, HPIV-2, HPIV-3, and HPIV-4.[30] Parainfluenza virus generally circulates from spring through winter, with different seasonality and peaks depending on serotypes.[31] In children, HPIV-1 and HPIV-2 cause croup and HPIV-3, the most prevalent serotype, is associated with bronchiolitis and pneumonia.

Epidemiology

Two reports describing large, population-based studies detail the morbidity and mortality of HPIV in older adults. Between 1976 and 1982, the Communicable Disease Surveillance Center in the United Kingdom received 5781 laboratory reports of HPIV infection.[32] Although just 2% of positive HPIV samples (121/5781) came from older adults, 46% (56/121) of those individuals had pneumonia or other lower respiratory tract infection. A population-based study of adults aged 65 or older in the Netherlands estimated the numbers of deaths attributable to HPIV between 1999 and 2007. The authors reported lower rates of mortality caused by HPIV (0.9%) compared with influenza A (1.5%) or RSV (1.4%).[33]

Several reports describe HPIV outbreaks in LTCFs, most owing to HPIV-3.[32,34,35] In 1993, 30% of residents (26/84) and 6% of staff (5/78) at an LTCF in Ontario, Canada, developed respiratory tract infections.[36] Paired sera from 6 of 10 ill residents showed a 4-fold or greater increase in antibodies to HPIV-3. One resident was hospitalized, although none died. In 1999, 51% of residents (25/49) at a 50-bed skilled nursing unit at a Wisconsin Veterans Home developed new respiratory symptoms.[37] Viral cultures from 4 of 10 residents tested grew HPIV-3. Because viral cultures are typically less sensitive than PCR-based detection methods, this likely underestimated the true prevalence of HPIV-3.[38] Three residents required hospitalization and 4 died. In 2016, 11 residents presented with respiratory symptoms in a 30-bed residential aged care facility in Australia. Nine of 10 nasopharyngeal swabs tested positive for HPIV-3 by PCR. Two residents were hospitalized and none died.[39] These outbreaks indicate that compared with RSV and HMPV, HPIV outbreaks in LTCF have similar rates of attack and morbidity.

Clinical Disease

In healthy immunocompetent adults, HPIV infections are usually asymptomatic or cause mild respiratory symptoms indistinguishable from other common respiratory viruses.[30] A prospective study of the etiology of community-acquired pneumonia among adults in the Netherlands identified HPIV in 6% of cases.[40] Reported in 1998, an investigation of an outbreak of lobar pneumonia at a 70-bed LTCF in Massachusetts suggests a possible association between *S pneumoniae* pneumonia and preceding HPIV infection.[35] Over 10 days, 10 residents developed lobar pneumonia; 9 had serum available. The study used 18 matched controls. Of those, 5 had both serologic evidence of recent HPIV-1 infection and upper respiratory infection symptoms in the preceding month, compared with 2 of 18 controls (matched odds ratio, 9.0; 95% CI, 1.2–208). Ultimately, 2 of the 10 residents with pneumonia died; both of them had evidence of *S pneumoniae* infection. The authors note that only 3 of the 67 residents had documentation of pneumococcal vaccination. After identification of the eighth case of pneumonia, all nursing home residents received influenza and pneumococcal vaccines.

RHINOVIRUS

A single-stranded, positive-sense RNA virus, the human rhinovirus (HRV) accounts for 30% to 50% of common colds each year.[41] There are more than 100 serotypes of HRV, which is divided into 3 genotypes, A, B, and C; the severity of illness does not seem to be associated with a particular genotype.[42] In temperate climates, HRV circulates year round and are more likely to cause illness in the warmer months; infections caused by influenza and RSV predominate in the winter months.[41] HRV causes respiratory infections in every age group, and recurrent infection can occur throughout life.[43]

Epidemiology

Rhinovirus infection is one of the most common noninfluenza respiratory viruses in older adults. A prospective study in the Netherlands evaluated community-dwelling older adults with acute respiratory symptoms for viral infections.[44] PCR on nasopharyngeal swabs or serology detected rhinovirus in 32% of cases (34/107), followed by coronavirus 17% (18/107) and influenza A 5% (5/107). Among symptom-free controls, these rates were 2% (2/91), 2% (2/91), and 0% (0/91), respectively. A similar prospective surveillance study in England found similar results with rhinovirus identified in 24% of respiratory infections (121/497) in adults aged 60 to 90 years.[45] Coronavirus (12%; 59/497) and influenza A or B (3%; 17/497) were the next most common pathogens. Multiple logistic regression analysis showed that current smoking (odds ratio, 1.47; 95% CI, 1.14–1.90) and chronic medical conditions (odds ratio, 1.40; 95% CI, 1.17–1.68) were independently associated with lower respiratory complications. Chronic medical conditions included regular treatment for heart disease, respiratory illness, or another high-risk condition designated by the Department of Health. Similarly, a prospective study in Italy assessed people over 65 years of age who presented to the emergency department with a fever and a respiratory illness in February and March of 2009 and 2010.[46] PCR performed on nasopharyngeal washes detected HRV in 16% of samples (17/103) in 2009 and 8% (11/135) in 2010. In comparison, influenza A was more prevalent than HRV in 2009 (24%, 25/103) and absent in 2010, likely because the pandemic H1N1 influenza circulated through the region in October through December 2009.

HRV is a frequent cause of outbreaks in LTCFs that are notable for high attack rates and mortality.[47–49] From July through December 2009, 269 LTCFs in Ontario, Canada, reported 297 respiratory outbreaks; all LTCFs submitted samples to the Ontario Public Health Laboratory.[50] Molecular-based methods implicated HRV as the cause of 59% of the outbreaks (174/297). The next most prevalent virus was influenza A, which cased 7.0% of the outbreaks (22/297).

In the summers of 2002 and 2003, two nursing homes in Pennsylvania reported severe respiratory disease outbreaks associated with HRV.[47] In facilities A and B, 24% (40/170) and 62% of residents (77/124) experienced a respiratory illness. Specimens collected from symptomatic residents at facility A and B tested positive for HRV in 4 of 10 and 6 of 19 samples, respectively. Of the 10 rhinovirus-positive cases, 5 residents had clinical and radiographic evidence of pneumonia. Between the 2 facilities, a total of 7 residents died of severe respiratory illness concurrent with the HRV. In June 2003, a 99-bed LTCF in California experienced a similar outbreak.[48] Notably, 21% of the residents (12/56) died, possibly owing to a secondary bacterial infection. Of 13 respiratory specimens collected, 7 (54%) were culture positive for rhinovirus. Furthermore, 2 of 3 sputum cultures grew nontypeable *Haemophilus influenza.* The high attack rate associated with HRV may render large numbers of residents vulnerable to secondary bacterial infection, ultimately resulting in both morbidity and mortality from a virus regarded as a cause of the common cold.

Clinical Disease

Usually regarded as a pathogen with low virulence, HRV may cause asymptomatic infection among younger adults.[51] Asymptomatic infection is less common in older adults. In addition to the common cold symptoms such as rhinorrhea, cough, and sore throat, HRV infection may cause asthma exacerbations in children and younger adults and, as discussed, may cause or predispose LTCF residents to bacterial pneumonia.[52,53]

HUMAN CORONAVIRUS

First described in 1965, human coronaviruses (HCoV) also cause common colds among all age groups, with infections occurring more often in winter and spring compared with summer and fall.[54] The Coronaviridae family, composed of single-stranded positive-sense RNA viruses, also includes severe acute respiratory syndrome coronavirus and Middle East respiratory syndrome coronavirus, both of which are beyond the scope of this review. Strains HCoV-229E and HCoV-OC43 seem to be most frequently associated with human respiratory diseases.

Epidemiology

HCoV causes upper respiratory infections in elderly people living in the community. Two prospective studies in Rochester, New York, and England used a 4-fold increase in antibody titers between the acute and convalescent phase to indicate infection[55,56] They found evidence for infection with HCoV-229E in 51% (31/61) and HCoV-229E or HCoV-OC43 in 30% (69/231), respectively, of community-dwelling older adults with acute respiratory illnesses.

Although HCoV is also one of the most common respiratory viruses in LTCFs to our knowledge, only 2 reports describe HCoV outbreaks in LTCFs.[57] Birch and colleagues[58] reported outbreaks of respiratory disease and influenza-like illness in August and September 2002 among 3 geographically distinct LTCFs in Melbourne, Australia. From 92 symptomatic residents at the 3 institutions, staff obtained 27 nasopharyngeal swabs. PCR-based tested detected HCoV-OC43 RNA in 59% of the specimens (16/27); no other viruses were isolated. Additionally, among 85 staff members,

37 developed respiratory symptoms, indicating an attack rate of 44%. Not surprisingly, epidemiologic investigations determined that LTCF staff members were the index case in 2 of the 3 LTCFs. The second report also describes an outbreak of HCoV-OC43. In the summer of 2003, an LTCF in British Columbia, Canada, reported that 67% of their residents (95/142) and 33% of their staff members (53/160) developed respiratory infections.[59] Eight residents died. Interestingly, the outbreak was initially attributed to severe acute respiratory syndrome coronavirus owing to cross-reactivity to antibodies against nucleocapsid proteins from both viruses. Subsequently, RT-PCR confirmed HCoV-OC43. Together, these 2 outbreaks suggest that HCoV-OC43 represents a virulent pathogen for older adults in LTCFs. Additionally, they also highlight the role that ill health care workers may have in transmitting illnesses to LCTF residents.

Clinical Disease

Similar to HMPV, HPIV, and HRV, HCoV infections often manifest as common colds without specific or defining characteristics. A large, prospective, cohort study by Walsh and colleagues[60] details clinical features of HCoV infection in adults. In Rochester, New York, adults who developed an acute respiratory illness in the winter months from 1999 to 2003 underwent surveillance with RT-PCR and serologic studies. The adults included 4 cohorts: healthy older adults (n = 611; age 75 $\pm$ 6 years), high-risk adults with underlying cardiopulmonary disease (n = 511; age 70 $\pm$ 11 years), healthy young adults (n = 291; age 33 $\pm$ 5 years), and a hospitalized group (n = 1388; age 75 $\pm$ 12 years). During the study period, testing identified 398 HCoV infections from all cohorts, 214 of which (54%) were symptomatic. Of those, 10% (21/214) of them had evidence of viral coinfection. Manifestations of HCoV infection among prospective cohorts excluding the hospitalized group were congestion (98%–100%), constitutional symptoms (53%–74%), and cough (40%–79%). Fever was not common; the mean temperature ranged 36.4°C to 36.8°C. Asymptomatic infection, defined as a 4-fold or greater increase in HCoV-specific serum IgG in the absence of respiratory symptoms, was common, ranging from 33% to 44% in prospective cohorts. Among 71 HCoV infections in the hospitalized group, 23 (32.3%) had infiltrate on chest radiography and 3 (4.2%) died. Although capable of causing acute exacerbations of chronic obstructive pulmonary disease or community-acquired pneumonia, most HCoV infections seem to be less severe than those caused by RSV, HMPV, and PIV.[61,62]

ADENOVIRUS

Human adenoviruses (HAdV), members of family Adenoviridae, was first isolated from human adenoid tissue in 1953. These double-stranded DNA viruses, of which there are now more than 50 serotypes identified, cause a variety of illnesses, most commonly respiratory infections, conjunctivitis, and gastroenteritis.[63]

Epidemiology

Only limited descriptions specifically focus on HAdV infection in older adults, Kandel and colleagues[64] reported an outbreak of HAdV type 4 among residents of an LTCF in Boston, Massachusetts, in April and May 2006. Acute respiratory infections developed in 30% of residents (12/40), and 4 of those 12 died. Nasopharyngeal aspirates from 7 specimens initially tested negative using a rapid antigen test. PCR-based testing subsequently confirmed HAdV type 4 in 3 of the 7 tests, highlighting the low sensitivity of the rapid test.

Clinical Disease

Although most people recover without complications, infection by some HAdV serotypes may cause severe pneumonia and significant morbidity and mortality, even among immunocompetent young adults.[62,65–69] From a population health perspective, however, HAdV is perhaps a less important pathogen in older adults compared with influenza and the other respiratory viruses described.

DIAGNOSTIC TESTING

A wide range of diagnostic tests may identify the cause of viral respiratory infections. Serologic testing compares acute and convalescent specimens collected weeks apart. Although useful for epidemiologic research, serologic testing is not practical for clinical care. Rapid antigen tests have an advantage of quick results, but are limited in their usefulness owing to poor sensitivity and specificity. When clinical suspicion of a disease is high, negative tests should be confirmed with another testing method.[70] Viral cultures are neither sensitive nor timely in their outcomes, rendering these unhelpful in clinical practice. Some laboratories may offer enzyme immunoassay testing. For most respiratory viruses, these also lack sensitivity.[38]

The US Food and Drug Administration has approved several nucleic acid amplification tests for clinical use, with tests for influenza representing the most commonly used single virus assay. Multiplex panels use PCR to test for several respiratory viruses at once, a practical strategy because clinical manifestations do not permit the identification of specific viral pathogens. The number of respiratory viruses tested, sensitivity, and specificity in detection of each virus are different depending on which multiplex PCR test is used.[71] Other than for influenza, the lack of effective antiviral medications combined with the costs associated with nucleic acid amplification test make routine use of these studies impractical for most clinical settings. A potential benefit to more routine use of nucleic acid amplification tests for acute respiratory infections, however, may be the early detection of viral outbreaks in LTCFs through active surveillance, which may confer further benefits by reducing unnecessary antibiotic use.[12] The Infectious Diseases Society of America endorsed this approach in their 2008 clinical practice guidelines addressing fever and infection in LTCF residents.[72] Finally, identification of viral pathogens among older adults with community-acquired pneumonia may support decisions to stop antibiotics and thus support antibiotic stewardship practices.[73]

PREVENTION AND MANAGEMENT

As demonstrated for influenza, vaccines are a safe and at least partially effective approach to preventing illness caused by respiratory viral pathogens. Although a detailed discussion of vaccines is beyond the scope of this article, of the pathogens discussed, RSV is a high priority for vaccine development, although none are yet available for clinical use. In the meantime, the most effective prevention measures include the use of transmission-based precautions, including hand hygiene and social distancing, as part of broader infection prevention and control activities.

Infection Prevention and Control

The prevalence and sheer number of respiratory viral pathogens means that, despite our best efforts, most adults will have 2 to 3 viral infections each year.[74] Understanding the transmission of respiratory viruses informs the foundation for infection prevention and control. We focus here on applying these principles to residents of LTCFs.[75]

Transmission

People may become infected with respiratory viruses through direct contact (person to person), indirect contact (via fomites), and droplets containing respiratory secretions. Direct physical contact with an infected person is the most common, efficient, and important form of noninfluenza respiratory virus transmission.[76] Indirect contact occurs via exposure to viable viral particles on fomites contaminated by infected individuals. Finally, susceptible individuals may breathe in droplets of respiratory secretions from an infected person who sneezes or coughs. The CDC defines droplets as respiratory secretions larger than 5 μm and advises using a surgical mask to prevent exposure.[77] Gralton and colleagues[78] evaluated the size of particles produced by 12 adults and 41 children with symptomatic respiratory infections. They reported that with breathing or coughing, 80% of the participants produced airborne particles less than 5 μm in diameter that contained viral RNA. These findings, and those of other investigators,[79,80] support consideration of airborne precautions for outbreaks with severe respiratory viral illnesses, including influenza. However, association with clinical outcomes is still lacking. In addition, airborne precautions are not possible outside of hospital settings and thus are not currently recommended.

Hand hygiene

Hand hygiene remains the most important measure to prevent infections in health care settings. Just as in acute care, health care workers in LTCFs demonstrate deficiencies in their hand hygiene practice[81,82] and alcohol-based hand rub improves adherence.[83] Schweon and colleagues[84] described a comprehensive hand hygiene program involving alcohol-based hand rub use by both health care workers and residents at an LTCF in Pennsylvania. Lower respiratory tract infections decreased among the residents. Although the outcomes did not differentiate between viral and bacterial infections, they clearly support the important role of basic hand hygiene practices to prevention infections.

Isolation precautions

In 2007, the CDC last updated guidelines for isolation precautions in health care setting including LTCFs.[77] In general, they recommend droplet precautions in addition to standard precautions during the care of individuals with a possible respiratory viral infection. Notably, they call for the use of personal protective equipment, including gowns, gloves, and a mask, for entry into rooms of people on droplet precautions. They also introduced respiratory hygiene and cough etiquette, asking symptomatic people to cover their mouth and nose when sneezing or coughing, to use tissues and dispose of them in no-touch receptacles, to perform hand hygiene after soiling of hands with respiratory secretions, and to wear a surgical mask if tolerated or maintain spatial separation of at least 3 feet when possible. Although not specifically mentioned in the 2007 CDC guidelines, social distancing also reduces the risk of respiratory virus transmission. Social distancing includes avoiding people who are sick, canceling group activities, and staying home from work when ill. This approach is readily implemented in long-term care and other communal settings.

Work restriction of health care personnel

Guidelines addressing infection control among health care personnel recognize that staff may transmit respiratory viral infections to others and indicate that people with acute viral respiratory infections should not care for high-risk individuals, particularly during community outbreaks of influenza and RSV.[85] The same document also acknowledges that restriction of infected health care personnel from all patient care duties may not be possible because large numbers of personnel may have viral respiratory illnesses during the winter. A prospective study of health care workers at a tertiary care children's hospital detected respiratory virus in 16.7% of nasal swabs collected from asymptomatic individuals during influenza season (November through April).[86] Perhaps of greater concern was that 46% of the subjects reported working while ill with an influenza-like illness. Although these findings may be representative of people working in long-term care, several of the descriptions of noninfluenza viral outbreaks in LTCFs suggest strong parallels. Accordingly, employers might consider strategies to help health care workers with respiratory illnesses minimize their contact with LTCF residents as part of resident safety. When this is not possible, cohorting sick staff and residents may help augment infection control efforts.[87]

Treatment

Unlike influenza, which may be treated with specific and effective antiviral agents, supportive care remains the mainstay of management for older adults with respiratory illnesses caused by the viruses discussed. Supportive care is an active process that includes frequent monitoring until the patient's clinical status improves.[88] Additional features of supportive care for people with respiratory viral infections include hydration, treatment of fever with acetaminophen, albuterol, supplemental oxygen, and perhaps nebulized saline.

Viral infections may precede or occur concurrently with bacterial pneumonia. When concomitant or secondary bacterial lower respiratory infection is suspected in patients with respiratory viral infection, empirical antibiotics should be used. Falsey and colleagues[89] investigated 771 adults hospitalized with respiratory illness, finding that 348 (41%) had a viral infection and, of those, 136 (39%) had evidence of bacterial coinfection, as assessed using procalcitonin and specific bacterial tests. Ideally, among older adults in whom a viral pneumonia is suspected, procalcitonin results that confirm the absence of a bacterial infection should help clinicians to stop antibiotics. A recent systematic review concluded that using procalcitonin to guide initiation and duration of antibiotic treatment in patients with acute respiratory infections reduced antibiotic consumption and was not associated with higher mortality rates or treatment failure.[90] Procalcitonin is not yet available as a point-of-care test and is, therefore, still relegated primarily for use in research and acute care settings.

Even with the recent introduction of procalcitonin, determining if a patient has a mixed viral-bacterial infection or bacterial superinfection after a viral respiratory illness presents a significant clinical challenge. In adults, typical clinical signs and symptoms suggestive of pneumonia (eg, temperature $\geq 38°C$ or $<35°C$, cough, dyspnea, tachypnea, hypoxia, abnormal percussion or altered breath sounds on auscultation, leukocytosis, or leukopenia) are not sufficient to accurately predict whether community-acquired pneumonia is owing to viral and/or bacterial etiologies.[91] Additional consideration of atypical signs and symptoms of infection common to frail older adults, such as decreased appetite, lethargy, delirium, and age-appropriate definitions of fever only adds to diagnostic uncertainty about pneumonia in general, let along the specific etiology. Molecular testing improves detection for bacterial and viral pathogens, but the implications of test results for clinical care are not yet clear. Gadsby and colleagues[92] collected sputum (96%) and endotracheal aspirates (4%) from 323 adults hospitalized for community-acquired pneumonia. Based on multiplex PCR, they detected viruses in 30% of patients (98/323), with 82% of viruses (80/98) codetected with bacteria. These results suggested potential deescalation of antibiotics in 77% of cases, but the authors did not specifically describe stopping antibiotic therapy.

The minimum criteria developed by Loeb and colleagues[93] for the initiation of antibiotics in residents of LTCFs may offer some guidance to help differentiate between viral and bacterial bronchitis and pneumonia. Developed mainly based on observational studies and expert opinion, the intent of these recommendations is to reduce unnecessary antibiotic use among LTCF residents. For residents with respiratory infections, the Loeb minimum criteria for initiation of antibiotics call for assessment of vital signs (temperature, heart rate, and respiratory rate), symptoms (cough, sputum, and rigors), delirium, and medical history of chronic obstructive pulmonary disease. These criteria do not require blood tests or imaging studies, permitting them to help inform clinical decisions about active monitoring versus initiating antibiotics in resource-limited settings. For settings with more robust resources, diagnostic tests may provide more specific guidance.

SUMMARY

The majority of clinical knowledge about noninfluenza respiratory viruses comes from pediatric studies. As demonstrated, these viral pathogens also have an important influence on the health of older adults. RSV, in particular, causes infections that rival the morbidity and mortality caused by influenza. Outbreaks of any of the viruses discussed, when they occur in LTCFs, also have grave consequences for frail older adults, especially among those with chronic cardiopulmonary diseases. Unlike influenza, effective vaccines and antiviral medications are not yet available, even for RSV. Accordingly, infection prevention and control measures remain the best protection against these pathogens. Hand hygiene is important in all settings; within health care facilities, the use of masks, gowns, and gloves may reduce the risk of infection transmission among health care workers and patients or residents.

Recent advances in rapid molecular diagnostic tests may permit greater recognition of the consequences of respiratory viral infections among older adults. In acute care settings, early recognition of viral infections among hospitalized patients may promote more judicious use of antibiotics. Within LTCFs, routine surveillance using multiplex PCR tests may rapidly identify viral outbreaks and foster swift implementation of infection prevention and control measures. Finally, a better assessment of the overall influence of noninfluenza respiratory pathogens may support innovations leading to effective antiviral therapy and vaccinations with the potential to improve the health of people of all ages.

REFERENCES

1. Heron M. Deaths: leading causes for 2014. Natl Vital Stat Rep 2016;65(5):1–96.
2. Quandelacy TM, Viboud C, Charu V, et al. Age- and sex-related risk factors for influenza-associated mortality in the United States between 1997-2007. Am J Epidemiol 2014;179(2):156–67.
3. Reed C, Kim IK, Singleton JA, et al. Estimated influenza illnesses and hospitalizations averted by vaccination–United States, 2013-14 influenza season. MMWR Morb Mortal Wkly Rep 2014;63(49):1151–4.
4. Widmer K, Zhu Y, Williams JV, et al. Rates of hospitalizations for respiratory syncytial virus, human metapneumovirus, and influenza virus in older adults. J Infect Dis 2012;206(1):56–62.
5. Falsey AR, McElhaney JE, Beran J, et al. Respiratory syncytial virus and other respiratory viral infections in older adults with moderate to severe influenza-like illness. J Infect Dis 2014;209(12):1873–81.

6. National Respiratory and Enteric Virus Surveillance System (NREVSS). Home. National Respiratory and Enteric Virus Surv System, CDC. Available at: https://www.cdc.gov/surveillance/nrevss/index.html. Accessed January 14, 2017.

7. Blount RE, Morris JA, Savage RE. Recovery of cytopathogenic agent from chimpanzees with coryza. Proc Soc Exp Biol Med 1956;92(3):544–9.

8. Centers for Disease Control and Prevention (CDC). Respiratory syncytial virus activity–United States, July 2011-January 2013. MMWR Morb Mortal Wkly Rep 2013;62(8):141–4.

9. Falsey AR, Hennessey PA, Formica MA, et al. Respiratory syncytial virus infection in elderly and high-risk adults. N Engl J Med 2005;352(17):1749–59.

10. Sorvillo FJ, Huie SF, Strassburg MA, et al. An outbreak of respiratory syncytial virus pneumonia in a nursing home for the elderly. J Infect 1984;9(3):252–6.

11. Ellis SE, Coffey CS, Mitchel EF, et al. Influenza– and respiratory syncytial virus–associated morbidity and mortality in the nursing home population. J Am Geriatr Soc 2003;51(6):761–7.

12. Caram LB, Chen J, Taggart EW, et al. Respiratory syncytial virus outbreak in a long-term care facility detected using reverse transcriptase polymerase chain reaction: an argument for real-time detection methods. J Am Geriatr Soc 2009;57(3):482–5.

13. Walsh EE, Peterson DR, Falsey AR. Is clinical recognition of respiratory syncytial virus infection in hospitalized elderly and high-risk adults possible? J Infect Dis 2007;195(7):1046–51.

14. Maggio M, Guralnik JM, Longo DL, et al. Interleukin-6 in aging and chronic disease: a magnificent pathway. J Gerontol A Biol Sci Med Sci 2006;61(6):575–84.

15. Walsh EE, Peterson DR, Kalkanoglu AE, et al. Viral shedding and immune responses to respiratory syncytial virus infection in older adults. J Infect Dis 2013;207(9):1424–32.

16. Duncan CB, Walsh EE, Peterson DR, et al. Risk factors for respiratory failure associated with respiratory syncytial virus infection in adults. J Infect Dis 2009;200(8):1242–6.

17. Lee N, Chan MCW, Lui GCY, et al. High viral load and respiratory failure in adults hospitalized for respiratory syncytial virus infections. J Infect Dis 2015;212(8): 1237–40.

18. Falsey AR, Walsh EE. Relationship of serum antibody to risk of respiratory syncytial virus infection in elderly adults. J Infect Dis 1998;177(2):463–6.

19. Walsh EE, Peterson DR, Falsey AR. Risk factors for severe respiratory syncytial virus infection in elderly persons. J Infect Dis 2004;189(2):233–8.

20. Falsey AR, Singh HK, Walsh EE. Serum antibody decay in adults following natural respiratory syncytial virus infection. J Med Virol 2006;78(11):1493–7.

21. Hall CB, Walsh EE, Long CE, et al. Immunity to and frequency of reinfection with respiratory syncytial virus. J Infect Dis 1991;163(4):693–8.

22. Agapov E, Sumino KC, Gaudreault-Keener M, et al. Genetic variability of human metapneumovirus infection: evidence of a shift in viral genotype without a change in illness. J Infect Dis 2006;193(3):396–403.

23. Boivin G, Serres GD, Hamelin ME, et al. An outbreak of severe respiratory tract infection due to human metapneumovirus in a long-term care facility. Clin Infect Dis 2007;44(9):1152–8.

24. Liao RS, Appelgate DM, Pelz RK. An outbreak of severe respiratory tract infection due to human metapneumovirus in a long-term care facility for the elderly in Oregon. J Clin Virol 2012;53(2):171–3.

25. Ibrahim S, Scott M, Bixler D, et al. Outbreaks of human metapneumovirus in two skilled nursing facilities -West Virginia and Idaho, 2011-2012. MMWR Morb Mortal Wkly Rep 2013;62(46):909–13.
26. Falsey AR, Erdman D, Anderson LJ, et al. Human metapneumovirus infections in young and elderly adults. J Infect Dis 2003;187(5):785–90.
27. Walsh EE, Peterson DR, Falsey AR. Another piece of the puzzle: human metapneumovirus infections in adults. Arch Intern Med 2008;168(22):2489–96.
28. Hamada N, Hara K, Matsuo Y, et al. Performance of a rapid human metapneumovirus antigen test during an outbreak in a long-term care facility. Epidemiol Infect 2014;142(2):424–7.
29. Johnstone J, Majumdar SR, Fox JD, et al. Human metapneumovirus pneumonia in adults: results of a prospective study. Clin Infect Dis 2008;46(4):571–4.
30. Henrickson KJ. Parainfluenza viruses. Clin Microbiol Rev 2003;16(2):242–64.
31. Fry AM, Curns AT, Harbour K, et al. Seasonal trends of human parainfluenza viral infections: United States, 1990–2004. Clin Infect Dis 2006;43(8):1016–22.
32. Parainfluenza infections in the elderly 1976-82. Br Med J (Clin Res Ed) 1983; 287(6405):1619.
33. van Asten L, van den Wijngaard C, van Pelt W, et al. Mortality attributable to 9 common infections: significant effect of influenza A, respiratory syncytial virus, influenza B, norovirus, and parainfluenza in elderly persons. J Infect Dis 2012; 206(5):628–39.
34. Yamakoshi M, Suzuki K, Yamamoto T, et al. An outbreak of parainfluenza 3 virus infection in the elderly in a ward. Kansenshogaku Zasshi 1999;73(4):298–304 [in Japanese].
35. Fiore AE, Iverson C, Messmer T, et al. Outbreak of pneumonia in a long-term care facility: antecedent human parainfluenza virus 1 infection may predispose to bacterial pneumonia. J Am Geriatr Soc 1998;46(9):1112–7.
36. Glasgow KW, Tamblyn SE, Blair G. A respiratory outbreak due to parainfluenza virus type 3 in a home for the aged–Ontario. Can Commun Dis Rep 1995;21(7): 57–61.
37. Faulks JT, Pharm R, Drinka PJ, et al. A serious outbreak of parainfluenza type 3 on a nursing unit. J Am Geriatr Soc 2000;48(10):1216–8.
38. Ginocchio CC. Detection of respiratory viruses using non-molecular based methods. J Clin Virol 2007;40(Suppl 1):S11–4.
39. Ryan S, Gillespie E, Stuart RL. A parainfluenza virus type 3 outbreak at a residential aged care facility: the role of microbiologic testing in early identification and antimicrobial stewardship. Am J Infect Control 2017;45(2):203–5.
40. Diederen BMW, van Der Eerden MM, Vlaspolder F, et al. Detection of respiratory viruses and Legionella spp. by real-time polymerase chain reaction in patients with community acquired pneumonia. Scand J Infect Dis 2009;41(1):45–50.
41. Jacobs SE, Lamson DM, George KS, et al. Human rhinoviruses. Clin Microbiol Rev 2013;26(1):135–62.
42. McCulloch DJ, Sears MH, Jacob JT, et al. Severity of rhinovirus infection in hospitalized adults is unrelated to genotype. Am J Clin Pathol 2014;142(2):165–72.
43. Zlateva KT, de Vries JJC, Coenjaerts FEJ, et al. Prolonged shedding of rhinovirus and re-infection in adults with respiratory tract illness. Eur Respir J 2014; 44(1):169–77.
44. Graat JM, Schouten EG, Heijnen M-LA, et al. A prospective, community-based study on virologic assessment among elderly people with and without symptoms of acute respiratory infection. J Clin Epidemiol 2003;56(12):1218–23.

45. Nicholson KG, Kent J, Hammersley V, et al. Risk factors for lower respiratory complications of rhinovirus infections in elderly people living in the community: prospective cohort study. BMJ 1996;313(7065):1119–23.

46. Pierangeli A, Scagnolari C, Selvaggi C, et al. Rhinovirus frequently detected in elderly adults attending an emergency department. J Med Virol 2011;83(11): 2043–7.

47. Hicks LA, Shepard CW, Britz PH, et al. Two outbreaks of severe respiratory disease in nursing homes associated with rhinovirus. J Am Geriatr Soc 2006;54(2): 284–9.

48. Louie JK, Yagi S, Nelson FA, et al. Rhinovirus outbreak in a long term care facility for elderly persons associated with unusually high mortality. Clin Infect Dis 2005; 41(2):262–5.

49. Wald TG, Shult P, Krause P, et al. A rhinovirus outbreak among residents of a long-term care facility. Ann Intern Med 1995;123(8):588–93.

50. Longtin J, Winter AL, Heng D, et al. Severe human rhinovirus outbreak associated with fatalities in a long-term care facility in Ontario, Canada. J Am Geriatr Soc 2010;58(10):2036–8.

51. Peltola V, Waris M, Österback R, et al. Rhinovirus transmission within families with children: incidence of symptomatic and asymptomatic infections. J Infect Dis 2008;197(3):382–9.

52. Teichtahl H, Buckmaster N, Pertnikovs E. The incidence of respiratory tract infection in adults requiring hospitalization for asthma. Chest 1997;112(3): 591–6.

53. Gern JE, Busse WW. Association of rhinovirus infections with asthma. Clin Microbiol Rev 1999;12(1):9–18.

54. Kahn JS, McIntosh K. History and recent advances in coronavirus discovery. Pediatr Infect Dis J 2005;24(11 Suppl):S223–7 [discussion: S226].

55. Falsey AR, McCann RM, Hall WJ, et al. The "common cold" in frail older persons: impact of rhinovirus and coronavirus in a senior daycare center. J Am Geriatr Soc 1997;45(6):706–11.

56. Nicholson KG, Kent J, Hammersley V, et al. Acute viral infections of upper respiratory tract in elderly people living in the community: comparative, prospective, population based study of disease burden. BMJ 1997;315(7115):1060–4.

57. Falsey AR, Dallal GE, Formica MA, et al. Long-term care facilities: a cornucopia of viral pathogens. J Am Geriatr Soc 2008;56(7):1281–5.

58. Birch CJ, Clothier HJ, Seccull A, et al. Human coronavirus OC43 causes influenza-like illness in residents and staff of aged-care facilities in Melbourne, Australia. Epidemiol Infect 2005;133(2):273–7.

59. Patrick DM, Petric M, Skowronski DM, et al. An outbreak of human coronavirus OC43 infection and serological cross-reactivity with SARS coronavirus. Can J Infect Dis Med Microbiol 2006;17(6):330–6.

60. Walsh EE, Shin JH, Falsey AR. Clinical impact of human coronaviruses 229E and OC43 infection in diverse adult populations. J Infect Dis 2013;208(10):1634–42.

61. Ko FWS, Ip M, Chan PKS, et al. Viral etiology of acute exacerbations of COPD in Hong Kong. Chest 2007;132(3):900–8.

62. Johnstone J, Majumdar SR, Fox JD, et al. Viral infection in adults hospitalized with community-acquired pneumonia: prevalence, pathogens, and presentation. Chest 2008;134(6):1141–8.

63. Echavarría M. Adenoviruses in immunocompromised hosts. Clin Microbiol Rev 2008;21(4):704–15.

64. Kandel R, Srinivasan A, D'Agata EMC, et al. Outbreak of adenovirus type 4 infection in a long-term care facility for the elderly. Infect Control Hosp Epidemiol 2010;31(7):755–7.

65. Klinger JR, Sanchez MP, Curtin LA, et al. Multiple cases of life-threatening adenovirus pneumonia in a mental health care center. Am J Respir Crit Care Med 1998;157(2):645–9.

66. Centers for Disease Control and Prevention (CDC). Acute respiratory disease associated with adenovirus serotype 14–four states, 2006-2007. MMWR Morb Mortal Wkly Rep 2007;56(45):1181–4.

67. Gu L, Liu Z, Li X, et al. Severe community-acquired pneumonia caused by adenovirus type 11 in immunocompetent adults in Beijing. J Clin Virol 2012; 54(4):295–301.

68. Sun B, He H, Wang Z, et al. Emergent severe acute respiratory distress syndrome caused by adenovirus type 55 in immunocompetent adults in 2013: a prospective observational study. Crit Care 2014;18:456.

69. Qu J-X, Gu L, Pu Z-H, et al. Viral etiology of community-acquired pneumonia among adolescents and adults with mild or moderate severity and its relation to age and severity. BMC Infect Dis 2015;15:89.

70. Baron EJ, Miller JM, Weinstein MP, et al. A guide to utilization of the microbiology laboratory for diagnosis of infectious diseases: 2013 recommendations by the Infectious Diseases Society of America (IDSA) and the American Society for Microbiology (ASM)a. Clin Infect Dis 2013;57(4):e22–121.

71. Popowitch EB, O'Neill SS, Miller MB. Comparison of the Biofire Filmarray RP, Genmark eSensor RVP, Luminex xTAG RVPv1, and Luminex xTAG RVP fast multiplex assays for detection of respiratory viruses. J Clin Microbiol 2013; 51(5):1528–33.

72. High KP, Bradley SF, Gravenstein S, et al. Clinical practice guideline for the evaluation of fever and infection in older adult residents of long-term care facilities: 2008 update by the Infectious Diseases Society of America. Clin Infect Dis 2009; 48(2):149–71.

73. Barlam TF, Cosgrove SE, Abbo LM, et al. Implementing an antibiotic stewardship program: guidelines by the Infectious Diseases Society of America and the Society for Healthcare Epidemiology of America. Clin Infect Dis 2016; 62(10):e51–77.

74. Monto AS. Studies of the community and family: acute respiratory illness and infection. Epidemiol Rev 1994;16(2):351–73.

75. Smith PW, Bennett G, Bradley S, et al. SHEA/APIC guideline: infection prevention and control in the long-term care facility. Am J Infect Control 2008;36(7): 504–35.

76. Hendley JO, Gwaltney JM. Mechanisms of transmission of rhinovirus infections. Epidemiol Rev 1988;10:243–58.

77. Siegel JD, Rhinehart E, Jackson M, et al. 2007 guideline for isolation precautions: preventing transmission of infectious agents in health care settings. Am J Infect Control 2007;35(10):S65–164.

78. Gralton J, Tovey ER, McLaws M-L, et al. Respiratory virus RNA is detectable in airborne and droplet particles. J Med Virol 2013;85(12):2151–9.

79. Lindsley WG, Blachere FM, Davis KA, et al. Distribution of airborne influenza virus and respiratory syncytial virus in an urgent care medical clinic. Clin Infect Dis 2010;50(5):693–8.

80. Bischoff WE, Swett K, Leng I, et al. Exposure to influenza virus aerosols during routine patient care. J Infect Dis 2013;207(7):1037–46.

81. Thompson BL, Dwyer DM, Ussery XT, et al. Handwashing and glove use in a long-term-care facility. Infect Control Hosp Epidemiol 1997;18(2):97–103.
82. Smith A, Carusone SC, Loeb M. Hand hygiene practices of health care workers in long-term care facilities. Am J Infect Control 2008;36(7):492–4.
83. Mody L, McNeil SA, Sun R, et al. Introduction of a waterless alcohol-based hand rub in a long-term–care facility. Infect Control Hosp Epidemiol 2003;24(3): 165–71.
84. Schweon SJ, Edmonds SL, Kirk J, et al. Effectiveness of a comprehensive hand hygiene program for reduction of infection rates in a long-term care facility. Am J Infect Control 2013;41(1):39–44.
85. Bolyard EA, Tablan OC, Williams WW, et al. Guideline for infection control in healthcare personnel, 1998. Hospital Infection Control Practices Advisory Committee. Infect Control Hosp Epidemiol 1998;19(6):407–63.
86. Esbenshade JC, Edwards KM, Esbenshade AJ, et al. Respiratory virus shedding in a cohort of on-duty healthcare workers undergoing prospective surveillance. Infect Control Hosp Epidemiol 2013;34(4):373–8.
87. Spires SS, Talbot HK, Pope CA, et al. Paramyxovirus outbreak in a long-term care facility: the challenges of implementing infection control practices in a congregate setting. Infect Control Hosp Epidemiol 2017;38(4):399–404.
88. Nace DA, Drinka PJ, Crnich CJ. Clinical uncertainties in the approach to long term care residents with possible urinary tract infection. J Am Med Dir Assoc 2014;15(2):133–9.
89. Falsey AR, Becker KL, Swinburne AJ, et al. Bacterial complications of respiratory tract viral illness: a comprehensive evaluation. J Infect Dis 2013;208(3): 432–41.
90. Schuetz P, Müller B, Christ-Crain M, et al. Procalcitonin to initiate or discontinue antibiotics in acute respiratory tract infections. Cochrane Database Syst Rev 2012;(9):CD007498.
91. Huijskens EGW, Koopmans M, Palmen FMH, et al. The value of signs and symptoms in differentiating between bacterial, viral and mixed aetiology in patients with community-acquired pneumonia. J Med Microbiol 2014;63(3):441–52.
92. Gadsby NJ, Russell CD, McHugh MP, et al. Comprehensive molecular testing for respiratory pathogens in community-acquired pneumonia. Clin Infect Dis 2016;62(7):817–23.
93. Loeb M, Bentley DW, Bradley S, et al. Development of minimum criteria for the initiation of antibiotics in residents of long-term-care facilities: results of a consensus conference. Infect Control Hosp Epidemiol 2001;22(2):120–4.
94. Garvie DG, Gray J. Outbreak of respiratory syncytial virus infection in the elderly. Br Med J 1980;281(6250):1253–4.
95. Meijer A, Overduin P, Hommel D, et al. Outbreak of respiratory syncytial virus infections in a nursing home and possible sources of introduction: the Netherlands, winter 2012/2013. J Am Geriatr Soc 2013;61(12):2230–1.
96. Doi I, Nagata N, Tsukagoshi H, et al. An outbreak of acute respiratory infections due to human respiratory syncytial virus in a nursing home for the elderly in Ibaraki, Japan, 2014. Jpn J Infect Dis 2014;67(4):326–8.
97. Honda H, Iwahashi J, Kashiwagi T, et al. Outbreak of human metapneumovirus infection in elderly inpatients in Japan. J Am Geriatr Soc 2006;54(1):177–80.
98. Omura T, Iizuka S, Tabara K, et al. Detection of human metapneumovirus genomes during an outbreak of bronchitis and pneumonia in a geriatric care home in Shimane, Japan, in autumn 2009. Jpn J Infect Dis 2011;64(1):85–7.

99. Te Wierik MJ, Nguyen DT, Beersma MF, et al. An outbreak of severe respiratory tract infection caused by human metapneumovirus in a residential care facility for elderly in Utrecht, the Netherlands, January to March 2010. Euro Surveill 2012;17(13) [pii:20132].

100. Mubareka S, Louie L, Wong H, et al. Co-circulation of multiple genotypes of human rhinovirus during a large outbreak of respiratory illness in a veterans' long-term care home. J Clin Virol 2013;58(2):455–60.

101. Lee N, Lui GC, Wong KT, et al. High morbidity and mortality in adults hospitalized for respiratory syncytial virus infections. Clin Infect Dis 2013;57(8):1069–77.

102. Falsey AR, Walsh EE, Hayden FG. Rhinovirus and coronavirus infection-associated hospitalizations among older adults. J Infect Dis 2002;185(9): 1338–41.

103. Wald TG, Miller BA, Shult P, et al. Can respiratory syncytial virus and influenza A be distinguished clinically in institutionalized older persons? J Am Geriatr Soc 1995;43(2):170–4.

104. Marx A, Gary HE, Marston BJ, et al. Parainfluenza virus infection among adults hospitalized for lower respiratory tract infection. Clin Infect Dis 1999;29(1): 134–40.

105. Falsey AR. Respiratory syncytial virus infection in adults. Semin Respir Crit Care Med 2007;28(2):171–81.

106. Falsey AR. Human metapneumovirus infection in adults. Pediatr Infect Dis J 2008;27(10 Suppl):S80–3.

Human Immunodeficiency Virus and Aging in the Era of Effective Antiretroviral Therapy

Puja Van Epps, MD[a,*], Robert C. Kalayjian, MD[a,b]

KEYWORDS

- Aging • HIV • Comorbidities • Telomere • Senescence • Frailty

KEY POINTS

- Persons living with HIV (PLWH) have accentuated risks for age-associated comorbidities.
- Compared to the general population, PLWH have a 2-fold higher risk of cardiovascular disease, a 3-fold increased risk of fracture, and a risk of kidney disease that is comparable to that in diabetes.
- Some comorbidities may present at younger ages than among the general population, suggesting the possibility of accelerated aging with HIV infection.

AGING WITH HUMAN IMMUNODEFICIENCY VIRUS

Advances in antiretroviral therapy (ART) have transformed infection with human immunodeficiency virus (HIV) into a chronic illness, in which the majority of persons living with HIV (PLWH) in the United States are now older than 50 years.[1] Despite substantial gains in health and survival that are now possible with ART, life expectancy in PLWH continues to lag by approximately 5 years, compared with the general population.[2–4]

PLWH have increased prevalence of age-related morbidities including: cardiovascular disease (CVD), hypertension, diabetes, bone fractures, neurocognitive impairment (NCI), cancer, and kidney and liver disease.[5–10] In a large, retrospective, cross-sectional study from Italy, polymorbidity (with at least 2 comorbidities) developed approximately 10 years earlier in PLWH compared with HIV-uninfected individuals.[9]

Disclosures: R.C. Kalayjian receives grant funding from Gilead (GS-US-292-1825); Geriatric Research, Education and Clinical Center, VISN 10; and CWRU Center for AIDS Research AI 036219.
[a] Division of Infectious Diseases, Geriatric Research, Education, and Clinical Center, Louis Stokes Cleveland Department of Veterans Affairs Medical Center, Case Western Reserve University School of Medicine, 10701 East Boulevard, Cleveland, OH 44106, USA; [b] Division of Infectious Diseases, MetroHealth Medical Center, Case Western Reserve University School of Medicine, 2500 MetroHealth Drive, Cleveland, OH 44109, USA
* Corresponding author.
E-mail address: puja.vanepps@va.gov

Furthermore, 84% of PLWH in a large study from the Netherlands were projected to have at least one comorbidity by 2030, up from 28% in 2010, and 29% were projected with at least 3 comorbidities by 2030.[11,12] These observations illustrate the accentuated risk of comorbidities in PLWH, and by virtue of younger ages at presentation compared to the general population, suggest that HIV may accelerate aging.[9,13] Evidence for such acceleration must take into account the increased prevalence of predisposing factors among PLWH including smoking, substance use disorders, viral coinfections (including hepatitis C virus [HCV] and human herpes viruses) and depression, and the possibility that HIV infection may accentuate these risk factors.[14,15] These analyses must also adjust for the younger age distribution of PLWH, compared with the general population.[16] Herein, we explore the clinical and experimental evidence for accentuated and accelerated age-associated comorbidities in HIV disease.

MECHANISMS OF AGING

Aging describes the time-dependent accumulation of cellular damage, leading to decreased function and increased vulnerability to death.[17] Hallmarks of mammalian aging, as proposed by Lopez-Otin and colleagues,[18] include those processes that are manifest during normal aging, whose experimental aggravation or amelioration accelerates or retards aging, with either premature death or a longer, healthier lifespan. Within this framework, these mechanisms may be characterized as primary, antagonistic, or integrative. Primary mechanisms are uniformly detrimental to cells including those that promote genetic instability or impair proteostasis (ie, protein homeostasis). Cellular senescence is an example of an antagonistic mechanism that protects cells from cancer while promoting aging. Integrative mechanisms emerge because of cumulative, uncompensated cell damage, resulting in dysregulated systems with diminished stem cell regenerative capacity, or altered intercellular communication from processes such as deregulated nutrient sensing or inflammation.

HIV infection, or its treatment, share many of these aging-associated hallmarks, including increased genetic instability, enhanced T-cell senescence, diminished naïve T-cell regeneration, and altered intracellular communication from deregulated nutrient sensing, heightened inflammation, and cytotoxic proteins (**Table 1**).

Genetic Instability

DNA methylation patterns of cytosine phosphate guanine residues change with age, and can be modeled to accurately predict chronologic age in healthy people.[19] Concentrated in sites that are under active regulation, these methylation patterns may alter the expression of genes that direct cellular differentiation and renewal.[20] The biological age that was estimated by this method accurately predicted increased mortality in persons with comorbidities. Older biological compared with chronologic

Table 1 Experimental evidence of age-accelerating mechanisms in HIV	
Genomic instability	Altered DNA methylation patterns Telomerase shortening Clonal expansion of mitochondrial DNA
Altered cellular regeneration and senescence	Impaired naive CD4 and CD8 cell regeneration Increased CD8 cell senescence
Altered intracellular communication	Heightened inflammation Insulin resistance

ages also were detected in individuals with Down syndrome, a disease that is associated with accelerated aging.[21,22] Such differences were similarly observed in studies of PLWH, wherein the average biological age was 4.9 years older than the chronologic age in 1 study of highly adherent ART-treated individuals.[20,23] In contrast with the mechanisms that follow, however, there is thus far no direct experimental evidence that alterations in DNA methylation can change the lifespan of an organism.

Telomeres are repeating DNA segments that protect the ends of chromosomes. Telomeres shorten with each cell division and are maintained by telomerase.[24] Telomere lengths indicate the cell's replicative history, where shorter lengths predicted increased mortality.[25] Correlates of shorter telomeres include chronic HIV and HCV infections, male sex, smoking, diabetes, atherosclerosis, and several cancers.[26–28] When measured in peripheral blood mononuclear cells, telomere shortening was detected within senescent CD8, but not CD4 cells of PLWH.[29–31] Nucleos(t)ide reverse transcriptase inhibitors including tenofovir also inhibit human telomerase reverse transcriptase, contributing to telomere shortening.[32] Telomere shortening was nevertheless observed in patients who did not receive ART.[31,33,34]

Age-associated mitochondrial DNA (mtDNA) changes arise from the clonal expansion of specific mtDNA deletion mutations that developed early in life, rather than from an accumulation of random mutations within the oxidative-rich mitochondrial environment, as was previously thought.[35] Preferential inhibition of mtDNA polymerase-γ by many nucleos(t)ide reverse transcriptase inhibitors leads to mtDNA depletion, impaired oxidative phosphorylation, and abnormal mitochondrial morphology.[36] Residual and cumulative toxicities by these agents are suggested by the demonstration of clonally expanded, age-related mtDNA deletion mutations in muscle fibers of patients with prior nucleos(t)ide exposure.[37] ART-naïve individuals also have evidence of mitochondrial dysfunction, with altered mtDNA content and reduced electron transfer complex gene expression and activity, suggesting independent, adverse mitochondrial effects by HIV infection.[38–41]

Immunosenesence

Both normal aging and HIV disease are associated with shifts in T-cell phenotypes, with an expansion of terminally differentiated senescent CD8 cells, and a depletion of naïve CD4 and CD8 T cells. Senescent CD8 cells expand in response of repetitive antigenic stimulation, particularly from chronic viral infections such as cytomegalovirus and Epstein–Barr virus.[42] They have reduced antigenic responsiveness and shortened telomeres, and are identified by loss of the costimulatory receptor CD28, and the gain of CD57 expression on their surface.[29,43,44] Senescent CD8 cells predicted increased mortality in ART-treated PLWH,[45] in whom the expansion of this phenotype also was associated with low CD4/CD8 ratios.[46] Low CD4/CD8 ratios also were associated with an increased risk of age-associated comorbidities, both in ART-treated PLWH, and in the elderly.[47,48]

Impaired Cellular Regeneration

In contrast with senescent cells, naïve T cells have abundant CD28 expression on their surface, which is necessary to generate a primary immune response to neoantigens. Their progenitors undergo thymic selection after leaving the bone marrow, but because of thymic involution that begins at puberty and is accelerated in HIV disease, adults rely on cytokine-driven homeostatic proliferation to maintain the naïve T-cell populations.[49] PLWH maintain fewer circulating naïve and total CD4 cells, and fewer naïve CD8 cells despite ART,[50,51] and the extent of this restoration was correlated positively with baseline naïve CD4 cell counts.[52]

Inflammation

Heightened inflammation is an independent predictor of mortality and morbidity, both in PLWH and in the general population.[53–55] Several studies have demonstrated contributions by immune activation and hypercoagulation to age-associated comorbidities in ART-treated PLWH. Included among these predictive circulating markers are D-dimer, C-reactive protein (CRP), IL-6, soluble tumor necrosis factor receptors-1 and -2, sCD14, markers of gut epithelial barrier dysfunction (zonulin and intestinal fatty acid binding protein), and the ratio of plasma kynurenine/tryptophan, a marker of the enzyme indolamine 2,3 dioxygenase-1 activity that has broad immunoregulatory activity.[53,56–61] The sources of inflammation in HIV disease are incompletely understood, but they are likely to include HIV reservoirs, chronic viral coinfections (particularly HCV and human herpes viruses), and gastrointestinal tract microbial translocation.[62] Although these markers typically remain elevated despite ART, many of these normalized when ART was initiated during acute HIV infection, except sCD14, CRP, and markers of fibrosis, in 1 study.[63]

DEREGULATED NUTRIENT SENSING

Insulin-like growth factor (IGF-1) is synthesized in response to growth hormone, and with insulin, engage IGF-1 receptors to activate intracellular signaling pathways that stimulate cellular proliferation, differentiation, and antioxidant formation while inhibiting apoptosis.[64] The action of insulin is impaired by inflammation, particularly involving macrophages that is mediated through the major nuclear factor-κB and JNK1 activation pathways, with release of proinflammatory cytokines including tumor necrosis factor-α, interleukin (IL)-1β, IL-6, and monocyte chemoattractant protein 1.[65] Chronically increased insulin levels in the face of insulin resistance may induce a maladaptive response with hyperactivity of IGF-1 pathways, leading to increased oxidative stress through the generation of reactive oxygen species by mitochondria and macrophages.[64]

IGF-1 activity decreases during normal aging, yet mutations that reduce IGF-1 signaling activity extend longevity.[66] This apparent contradiction might be understood as a defensive response by aging cells to an environment of heightened immune activation and oxidative stress, where cell damage is limited by reducing cellular metabolism. Caloric restriction with adequate nutrition also extends the life span of laboratory animals, in association with lower plasma insulin levels, increased insulin sensitivity, and reduced mitochondrial reactive oxygen species formation.[66]

Insulin resistance is a major metabolic feature of obesity and a central feature of the metabolic syndrome that includes obesity, hypertension, and dyslipidemia. The prevalence of insulin resistance is high among PLWH receiving ART (between 14% and 25%), but comparable with that of the general US population; protease inhibitor and stavudine use increase this risk.[67–69]

AGE-ASSOCIATED COMORBIDITIES AND HUMAN IMMUNODEFICIENCY VIRUS: CURRENT KNOWLEDGE OF EPIDEMIOLOGY AND MECHANISMS
Cardiovascular Disease

ART-treated PLWH in the United States have nearly twice the risk for myocardial infarction (MI), sudden death, and heart failure compared with the general population (**Table 2**).[70–72] In addition to an overrepresentation of traditional risk factors, heightened inflammation, increased T-cell senescence, ART toxicities, and HIV-specific factors contribute to these risks.

Markers of inflammation, coagulation, renal function, and N-terminal pro-brain natriuretic factor predicted all-cause mortality and/or MI in both the general population and

Table 2
Clinical evidence of age-accentuated and age-accelerated associations in people living with human immunodeficiency virus

	Age Accentuated	Age Accelerated
Cardiovascular disease	√	
Cancer[a]	√	√
Kidney disease	√	√
Liver disease	√	
Cognitive impairment	√	
Frailty	√	√
Bone disease	√	

[a] Myeloma, lung, and anal cancers.

in PLWH.[53,54,59,73–77] Subclinical atherosclerosis was also associated with markers of monocyte activation (CCL2, sCD14, and sCD163), endothelial dysfunction (soluble vascular adhesion molecule-1 and myeloperoxidase) and T-cell senescence in PLWH.[78–80]

Longer durations of ART use and lower nadir CD4 cell counts were associated with increased MI risk, as was higher time-updated (repeated measurements within the same individuals over time) HIV viral load, and lower CD4 cell counts.[81] HIV infection was associated with a greater prevalence of both coronary artery calcium and noncalcified atherosclerotic plaques, determined using noncontrast cardiac computed tomography in the Multicenter AIDS Cohort Study.[82] Despite these differences, HIV-specific variables did not improve predictive models of CVD when included in the Pooled Cohort Equations that were derived from the general population.[83]

Although PLWH had a higher incidence of MI (IR, 2.02 vs 1.28 per 1000 person-years), the mean age at initial MI diagnosis did not differ (56.2 vs 56.0 years for HIV-infected vs uninfected veterans, respectively) in the multisite Veterans Aging Cohort Study (VACS).[84]

Malignancy

HIV disease portends a higher risk of infection-related cancers that are both AIDS-defining, including Kaposi sarcoma, cervical cancer and non-Hodgkin lymphoma, and non–AIDS–defining cancers, including rectal and liver cancers. Infection-unrelated cancers are also increased in ART-treated individuals, including Hodgkin disease, melanoma, and lung cancer.[85–87] By contrast, the risk of prostate and breast cancer, two of the most prevalent age-associated malignancies in the general population, were not increased and may be lower in PLWH.[88–91]

In addition to a higher prevalence of carcinogenic exposure, including smoking and possibly alcohol use, immunosuppression and chronic inflammation were associated with increased risk for both infection-related and infection-unrelated cancers in PLWH.[88,92,93] In a large cohort from 3 randomized clinical trials, increased risk of any cancer was associated with higher levels of IL-6 (hazard ratio [HR], 1.38), CRP (HR, 1.16) and D-dimer (HR, 1.17) and these significant associations were evident for both infection-related and infection-unrelated cancers.[89,94] Among non–AIDS–defining cancers, the risk for melanoma, lung, and liver cancers were increased in association with low CD4 cell counts. Although ART clearly mitigates the risk of AIDS-defining cancers, immediate initial ART in persons with CD4 cell counts of greater than 500 cells/µL was associated with reduced incidences of infection-related cancers (HR, 0.26; 95% CI, 0.11–0.64), and with nonsignificant decreases in non infectious cancers (HR, 0.49; 95% CI, 0.21–1.15) in the Strategic Timing of Antiretroviral Treatment trial.[95]

Data are conflicting as to whether cancer presents at younger ages in PLWH. Shiels and colleagues[96,97] identified significantly younger median ages of onset for myeloma (52 years vs 56 years), lung (50 years vs 54 years), and anal cancers (42 years vs 45 years) in PLWH, compared with the general population. In the VACS cohort, however, there were no differences in the age at presentation of non–AIDS–defining cancers, including myeloma, lung, and anal cancers.[84,96,98,99]

Kidney Disease

PLWH have a higher risk of kidney disease that is comparable with diabetes.[100] As with CVD, an overrepresentation of traditional risk factors, such as HCV coinfection as well as ART toxicities and HIV-specific factors contribute to this risk.[101]

As in the general population, kidney disease in PLWH is associated with greater all-cause mortality and with increased risks of CVD and cognitive impairment.[64,73,102–105] Markers of inflammation, including elevated plasma: soluble tumor necrosis factor receptors-1 and 2, CCL2, and sCD27 levels were associated with kidney damage (defined by either proteinuria or reduced glomerular filtration rates) both in PLWH and in the general population.[106–111] HIV-specific factors that are associated with kidney damage include higher baseline and time-updated viral load, and lower time-updated CD4 cell counts.[112] The incidence of end-stage renal disease in PLWH was significantly higher (2.56 per 1000 person-years vs 1.68 per 1000 person-years), and the age at presentation was significantly younger than in HIV-uninfected veterans in the VACS cohort (56.0 years vs 59.4 years; adjusted mean age difference, −0.46 years [95% CI, −0.86 to −0.07]).[84]

HIV-associated nephropathy is a specific clinicopathologic manifestation that occurs almost exclusively in persons of recent African descent. It is characterized by collapsing focal glomerulosclerosis, nephrotic range proteinuria, and rapid progression to end-stage renal disease.[101] Direct viral effects are implicated by the demonstration of a productive HIV infection in renal epithelial cells from patients with HIV-associated nephropathy, and by the dramatic decline in incidence of this syndrome with effective ART.[113,114] Allelic mutations in the apolipoprotein L1 gene (APOL1) that are prevalent among persons of recent African descent, account for the striking racial associations with HIV-associated nephropathy and contribute to increased risk of progressive nondiabetic kidney disease among African Americans in the general US population.[115–117] The magnitude of this association was markedly increased among PLWH, such that HIV-infected African Americans with 2 allelic mutations had a 50% estimated lifetime risk of end-stage kidney disease in the absence of ART, compared with a 4% lifetime risk for this outcome among HIV-uninfected African Americans.[117]

APOL1 encodes a circulating protein that lyses the African trypanosome T brucei brucei, sharing homology with BcL-2 proteins involved in autophagy.[118] Although the mechanisms of cell damage are incompletely understood, recent studies of cultured human embryonic kidney cells that expressed these allelic mutations implicate altered intracellular communication, with net efflux of intracellular potassium, resulting in activation of stress-activated protein kinases and cell death.[119]

Liver Disease

Liver disease, largely owing to coinfection with hepatitis B and C, has emerged as a leading cause of morbidity and mortality in PLWH. Accounting for 13% of deaths in the Data collection on adverse events of anti-HIV drugs (D:A:D),[5] liver disease was included among the top 3 causes of death in the longitudinal HIV Outpatient Study cohort. The attributable mortality from liver disease has increased from 0.09 to 0.16 per 100 person-years from 1996 to 2004.[120] Compared with HIV-uninfected individuals, PLWH who are coinfected with HCV or HBV have significantly more liver fibrosis, more hepatic steatosis, and more rapid progression to cirrhosis with hepatic decompensation.[121–123] Hepatic steatosis or nonalcoholic fatty liver disease, in the absence of viral coinfection, is associated with metabolic syndrome and may be more common in PLWH than in the general population. Crum-Cianflone and colleagues[124] have detected hepatic steatosis at 31% in a cross-sectional HIV cohort in a large urban US clinic.

Older age at HCV acquisition and alcohol consumption are strong predictors of liver fibrosis in both HIV-infected and HIV-uninfected individuals; low CD4 count also is associated with fibrosis in PLWH.[125]

Neurocognitive Impairment

ART has dramatically reduced the prevalence of AIDS dementia complex, but NCI, as determined by neuropsychological testing, is common in PLWH despite viral suppressive ART in both plasma and cerebrospinal fluid.[126] Often asymptomatic, the natural history of NCI is incompletely understood. In the multicenter prospective CHARTER study, neurocognitive stability was observed over a mean of 35 months in 60.8%, whereas 22.7% and 16.5% either declined or improved, respectively.[127] Compared with individuals without NCI, asymptomatic NCI was associated with higher risk of subsequent impairment in activities of daily living.[128] Furthermore, NCI (symptomatic or not) was associated with higher risk of frailty and with a higher VACS Index, a composite marker of HIV disease severity that predicts mortality.[129,130]

The role of inflammation in the pathogenesis of NCI is implicated by associations with markers of monocyte activation (sCD14 and sCD163).[131] Endovascular disease is also likely to contribute to this pathogenesis, as suggested by associations with preexisting cardiovascular comorbidities (including carotid intima media thickness, low-density lipoprotein cholesterol, and markers of kidney disease) in longitudinal cohort studies.[105,132,133]

GERIATRIC SYNDROMES AND FRAILTY

Frailty is a geriatric syndrome that implies decreased physiologic reserve and diminished resistance to stressors, and is predictive of adverse health outcomes including falls, disability, and death in older adults (>60 years).[134] HIV infection is associated with a functional decline that is reminiscent of frailty in the elderly, but manifests at younger ages in PLWH.[135] The prevalence of frailty in PLWH ranged from 5% to 20% in large cohorts with mean ages between 40 and 55 years.[136,137] Frailty was an independent predictor of death in the AIDS Linked to the IntraVenous Experience (ALIVE) cohort of HIV-infected injection drug users with a mean age of 49 years.[138] Frailty was associated with an increased prevalence of comorbidities[139] and predicted increased hospitalization rates and mortality in PLWH.[140]

Heightened inflammation, including elevated plasma IL-6, tumor necrosis factor-α, and CRP, were associated with frailty in both geriatric populations and in PLWH.[141–145] Among the latter, frailty also was associated with low CD4; high CD8 cell counts and increased T-cell activation (as HLA-DR/CD38).[146–151]

As with frailty, falls are also more common in PLWH, in whom they also occur at younger ages. In 1 study, 30% of virally suppressed PLWH between the ages of

45 to 65 years, reported at least 1 fall during the previous year, an event rate that was comparable with that of HIV-uninfected adults greater than 65 years old.[152]

Bone Disease

PLWH have reduced bone mineral density and increased risk of fractures.[153–156] In a metaanalysis of 11 studies, 67% of PLWH had reduced bone mineral density and 15% had osteoporosis.[157] Several studies have documented increased fracture risk in PLWH, where the incidence of fractures was up to 3-fold higher compared with the age-adjusted general population. Similar fracture rates were evident between men and women.[156,158–160]

In addition to the traditional risk factors for osteoporosis, including low body mass index,[161,162] smoking, hypogonadism, and low vitamin D, HCV coinfection was also associated with low bone mineral density in PLWH.[92,163–166] Direct effects on osteoblast and osteoclasts by HIV proteins also may contribute to bone loss.[167,168]

In contrast with the most other comorbidities, ART exacerbates bone loss, particularly during the first year of ART initiation. The magnitude of ART-associated bone loss was greater in association with tenofovir disoproxil fumarate or protease inhibitor-containing regimens. Other correlates of ART-associated bone loss include increased CD4 cell restoration and greater bone turnover, with heightened osteoclast mediated bone resorption and corresponding increases in osteoblast mediated new bone formation.[169–172]

CLINICAL IMPLICATIONS

PLWH have accentuated risk of age-associated comorbidities with polymorbidity, which in part is associated with heightened inflammation and immune suppression. There is growing experimental evidence of accelerated aging with HIV, whereas clinical evidence for this process includes chronic kidney disease, frailty, and some non–AIDS–defining cancers (including lung and anal cancers, and myeloma). Early and continuous ART reduces the risk of most comorbidities, including kidney disease and cancer, suggesting that age-accelerating or age-accentuating effects by HIV infection may be reversible.[6,7,95] Nevertheless, the prospects of increasing rates of polymorbidity in PLWH argue for interdisciplinary model of comprehensive care delivery that incorporates geriatric principles of care (discussed elsewhere in this article), prevention, and cancer screening.

Beginning with early HIV diagnosis and prompt treatment,[7] once ART-mediated viral suppression is achieved, care should focus on screening for age-associated illnesses as supported by current evidence. Whenever possible, age-appropriate screening for malignancy should be based on HIV-specific evidence. This includes a special focus on cervical and anal cancers and possibly lung cancers.[173,174] The Infectious Diseases Society of America and HIV Medicine Association recommends that HIV-infected women undergo a cervical Pap test upon entry into of care, and this test should be repeated at 6 months and annually thereafter if results are normal. Women with abnormal results including, atypical squamous cells, atypical glandular cells, low-grade or high-grade squamous intraepithelial lesion, or squamous carcinoma noted by Pap testing, should undergo colposcopy and biopsy. Men who have sex with men, women with a history of receptive anal intercourse or abnormal cervical Pap test results, and all HIV-infected persons with genital warts should have anal Pap tests. Abnormal cytologic examinations should be investigated with a high-resolution anoscopy and biopsy of suspicious lesions.

For lung cancer, current guidelines for general population target individuals with heavy, long-standing smoking history.[175] The US Preventative Services Task Force recommends annual screening for lung cancer with low-dose computed tomography in adults aged 55 to 80 years who have a 30 pack-year smoking history and currently smoke or have quit within the past 15 years. Further research is needed in the use of low-dose computed tomography for the screening of lung cancer in PLWH, because there does seem to be both an accentuated risk and a modest premature onset in this population.

Based on lack of increased risks, breast cancer and colorectal cancer screening should follow guidelines established for the general population. Outside of those with higher risk of prostate cancer (ie, those with family history, particularly among African Americans),[176] enhanced screening for prostate cancer in PLWH is not supported by evidence.

In terms of prevention, a focus on correcting modifiable risk factors for major chronic illnesses has become increasingly vital as the PLWH age. Based on the well-established excess mortality risk owing to tobacco use in PLWH, smoking cessation is a high priority in this population.[177,178] In addition, clinicians should actively address alcohol and substance use dependence in the clinic. Key challenge facing clinicians is how to translate our understanding of HIV-mediated liver damage into approaches for detection and treatment. The strongest case thus far has been for treatment of coviral infections to prevent progression of fibrosis.[121] In the setting of monoinfection, clinicians should focus efforts on correcting traditional risk factors for nonalcoholic fatty liver disease, including adiposity and dyslipidemia.

Focus on physical activity and obesity management may not only help to alleviate the metabolic syndrome[179] and associated complications, but also impede age-associated functional decline.[180] And last, integrating geriatric principles of care to include polypharmacy management, neurocognitive and functional assessments, and addressing end-of-life issues, will become increasingly important with this aging population in which geriatric syndromes are common.[181,182] Such an approach should involve both management of debility in any of the geriatric domains as well as preventing further decline. An important element of geriatric care is prevention of falls, which is intricately linked to prevention of bone loss and osteoporosis.[183] Fracture Risk Assessment Tool (FRAX) is an algorithm developed by the World Health Organization that takes into account traditional risk factors for bone loss to help predict the 10-year probability of a major fracture.[184] However, FRAX score was developed for the general population may underestimate fracture risk in PLWH.[185] Presently, the Infectious Diseases Society of America recommends dual-energy x-ray absorptiometry screening for osteoporosis in PLWH 50 years of age or older.[174] Owing to the heightened risk of osteoporosis, some experts go a step further in recommending dual-energy x-ray absorptiometry in HIV-infected individuals aged 40 to 49 years who have an FRAX score of greater than 10%.[186]

SUMMARY

Effective care of older HIV-infected adults that focuses on quality of life will need to span from effective treatment of HIV to preventing and managing polymorbidity to appraisal of social determinants of health and more seamlessly integrate community and social services into health care delivery.[187]

REFERENCES

1. Centers for Disease Control and Prevention (CDC). HIV surveillance–United States, 1981-2008. MMWR Morb Mortal Wkly Rep 2011;60:689–93.

2. Gueler A, Moser A, Calmy A, et al. Life expectancy in HIV-positive persons in Switzerland: matched comparison with general population. AIDS 2017;31:427–36.

3. Walensky RP, Paltiel AD, Losina E, et al. The survival benefits of AIDS treatment in the United States. J Infect Dis 2006;194:11–9.

4. Teeraananchai S, Kerr SJ, Amin J, et al. Life expectancy of HIV-positive people after starting combination antiretroviral therapy: a meta-analysis. HIV Med 2017; 18(4):256–66.

5. Smith CJ, Ryom L, Weber R, et al. Trends in underlying causes of death in people with HIV from 1999 to 2011 (D: A:D): a multicohort collaboration. Lancet 2014;384:241–8.

6. Strategies for Management of Antiretroviral Therapy (SMART) Study Group, El-Sadr WM, Lundgren J, et al. CD4+ count-guided interruption of antiretroviral treatment. N Engl J Med 2006;355:2283–96.

7. Group ISS, Lundgren JD, Babiker AG, et al. Initiation of antiretroviral therapy in early asymptomatic HIV infection. N Engl J Med 2015;373:795–807.

8. Weber R, Ruppik M, Rickenbach M, et al. Decreasing mortality and changing patterns of causes of death in the Swiss HIV cohort study. HIV Med 2013;14: 195–207.

9. Guaraldi G, Orlando G, Zona S, et al. Premature age-related comorbidities among HIV-infected persons compared with the general population. Clin Infect Dis 2011;53:1120–6.

10. Guaraldi G, Zona S, Brothers TD, et al. Aging with HIV vs. HIV seroconversion at older age: a diverse population with distinct comorbidity profiles. PLoS One 2015;10:e0118531.

11. Smit M, Brinkman K, Geerlings S, et al. Future challenges for clinical care of an ageing population infected with HIV: a modelling study. Lancet Infect Dis 2015; 15:810–8.

12. Schouten J, Wit FW, Stolte IG, et al. Cross-sectional comparison of the prevalence of age-associated comorbidities and their risk factors between HIV-infected and uninfected individuals: the AGEhIV cohort study. Clin Infect Dis 2014;59:1787–97.

13. Pathai S, Bajillan H, Landay AL, et al. Is HIV a model of accelerated or accentuated aging? J Gerontol A Biol Sci Med Sci 2014;69:833–42.

14. Shirley DK, Kaner RJ, Glesby MJ. Effects of smoking on non-AIDS-related morbidity in HIV-infected patients. Clin Infect Dis 2013;57:275–82.

15. Goulet JL, Fultz SL, Rimland D, et al. Aging and infectious diseases: do patterns of comorbidity vary by HIV status, age, and HIV severity? Clin Infect Dis 2007; 45:1593–601.

16. Martin J, Volberding P. HIV and premature aging: a field still in its infancy. Ann Intern Med 2010;153:477–9.

17. Gems D, Partridge L. Genetics of longevity in model organisms: debates and paradigm shifts. Annu Rev Physiol 2013;75:621–44.

18. Lopez-Otin C, Blasco MA, Partridge L, et al. The hallmarks of aging. Cell 2013; 153:1194–217.

19. Horvath S. DNA methylation age of human tissues and cell types. Genome Biol 2013;14:R115.

20. Gross AM, Jaeger PA, Kreisberg JF, et al. Methylome-wide analysis of chronic HIV infection reveals five-year increase in biological age and epigenetic targeting of HLA. Mol Cell 2016;62:157–68.

21. Marioni RE, Shah S, McRae AF, et al. DNA methylation age of blood predicts all-cause mortality in later life. Genome Biol 2015;16:25.

22. Horvath S, Garagnani P, Bacalini MG, et al. Accelerated epigenetic aging in Down syndrome. Aging Cell 2015;14:491–5.
23. Horvath S, Levine AJ. HIV-1 Infection accelerates age according to the epigenetic clock. J Infect Dis 2015;212:1563–73.
24. Blackburn EH. Telomeres and telomerase: their mechanisms of action and the effects of altering their functions. FEBS Lett 2005;579:859–62.
25. Cawthon RM, Smith KR, O'Brien E, et al. Association between telomere length in blood and mortality in people aged 60 years or older. Lancet 2003;361:393–5.
26. Kitay-Cohen Y, Goldberg-Bittman L, Hadary R, et al. Telomere length in Hepatitis C. Cancer Genet Cytogenet 2008;187:34–8.
27. Oeseburg H, de Boer RA, van Gilst WH, et al. Telomere biology in healthy aging and disease. Pflugers Arch 2010;459:259–68.
28. Moller P, Mayer S, Mattfeldt T, et al. Sex-related differences in length and erosion dynamics of human telomeres favor females. Aging (Albany NY) 2009;1:733–9.
29. Effros RB, Allsopp R, Chiu CP, et al. Shortened telomeres in the expanded CD28-CD8+ cell subset in HIV disease implicate replicative senescence in HIV pathogenesis. AIDS 1996;10:F17–22.
30. Palmer LD, Weng N, Levine BL, et al. Telomere length, telomerase activity, and replicative potential in HIV infection: analysis of CD4+ and CD8+ T cells from HIV-discordant monozygotic twins. J Exp Med 1997;185:1381–6.
31. Wolthers KC, Bea G, Wisman A, et al. T cell telomere length in HIV-1 infection: no evidence for increased CD4+ T cell turnover. Science 1996;274:1543–7.
32. Leeansyah E, Cameron PU, Solomon A, et al. Inhibition of telomerase activity by human immunodeficiency virus (HIV) nucleos(t)ide reverse transcriptase inhibitors: a potential factor contributing to HIV-associated accelerated aging. J Infect Dis 2013;207:1157–65.
33. Zanet DL, Thorne A, Singer J, et al. Association between short leukocyte telomere length and HIV infection in a cohort study: no evidence of a relationship with antiretroviral therapy. Clin Infect Dis 2014;58:1322–32.
34. Pathai S, Lawn SD, Gilbert CE, et al. Accelerated biological ageing in HIV-infected individuals in South Africa: a case-control study. AIDS 2013;27:2375–84.
35. Bratic A, Larsson NG. The role of mitochondria in aging. J Clin Invest 2013;123:951–7.
36. Dagan T, Sable C, Bray J, et al. Mitochondrial dysfunction and antiretroviral nucleoside analog toxicities: what is the evidence? Mitochondrion 2002;1:397–412.
37. Payne BA, Wilson IJ, Hateley CA, et al. Mitochondrial aging is accelerated by anti-retroviral therapy through the clonal expansion of mtDNA mutations. Nat Genet 2011;43:806–10.
38. Garrabou G, Lopez S, Moren C, et al. Mitochondrial damage in adipose tissue of untreated HIV-infected patients. AIDS 2011;25:165–70.
39. Miro O, Lopez S, Martinez E, et al. Mitochondrial effects of HIV infection on the peripheral blood mononuclear cells of HIV-infected patients who were never treated with antiretrovirals. Clin Infect Dis 2004;39:710–6.
40. Miura T, Goto M, Hosoya N, et al. Depletion of mitochondrial DNA in HIV-1-infected patients and its amelioration by antiretroviral therapy. J Med Virol 2003;70:497–505.
41. Morse CG, Voss JG, Rakocevic G, et al. HIV infection and antiretroviral therapy have divergent effects on mitochondria in adipose tissue. J Infect Dis 2012;205:1778–87.

42. Papagno L, Spina CA, Marchant A, et al. Immune activation and CD8+ T-cell differentiation towards senescence in HIV-1 infection. PLoS Biol 2004;2:E20.

43. Cobos Jimenez V, Wit FW, Joerink M, et al. T-cell activation independently associates with immune senescence in HIV-infected recipients of long-term antiretroviral treatment. J Infect Dis 2016;214:216–25.

44. Wikby A, Maxson P, Olsson J, et al. Changes in CD8 and CD4 lymphocyte subsets, T cell proliferation responses and non-survival in the very old: the Swedish longitudinal OCTO-immune study. Mech Ageing Dev 1998;102:187–98.

45. Lee SA, Sinclair E, Jain V, et al. Low proportions of CD28- CD8+ T cells expressing CD57 can be reversed by early ART initiation and predict mortality in treated HIV infection. J Infect Dis 2014;210:374–82.

46. Serrano Villar S, Porta-Etessam J. Reply. Med Clin (Barc) 2015;144:238 [in Spanish].

47. Ferguson FG, Wikby A, Maxson P, et al. Immune parameters in a longitudinal study of a very old population of Swedish people: a comparison between survivors and nonsurvivors. J Gerontol A Biol Sci Med Sci 1995;50:B378–82.

48. Castilho JL, Shepherd BE, Koethe J, et al. CD4+/CD8+ ratio, age, and risk of serious noncommunicable diseases in HIV-infected adults on antiretroviral therapy. AIDS 2016;30:899–908.

49. Jameson SC. Maintaining the norm: T-cell homeostasis. Nat Rev Immunol 2002; 2:547–56.

50. Kalayjian RC, Spritzler J, Matining RM, et al. Older HIV-infected patients on antiretroviral therapy have B-cell expansion and attenuated CD4 cell increases with immune activation reduction. AIDS 2013;27:1563–71.

51. Althoff KN, Justice AC, Gange SJ, et al. Virologic and immunologic response to HAART, by age and regimen class. AIDS 2010;24:2469–79.

52. Schacker TW, Bosch RJ, Bennett K, et al. Measurement of naive CD4 cells reliably predicts potential for immune reconstitution in HIV. J Acquir Immune Defic Syndr 2010;54:59–62.

53. Kuller LH, Tracy R, Belloso W, et al. Inflammatory and coagulation biomarkers and mortality in patients with HIV infection. PLoS Med 2008;5:e203.

54. Pai JK, Pischon T, Ma J, et al. Inflammatory markers and the risk of coronary heart disease in men and women. N Engl J Med 2004;351:2599–610.

55. Proctor MJ, McMillan DC, Horgan PG, et al. Systemic inflammation predicts all-cause mortality: a Glasgow Inflammation Outcome Study. PLoS One 2015;10: e0116206.

56. Hunt PW, Lee SA, Siedner MJ. Immunologic biomarkers, morbidity, and mortality in treated HIV infection. J Infect Dis 2016;214(Suppl 2):S44–50.

57. Kalayjian RC, Machekano RN, Rizk N, et al. Pretreatment levels of soluble cellular receptors and interleukin-6 are associated with HIV disease progression in subjects treated with highly active antiretroviral therapy. J Infect Dis 2010;201: 1796–805.

58. Hunt PW, Sinclair E, Rodriguez B, et al. Gut epithelial barrier dysfunction and innate immune activation predict mortality in treated HIV infection. J Infect Dis 2014;210:1228–38.

59. Tenorio AR, Zheng Y, Bosch RJ, et al. Soluble markers of inflammation and coagulation but not T-cell activation predict non-AIDS-defining morbid events during suppressive antiretroviral treatment. J Infect Dis 2014;210:1248–59.

60. Justice AC, Freiberg MS, Tracy R, et al. Does an index composed of clinical data reflect effects of inflammation, coagulation, and monocyte activation on mortality among those aging with HIV? Clin Infect Dis 2012;54:984–94.

61. Sandler NG, Wand H, Roque A, et al. Plasma levels of soluble CD14 independently predict mortality in HIV infection. J Infect Dis 2011;203:780–90.
62. Brenchley JM, Price DA, Schacker TW, et al. Microbial translocation is a cause of systemic immune activation in chronic HIV infection. Nat Med 2006;12:1365–71.
63. Sereti I, Krebs SJ, Phanuphak N, et al. Persistent, albeit reduced, chronic inflammation in persons starting antiretroviral therapy in acute HIV infection. Clin Infect Dis 2017;64:124–31.
64. Avogaro A, de Kreutzenberg SV, Fadini GP. Insulin signaling and life span. Pflugers Arch 2010;459:301–14.
65. Schenk S, Saberi M, Olefsky JM. Insulin sensitivity: modulation by nutrients and inflammation. J Clin Invest 2008;118:2992–3002.
66. Junnila RK, List EO, Berryman DE, et al. The GH/IGF-1 axis in ageing and longevity. Nat Rev Endocrinol 2013;9:366–76.
67. Samaras K, Wand H, Law M, et al. Prevalence of metabolic syndrome in HIV-infected patients receiving highly active antiretroviral therapy using International Diabetes Foundation and Adult Treatment Panel III criteria: associations with insulin resistance, disturbed body fat compartmentalization, elevated C-reactive protein, and [corrected] hypoadiponectinemia. Diabetes Care 2007;30:113–9.
68. Mondy K, Overton ET, Grubb J, et al. Metabolic syndrome in HIV-infected patients from an urban, midwestern US outpatient population. Clin Infect Dis 2007;44:726–34.
69. Jerico C, Knobel H, Montero M, et al. Metabolic syndrome among HIV-infected patients: prevalence, characteristics, and related factors. Diabetes Care 2005;28:132–7.
70. Freiberg MS, Chang CC, Kuller LH, et al. HIV infection and the risk of acute myocardial infarction. JAMA Intern Med 2013;173:614–22.
71. Butt AA, Chang CC, Kuller L, et al. Risk of heart failure with human immunodeficiency virus in the absence of prior diagnosis of coronary heart disease. Arch Intern Med 2011;171:737–43.
72. Wester CW, Koethe JR, Shepherd BE, et al. Non-AIDS-defining events among HIV-1-infected adults receiving combination antiretroviral therapy in resource-replete versus resource-limited urban setting. AIDS 2011;25:1471–9.
73. George E, Lucas GM, Nadkarni GN, et al. Kidney function and the risk of cardiovascular events in HIV-1-infected patients. AIDS 2010;24:387–94.
74. Kragelund C, Gronning B, Kober L, et al. N-terminal pro-B-type natriuretic peptide and long-term mortality in stable coronary heart disease. N Engl J Med 2005;352:666–75.
75. Gingo MR, Zhang Y, Ghebrehawariat KB, et al. Elevated NT-pro-brain natriuretic peptide level is independently associated with all-cause mortality in HIV-infected women in the early and recent HAART eras in the Women's Interagency HIV Study cohort. PLoS One 2015;10:e0123389.
76. Duprez DA, Neuhaus J, Tracy R, et al. N-terminal-proB-type natriuretic peptide predicts cardiovascular disease events in HIV-infected patients. AIDS 2011;25:651–7.
77. Zethelius B, Berglund L, Sundstrom J, et al. Use of multiple biomarkers to improve the prediction of death from cardiovascular causes. N Engl J Med 2008;358:2107–16.
78. Kaplan RC, Sinclair E, Landay AL, et al. T cell activation predicts carotid artery stiffness among HIV-infected women. Atherosclerosis 2011;217:207–13.

79. McKibben RA, Margolick JB, Grinspoon S, et al. Elevated levels of monocyte activation markers are associated with subclinical atherosclerosis in men with and those without HIV infection. J Infect Dis 2015;211:1219–28.

80. Ross AC, Rizk N, O'Riordan MA, et al. Relationship between inflammatory markers, endothelial activation markers, and carotid intima-media thickness in HIV-infected patients receiving antiretroviral therapy. Clin Infect Dis 2009;49: 1119–27.

81. Salinas JL, Rentsch C, Marconi VC, et al. Baseline, time-updated, and cumulative HIV care metrics for predicting acute myocardial infarction and all-cause mortality. Clin Infect Dis 2016;63:1423–30.

82. Shaw LJ, Giambrone AE, Blaha MJ, et al. Long-term prognosis after coronary artery calcification testing in asymptomatic patients: a cohort study. Ann Intern Med 2015;163:14–21.

83. Feinstein MJ, Kim JH, Bibangambah P, et al. Ideal cardiovascular health and carotid atherosclerosis in a mixed cohort of HIV-infected and uninfected Ugandans. AIDS Res Hum Retroviruses 2017;33:49–56.

84. Althoff KN, McGinnis KA, Wyatt CM, et al. Comparison of risk and age at diagnosis of myocardial infarction, end-stage renal disease, and non-AIDS-defining cancer in HIV-infected versus uninfected adults. Clin Infect Dis 2015;60:627–38.

85. Clifford GM, Polesel J, Rickenbach M, et al. Cancer risk in the Swiss HIV Cohort Study: associations with immunodeficiency, smoking, and highly active antiretroviral therapy. J Natl Cancer Inst 2005;97:425–32.

86. Biggar RJ, Chaturvedi AK, Goedert JJ, et al. AIDS-related cancer and severity of immunosuppression in persons with AIDS. J Natl Cancer Inst 2007;99: 962–72.

87. Calabresi A, Ferraresi A, Festa A, et al. Incidence of AIDS-defining cancers and virus-related and non-virus-related non-AIDS-defining cancers among HIV-infected patients compared with the general population in a large health district of Northern Italy, 1999-2009. HIV Med 2013;14:481–90.

88. Brickman C, Palefsky JM. Cancer in the HIV-infected host: epidemiology and pathogenesis in the antiretroviral era. Curr HIV/AIDS Rep 2015;12:388–96.

89. Borges AH, Silverberg MJ, Wentworth D, et al. Predicting risk of cancer during HIV infection: the role of inflammatory and coagulation biomarkers. AIDS 2013; 27:1433–41.

90. Hleyhel M, Hleyhel M, Bouvier AM, et al. Risk of non-AIDS-defining cancers among HIV-1-infected individuals in France between 1997 and 2009: results from a French cohort. AIDS 2014;28:2109–18.

91. Silverberg MJ, Chao C, Leyden WA, et al. HIV infection, immunodeficiency, viral replication, and the risk of cancer. Cancer Epidemiol Biomarkers Prev 2011;20: 2551–9.

92. Mdodo R, Frazier EL, Dube SR, et al. Cigarette smoking prevalence among adults with HIV compared with the general adult population in the United States: cross-sectional surveys. Ann Intern Med 2015;162:335–44.

93. McGinnis KA, Fultz SL, Skanderson M, et al. Hepatocellular carcinoma and non-Hodgkin's lymphoma: the roles of HIV, hepatitis C infection, and alcohol abuse. J Clin Oncol 2006;24:5005–9.

94. Shiels MS, Pfeiffer RM, Hildesheim A, et al. Circulating inflammation markers and prospective risk for lung cancer. J Natl Cancer Inst 2013;105:1871–80.

95. Borges AH, Neuhaus J, Babiker AG, et al. Immediate antiretroviral therapy reduces risk of infection-related cancer during early HIV infection. Clin Infect Dis 2016;63:1668–76.

96. Shiels MS, Pfeiffer RM, Engels EA. Age at cancer diagnosis among persons with AIDS in the United States. Ann Intern Med 2010;153:452–60.

97. Shiels MS, Althoff KN, Pfeiffer RM, et al. HIV infection, immunosuppression, and age at diagnosis of non-AIDS-defining cancers. Clin Infect Dis 2017;64(4):468–75.

98. Intra M, Gentilini O, Brenelli F, et al. Breast cancer among HIV-infected patients: the experience of the European Institute of Oncology. J Surg Oncol 2005;91:141–2.

99. Shiels MS, Cole SR, Kirk GD, et al. A meta-analysis of the incidence of non-AIDS cancers in HIV-infected individuals. J Acquir Immune Defic Syndr 2009;52:611–22.

100. Medapalli RK, Parikh CR, Gordon K, et al. Comorbid diabetes and the risk of progressive chronic kidney disease in HIV-infected adults: data from the Veterans Aging Cohort Study. J Acquir Immune Defic Syndr 2012;60:393–9.

101. Lucas GM, Ross MJ, Stock PG, et al. Clinical practice guideline for the management of chronic kidney disease in patients infected with HIV: 2014 update by the HIV Medicine Association of the Infectious Diseases Society of America. Clin Infect Dis 2014;59:e96–138.

102. Choi AI, Li Y, Deeks SG, et al. Association between kidney function and albuminuria with cardiovascular events in HIV-infected persons. Circulation 2010;121:651–8.

103. Hemmelgarn BR, Manns BJ, Lloyd A, et al. Relation between kidney function, proteinuria, and adverse outcomes. JAMA 2010;303:423–9.

104. Jassal SK, Kritz-Silverstein D, Barrett-Connor E. A prospective study of albuminuria and cognitive function in older adults: the Rancho Bernardo study. Am J Epidemiol 2010;171:277–86.

105. Kalayjian RC, Wu K, Evans S, et al. Proteinuria is associated with neurocognitive impairment in antiretroviral therapy treated HIV-infected individuals. J Acquir Immune Defic Syndr 2014;67:30–5.

106. Abraham AG, Darilay A, McKay H, et al. Kidney dysfunction and markers of inflammation in the multicenter AIDS cohort study. J Infect Dis 2015;212:1100–10.

107. Bruggeman LA, O'Toole JF, Ross MD, et al. Plasma apolipoprotein L1 levels do not correlate with CKD. J Am Soc Nephrol 2014;25:634–44.

108. Shinha T, Mi D, Liu Z, et al. Relationships between renal parameters and serum and urine markers of inflammation in those with and without HIV infection. AIDS Res Hum Retroviruses 2015;31:375–83.

109. Nakatsuji T. High levels of serum soluble CD27 correlated with renal dysfunction. Clin Exp Med 2003;2:192–6.

110. Niewczas MA, Gohda T, Skupien J, et al. Circulating TNF receptors 1 and 2 predict ESRD in type 2 diabetes. J Am Soc Nephrol 2012;23:507–15.

111. Tesch GH. MCP-1/CCL2: a new diagnostic marker and therapeutic target for progressive renal injury in diabetic nephropathy. Am J Physiol Renal Physiol 2008;294:F697–701.

112. Kalayjian RC, Lau B, Mechekano RN, et al. Risk factors for chronic kidney disease in a large cohort of HIV-1 infected individuals initiating antiretroviral therapy in routine care. AIDS 2012;26:1907–15.

113. Marras D, Bruggeman LA, Gao F, et al. Replication and compartmentalization of HIV-1 in kidney epithelium of patients with HIV-associated nephropathy. Nat Med 2002;8:522–6.

114. Lucas GM, Eustace JA, Sozio S, et al. Highly active antiretroviral therapy and the incidence of HIV-1-associated nephropathy: a 12-year cohort study. AIDS 2004;18:541–6.

115. Foster MC, Coresh J, Fornage M, et al. APOL1 variants associate with increased risk of CKD among African Americans. J Am Soc Nephrol 2013;24:1484–91.

116. Genovese G, Friedman DJ, Ross MD, et al. Association of trypanolytic ApoL1 variants with kidney disease in African Americans. Science 2010;329:841–5.

117. Kopp JB, Nelson GW, Sampath K, et al. APOL1 genetic variants in focal segmental glomerulosclerosis and HIV-associated nephropathy. J Am Soc Nephrol 2011;22:2129–37.

118. Wan G, Zhaorigetu S, Liu Z, et al. Apolipoprotein L1, a novel Bcl-2 homology domain 3-only lipid-binding protein, induces autophagic cell death. J Biol Chem 2008;283:21540–9.

119. Olabisi OA, Zhang JY, VerPlank L, et al. APOL1 kidney disease risk variants cause cytotoxicity by depleting cellular potassium and inducing stress-activated protein kinases. Proc Natl Acad Sci U S A 2016;113:830–7.

120. Palella FJ Jr, Baker RK, Moorman AC, et al. Mortality in the highly active antiretroviral therapy era: changing causes of death and disease in the HIV outpatient study. J Acquir Immune Defic Syndr 2006;43:27–34.

121. Macias J, Berenguer J, Japon MA, et al. Fast fibrosis progression between repeated liver biopsies in patients coinfected with human immunodeficiency virus/hepatitis C virus. Hepatology 2009;50:1056–63.

122. Macias J, Berenguer J, Japon MA, et al. Hepatic steatosis and steatohepatitis in human immunodeficiency virus/hepatitis C virus-coinfected patients. Hepatology 2012;56:1261–70.

123. Vinikoor MJ, Sinkala E, Chilengi R, et al. Impact of antiretroviral therapy on liver fibrosis among human immunodeficiency virus-infected adults with and without HBV coinfection in Zambia. Clin Infect Dis 2017;64(10):1343–9.

124. Crum-Cianflone N, Dilay A, Collins G, et al. Nonalcoholic fatty liver disease among HIV-infected persons. J Acquir Immune Defic Syndr 2009;50:464–73.

125. Benhamou Y, Bochet M, Di Martino V, et al. Liver fibrosis progression in human immunodeficiency virus and hepatitis C virus coinfected patients. The Multivirc Group. Hepatology 1999;30:1054–8.

126. Clifford DB, Ances BM. HIV-associated neurocognitive disorder. Lancet Infect Dis 2013;13:976–86.

127. Heaton RK, Franklin DR Jr, Deutsch R, et al. Neurocognitive change in the era of HIV combination antiretroviral therapy: the longitudinal CHARTER study. Clin Infect Dis 2015;60:473–80.

128. Grant I, Franklin DR Jr, Deutsch R, et al. Asymptomatic HIV-associated neurocognitive impairment increases risk for symptomatic decline. Neurology 2014;82:2055–62.

129. Marquine MJ, Montoya JL, Umlauf A, et al. The Veterans Aging Cohort Study (VACS) index and neurocognitive change: a longitudinal study. Clin Infect Dis 2016;63:694–702.

130. Erlandson KM, Wu K, Koletar SL, et al. Frailty and components of the frailty phenotype are associated with modifiable risk factors and antiretroviral therapy. J Infect Dis 2017;215(6):933–7.

131. Imp BM, Rubin LH, Tien PC, et al. Monocyte activation is associated with worse cognitive performance in HIV-infected women with virologic suppression. J Infect Dis 2017;215:114–21.

132. Aaboud M, Aad G, Abbott B, et al. Measurement of the prompt J/[Formula: see text] pair production cross-section in pp collisions at [Formula: see text] TeV with the ATLAS detector. Eur Phys J C Part Fields 2017;77:76.

133. Becker JT, Kingsley L, Mullen J, et al. Vascular risk factors, HIV serostatus, and cognitive dysfunction in gay and bisexual men. Neurology 2009;73:1292–9.
134. Fried LP, Tangen CM, Walston J, et al. Frailty in older adults: evidence for a phenotype. J Gerontol A Biol Sci Med Sci 2001;56:M146–56.
135. Erlandson KM, Schrack JA, Jankowski CM, et al. Functional impairment, disability, and frailty in adults aging with HIV-infection. Curr HIV/AIDS Rep 2014;11:279–90.
136. Ruiz M, Cefalu C. Characteristics of frail patients in a geriatric-HIV program: the experience of an urban academic center at one year follow-up. J Int Assoc Physicians AIDS Care (Chic) 2011;10:138–43.
137. Onen NF, Agbebi A, Shacham E, et al. Frailty among HIV-infected persons in an urban outpatient care setting. J Infect 2009;59:346–52.
138. Piggott DA, Muzaale AD, Mehta SH, et al. Frailty, HIV infection, and mortality in an aging cohort of injection drug users. PLoS One 2013;8:e54910.
139. Oursler KK, Goulet JL, Leaf DA, et al. Association of comorbidity with physical disability in older HIV-infected adults. AIDS Patient Care STDS 2006;20: 782–91.
140. Akgun KM, Tate JP, Crothers K, et al. An adapted frailty-related phenotype and the VACS Index as predictors of hospitalization and mortality in HIV-infected and uninfected individuals. J Acquir Immune Defic Syndr 2014;67(4):397–404.
141. Saum KU, Dieffenbach AK, Jansen EH, et al. Association between oxidative stress and frailty in an elderly German population: results from the ESTHER cohort study. Gerontology 2015;61:407–15.
142. Kanapuru B, Ershler WB. Inflammation, coagulation, and the pathway to frailty. Am J Med 2009;122:605–13.
143. Leng SX, Tian X, Matteini A, et al. IL-6-independent association of elevated serum neopterin levels with prevalent frailty in community-dwelling older adults. Age Ageing 2011;40:475–81.
144. Desquilbet L, Jacobson LP, Fried LP, et al. HIV-1 infection is associated with an earlier occurrence of a phenotype related to frailty. J Gerontol A Biol Sci Med Sci 2007;62:1279–86.
145. Mitnitski A, Collerton J, Martin-Ruiz C, et al. Age-related frailty and its association with biological markers of ageing. BMC Med 2015;13:161.
146. Desquilbet L, Margolick JB, Fried LP, et al. Relationship between a frailty-related phenotype and progressive deterioration of the immune system in HIV-infected men. J Acquir Immune Defic Syndr 2009;50:299–306.
147. Levett TJ, Cresswell FV, Malik MA, et al. Systematic review of prevalence and predictors of frailty in individuals with human immunodeficiency virus. J Am Geriatr Soc 2016;64:1006–14.
148. Erlandson KM, Allshouse AA, Jankowski CM, et al. Association of functional impairment with inflammation and immune activation in HIV type 1-infected adults receiving effective antiretroviral therapy. J Infect Dis 2013;208:249–59.
149. Buggert M, Tauriainen J, Yamamoto T, et al. T-bet and Eomes are differentially linked to the exhausted phenotype of CD8+ T cells in HIV infection. PLoS Pathog 2014;10:e1004251.
150. Bartovska Z, Beran O, Rozsypal H, et al. Antiretroviral treatment of HIV infection does not influence HIV-specific immunity but has an impact on non-specific immune activation. Curr HIV Res 2011;9:88–94.
151. Margolick JB, Bream JH, Martinez-Maza O, et al. Frailty and circulating markers of inflammation in HIV+ and HIV- men in the multicenter AIDS cohort study. J Acquir Immune Defic Syndr 2017;74:407–17.

152. Tinetti ME, Speechley M, Ginter SF. Risk factors for falls among elderly persons living in the community. N Engl J Med 1988;319:1701–7.
153. Grund B, Peng G, Gibert CL, et al. Continuous antiretroviral therapy decreases bone mineral density. AIDS 2009;23:1519–29.
154. Cazanave C, Dupon M, Lavignolle-Aurillac V, et al. Reduced bone mineral density in HIV-infected patients: prevalence and associated factors. AIDS 2008;22: 395–402.
155. Brown TT, Ruppe MD, Kassner R, et al. Reduced bone mineral density in human immunodeficiency virus-infected patients and its association with increased central adiposity and postload hyperglycemia. J Clin Endocrinol Metab 2004; 89:1200–6.
156. Triant VA, Brown TT, Lee H, et al. Fracture prevalence among human immunodeficiency virus (HIV)-infected versus non-HIV-infected patients in a large U.S. healthcare system. J Clin Endocrinol Metab 2008;93:3499–504.
157. Brown TT, Qaqish RB. Antiretroviral therapy and the prevalence of osteopenia and osteoporosis: a meta-analytic review. AIDS 2006;20:2165–74.
158. Sharma A, Shi Q, Hoover DR, et al. increased fracture incidence in middle-aged HIV-infected and HIV-uninfected women: updated results from the women's interagency HIV study. J Acquir Immune Defic Syndr 2015;70:54–61.
159. Young B, Dao CN, Buchacz K, et al. Increased rates of bone fracture among HIV-infected persons in the HIV Outpatient Study (HOPS) compared with the US general population, 2000-2006. Clin Infect Dis 2011;52:1061–8.
160. Prieto-Alhambra D, Guerri-Fernandez R, De Vries F, et al. HIV infection and its association with an excess risk of clinical fractures: a nationwide case-control study. J Acquir Immune Defic Syndr 2014;66:90–5.
161. Bolland MJ, Grey AB, Gamble GD, et al. CLINICAL Review #: low body weight mediates the relationship between HIV infection and low bone mineral density: a meta-analysis. J Clin Endocrinol Metab 2007;92:4522–8.
162. Kooij KW, Wit FW, Bisschop PH, et al. Low bone mineral density in patients with well-suppressed HIV infection: association with body weight, smoking, and prior advanced HIV disease. J Infect Dis 2015;211:539–48.
163. Staples CT Jr, Rimland D, Dudas D. Hepatitis C in the HIV (human immunodeficiency virus) Atlanta V.A. (Veterans Affairs Medical Center) cohort study (HAVACS): the effect of coinfection on survival. Clin Infect Dis 1999;29:150–4.
164. Wunder DM, Bersinger NA, Fux CA, et al. Hypogonadism in HIV-1-infected men is common and does not resolve during antiretroviral therapy. Antivir Ther 2007; 12:261–5.
165. Teichmann J, Lange U, Discher T, et al. Bone mineral density in human immunodeficiency virus-1 infected men with hypogonadism prior to highly-active-antiretroviral-therapy (HAART). Eur J Med Res 2009;14:59–64.
166. Allavena C, Delpierre C, Cuzin L, et al. High frequency of vitamin D deficiency in HIV-infected patients: effects of HIV-related factors and antiretroviral drugs. J Antimicrob Chemother 2012;67:2222–30.
167. Beaupere C, Garcia M, Larghero J, et al. The HIV proteins Tat and Nef promote human bone marrow mesenchymal stem cell senescence and alter osteoblastic differentiation. Aging Cell 2015;14:534–46.
168. Chew N, Tan E, Li L, et al. HIV-1 tat and rev upregulates osteoclast bone resorption. J Int AIDS Soc 2014;17:19724.
169. Brown TT, McComsey GA, King MS, et al. Loss of bone mineral density after antiretroviral therapy initiation, independent of antiretroviral regimen. J Acquir Immune Defic Syndr 2009;51:554–61.

170. Brown TT, Moser C, Currier JS, et al. Changes in bone mineral density after initiation of antiretroviral treatment with tenofovir disoproxil fumarate/emtricitabine plus atazanavir/ritonavir, darunavir/ritonavir, or raltegravir. J Infect Dis 2015; 212:1241–9.

171. McComsey GA, Kitch D, Daar ES, et al. Bone mineral density and fractures in antiretroviral-naive persons randomized to receive abacavir-lamivudine or tenofovir disoproxil fumarate-emtricitabine along with efavirenz or atazanavir-ritonavir: AIDS Clinical Trials Group A5224s, a substudy of ACTG A5202. J Infect Dis 2011;203:1791–801.

172. Bernardino JI, Mocroft A, Mallon PW, et al. Bone mineral density and inflammatory and bone biomarkers after darunavir-ritonavir combined with either raltegravir or tenofovir-emtricitabine in antiretroviral-naive adults with HIV-1: a substudy of the NEAT001/ANRS143 randomised trial. Lancet HIV 2015;2:e464–73.

173. Mofenson LM, Brady MT, Danner SP, et al. Guidelines for the prevention and treatment of opportunistic infections among HIV-exposed and HIV-infected children: recommendations from CDC, the National Institutes of Health, the HIV Medicine Association of the Infectious Diseases Society of America, the Pediatric Infectious Diseases Society, and the American Academy of Pediatrics. MMWR Recomm Rep 2009;58:1–166.

174. Aberg JA, Gallant JE, Ghanem KG, et al. Primary care guidelines for the management of persons infected with HIV: 2013 update by the HIV Medicine Association of the Infectious Diseases Society of America. Clin Infect Dis 2014;58: 1–10.

175. Moyer VA, U.S. Preventive Services Task Force. Screening for lung cancer: U.S. Preventive Services Task Force recommendation statement. Ann Intern Med 2014;160:330–8.

176. Moyer VA, U.S. Preventive Services Task Force. Screening for prostate cancer: U.S. Preventive Services Task Force recommendation statement. Ann Intern Med 2012;157:120–34.

177. Reddy KP, Parker RA, Losina E, et al. Impact of cigarette smoking and smoking cessation on life expectancy among people with HIV: a US-based modeling study. J Infect Dis 2016;214:1672–81.

178. Helleberg M, May MT, Ingle SM, et al. Smoking and life expectancy among HIV-infected individuals on antiretroviral therapy in Europe and North America. AIDS 2015;29:221–9.

179. Forde C, Loy A, O'Dea S, et al. Physical activity is associated with metabolic health in men living with HIV. AIDS Behav 2017. [Epub ahead of print].

180. Fazeli PL, Marquine MJ, Dufour C, et al. Physical activity is associated with better neurocognitive and everyday functioning among older adults with HIV disease. AIDS Behav 2015;19:1470–7.

181. Greene M, Covinsky KE, Valcour V, et al. Geriatric syndromes in older HIV-infected adults. J Acquir Immune Defic Syndr 2015;69:161–7.

182. Greene M, Justice AC, Lampiris HW, et al. Management of human immunodeficiency virus infection in advanced age. JAMA 2013;309:1397–405.

183. Erlandson KM, Guaraldi G, Falutz J. More than osteoporosis: age-specific issues in bone health. Curr Opin HIV AIDS 2016;11:343–50.

184. Kanis JA, Oden A, Johansson H, et al. FRAX and its applications to clinical practice. Bone 2009;44:734–43.

185. Calmy A, Fux CA, Norris R, et al. Low bone mineral density, renal dysfunction, and fracture risk in HIV infection: a cross-sectional study. J Infect Dis 2009; 200:1746–54.

186. Brown TT, Hoy J, Borderi M, et al. Recommendations for evaluation and management of bone disease in HIV. Clin Infect Dis 2015;60:1242–51.
187. Niderost S, Imhof C. Aging with HIV in the era of antiretroviral treatment: living conditions and the quality of life of people aged above 50 living with HIV/AIDS in Switzerland. Gerontol Geriatr Med 2016;2. 2333721416636300.

Herpes Zoster in the Older Adult

Amrita R. John, MBBS[a], David H. Canaday, MD[b],*

KEYWORDS

- Older adults • Shingles • Zoster • Postherpetic neuralgia • Vaccination

KEY POINTS

- The incidence of herpes zoster has been increasing over the past several decades, with older adults disproportionately affected.
- Although postherpetic neuralgia gradually resolves in most older adults, there is a subset of patients who are refractory to pain management and in whom the pain continues to worsen over time.
- For 3 to 12 months after an episode of herpes zoster, individuals older than 50 years are at higher risk for stroke or myocardial infarction compared with the general population.
- Antiviral therapy is indicated in patients greater than 50 years of age.
- The current commercially available live-attenuated vaccine for the prevention of shingles shows significant declines in efficacy 7 to 10 years after vaccination.

INTRODUCTION

Primary infection with varicella zoster virus (VZV) causes chicken pox, a self-limited disease that is characterized by disseminated skins lesions and occurs mostly in childhood. Herpes zoster (HZ), which is also known as shingles, is the result of reactivation of latent VZV and occurs more frequently in older adults and immunocompromised individuals.

EPIDEMIOLOGY

The incidence of HZ has been increasing over the past several decades. Some studies indicate more than a 4-fold increase since the 1940s affecting elderly people and

Disclosure Statement: A. John: None. D.H. Canaday: Seqirus, Merck, Sanofi Pasteur: Grant investigator/recipient.
[a] Division of Infectious Diseases and HIV Medicine, Department of Medicine, Case Western Reserve University, Cleveland, OH 44106, USA; [b] Geriatric Research Education and Clinical Center (GRECC), Louis Stokes Cleveland Department of Veterans Affairs Medical Center (LSCVAMC), Cleveland, OH 44106, USA
* Corresponding author. GRECC Louis Stokes Cleveland VA Medical Center, 10701 East Boulevard, Cleveland, OH 44106.
E-mail address: David.Canaday@case.edu

women disproportionately.[1] The rising incidence rate appears to be a global phenomenon, occurring independent of demographic shifts seen with a growing elderly population and increasing prevalence of immunocompromised individuals.[1–3]

North American database studies indicate that this increase in incidence of HZ started even before the introduction of the varicella vaccine, debunking the theory that the increase was due to older individuals no longer having the immunologic boosting from periodic community exposure to children with chickenpox (Hope-Simpson hypothesis).[2,4,5]

The lifetime risk of HZ in the general population ranges from 20% to 30%, but the risk increases dramatically after 50 years of age with a lifetime risk of HZ reaching 50% at age 85 years. Current estimates point to more than 1 million cases of HZ in the United States every year, costing the US health care system 5 billion USD annually.[6–8] HZ, originally not thought to occur more than once in an individual, is now estimated to recur in approximately 6.4% of immunocompetent people. The recurrence rate is higher among the immunocompromised population.[2,6,9,10]

PATHOGENESIS

VZV is a double-stranded DNA human neurotrophic alphaherpesvirus. The primary infection, or chickenpox, might be subclinical or present with fever and vesicular lesions. At this time, VZV establishes a latent state in dorsal root ganglia of peripheral neurons, cranial nerve ganglia, and autonomic nerve ganglia along the entire neuroaxis through retrograde axonal transport from the cutaneous lesions or by hematogenous spread during the viremic phase.[7,11] Months to years later, reactivation of VZV manifests clinically as HZ, with the spectrum of disease ranging from disseminated zoster to the more commonly seen typical dermatomal HZ.

During the period of latency, VZV downregulates gene expression and in turn the production of major histocompatibility complex I antigen on the surface of infected cells.[12] Reactivation occurs when VZV is able to overpower immune controls and spreads through the affected ganglions and nerves to reach the skin and manifest as HZ.[7,12,13]

Risk factors for reactivation of VZV include older age and immunocompromised status from such conditions as HIV-1 infection, lymphoma, leukemia, bone marrow transplant, solid organ transplant, and immunosuppressive medications. One mechanism of reactivation from these risk factors is decreased VZV-specific cell-mediated immunity.[14] There are data associating depression with development of HZ. Weight loss and sleep disturbances were also found to be associated with risk of VZV recurrence independent of depression as a risk factor. Other risk factors include Caucasian race, female sex, physical trauma, diabetes mellitus, and a prior history of HZ. Finally, a family history of HZ increases risk in a dose-dependent manner; the greater the number of relatives affected, particularly first-degree relatives, the higher the risk of HZ for an individual in that family.[5,6,15]

CLINICAL FEATURES

Classically, reactivation of VZV presents as a unilateral dermatomal rash (ie, does not cross the midline), which is initially maculopapular on an erythematous base, evolves into a vesicular-pustular appearance, which after 7 to 10 days begins to crust over and heals within 2 to 4 weeks. It can either be limited to a single dermatome or occur over adjacent dermatomes depending on the distribution of the sensory ganglia where reactivation occurs.[16] In older adults, the rash may have an atypical appearance and may be limited to a small patch within the dermatome, or have a maculopapular appearance without evolving into vesicles.[6] The onset of the rash is often preceded by neuropathic pain (aching, burning, lancinating) over the involved dermatome or dermatomes. This prodromal phase can result in a diagnostic dilemma for the physician because it may mimic other painful conditions in older adults, such as migraine headaches, trigeminal neuralgia, myocardial infarction, biliary or renal colic, appendicitis, lumbosacral pain, or muscle strain. The presence of very sensitive skin could clue the physician that this is HZ. This prodromal phase may be associated with systemic symptoms of fever, fatigue, headache, malaise, and photophobia. In some cases, the prodromal phase is not followed by the development of rash; this is termed zoster sine herpete.[16,17]

Between 2.5% and 20% of people with HZ present as herpes zoster ophthalmicus (HZO), which occurs when the VZV reactivation involves the ophthalmic branch of the trigeminal nerve.[18,19] Because the cranial nerve V1 also innervates the skin over the nose, the presence of a cutaneous lesion at the tip of the nose, referred to as Hutchinson sign, is highly predictive of ocular involvement.[7] Eye manifestations include periorbital cutaneous lesions, conjunctival injection and chemosis, keratitis, corneal ulceration, uveitis, scleritis, episcleritis, glaucoma, retinal necrosis, and optic neuritis. Keratitis remains the most commonly seen complication. Acute retinal necrosis (ARN), however, is associated with greater morbidity and occurs in both immunocompetent and immunocompromised hosts. ARN is a full-thickness patchy rapid necrosis of the retina presenting with periorbital pain, floaters, and almost always permanent peripheral vision loss. In the immunocompromised host, progressive outer retinal necrosis (PORN) occurs and, although similar to ARN, often presents as sudden onset of painless vision loss, floaters, and constricted visual fields with retinal detachment. PORN may be preceded by zoster ophthalmicus, retrobulbar neuritis, aseptic meningitis, and/or central retinal artery occlusion. PORN may present concurrently with VZV vasculopathy, which is discussed in greater detail in later discussion.[7,19]

HZ may manifest as cranial neuritis, with an array of clinical presentations depending on the cranial nerve affected. HZ neuritis involving cranial nerves III, IV, and VI may present with ophthalmoplegia and/or ptosis; involvement of branches V2 and V3 of the trigeminal nerve may rarely present with osteonecrosis and spontaneous tooth loss. Ramsey-Hunt syndrome describes involvement of cranial nerve VII, which presents as an ipsilateral facial palsy with lesions in the external auditory meatus and tympanic membrane or on the ipsilateral anterior two-thirds of the tongue and hard palate. Involvement of cranial nerve VIII may occur simultaneously, with symptoms of nausea, vomiting, hearing loss, tinnitus, vertigo, and nystagmus.[7,13] HZ of cranial nerves XI, X, and IX presents as odynophagia, dysphagia, hoarseness, dysgeusia, hemilaryngeal or hemipharyngeal paresis.[20] HZ involving the cervical or lumbar nerve roots may result in radiculopathy. Rarely, cervical zoster may result in diaphragmatic weakness, and thoracic zoster can result in abdominal wall weakness and herniation.[7]

VZV myelitis, which is characterized by paresis of the extremities, bowel and/or bladder incontinence, and sensory deficits, has 2 types of clinical presentation. In immunocompetent hosts, it is usually self-limited and occurs days to weeks after acute varicella or zoster. In the immunocompromised host, VZV myelitis is more likely have a poor outcome associated with disability and even death.[7,13]

VZV recurrence can also present as encephalitis and meningitis. Patients usually present with altered mental status and focal neurologic deficits. Seizures are rarely seen, and a third of patients may not have a rash. Even with effective treatment, the mortality ranges from 9% to 20%, and survivors might be left with residual deficits, such as slowing of cognitive processes, memory loss, and emotional disturbances.[13]

There are also instances of VZV recurrence affecting viscera resulting in pancreatitis, hepatitis, and gastritis. Visceral zoster is thought to be due to reactivation in dorsal root and/or autonomic ganglia followed by transaxonal spread via post–ganglionic fibers to the organ being supplied. It should be considered in persons with current or recent cutaneous zoster if their clinical or laboratory parameters suggest internal organ involvement and polymerase chain reaction (PCR) in blood, histologic, or culture data supports the presence of VZV.[11,21–24]

Disseminated HZ is defined as the presence of 20 or more vesicles outside the area of the primary and adjacent dermatomes or the involvement of 3 or more dermatomes. Both disseminated and visceral zosters are more common in immunocompromised individuals; however, there have been case reports of visceral VZV in the immunocompetent host as well.[22]

POSTZOSTER SEQUELAE

One of the hallmarks of HZ is that after resolution of the vesicular rash, individuals may experience additional sequelae. For older adults in particular, these may have adverse effects on functional status, independence, and quality of life. The postzoster sequelae are discussed later.

Postherpetic Neuralgia

A consensus definition for postherpetic neuralgia (PHN) is still to be determined, because definitions to date have been arbitrary ranging from 1 month to 6 months after rash onset. The conventional definition is "pain continuing 90 days past the diagnosis of HZ or rash onset."[25] Because of this lack of a consensus definition and the varying age ranges of the populations being studied, the incidence of PHN after HZ ranges from 5% to 30% and occurs in 50% of HZ affected individuals greater than 85 years.[2,3,5,26–28] It is considered the most debilitating sequelae of HZ because it impairs the affected individual's quality of life across all 4 health domains: physical, psychological, functional, and social.[27]

Risk factors for the development of PHN include prodromal symptoms, severity of pain and rash extent, older age, immunosuppression, diabetes, and presence of zoster ophthalmicus. Although PHN gradually resolves in most older adults, there is a subset of patients who are refractory to pain management and in whom the pain lingers or even continues to worsen over time. Some might have a temporary cessation of pain only to have it return weeks to months later.[29,30]

The pain might be constant, intermittent, or stimulus driven. Some describe it as burning, throbbing, stabbing, or shooting. The most debilitating is allodynia, which occurs when normal tactile experiences (clothes, wind, and so forth) cause severe pain. Besides suffering from the various subtypes of pain, the person may also develop anxiety, depression, weight loss, sleep disturbances, or social isolation and have difficulty with their activities of daily living. The Zoster Brief Pain Inventory is a useful tool in the evaluation of PHN.[12,31]

Secondary Bacterial Infection

Secondary bacterial infection needs to be suspected if there is no resolution of clinical symptoms within 1 to 2 weeks and the rash appears to worsen. Secondary bacterial infection is often due to Staphylococcal or Streptococcal infection, and if not diagnosed early, can rarely lead to septicemia.[16,32] In HZO, this may present with yellowish drainage and crusting from the eye.[33]

Other Dermatologic Complications

A wide range of benign and malignant lesions rarely can develop months to years later at the site of previous cutaneous HZ. These dermatological complications include postzoster granulomatous dermatitis, granulomatous vasculitis, atypical lymphoid proliferation, dermatophytosis, lymphoplasmacytoid lymphoma, T-cell lymphoma, leukemia cutis, Kaposi sarcoma, and pseudolymphoma.[34]

Residual Neurologic Manifestations of Varicella Zoster Virus

Neurologic signs and symptoms can present during the active phase of the VZV primary infection (chickenpox) or reactivation disease (HZ) and as chronic residual deficits after an episode of VZV encephalitis or meningitis. Central nervous system (CNS) manifestations of HZ in adults can result in outcomes ranging from complete recovery to deficits, such as loss of memory, impaired executive functioning, learning difficulties with severe disability, and death. Transverse myelitis can occur either during the acute infection or as postinfectious sequelae. Mortality from transverse myelitis is reported at 23% and almost always occurs in the immunocompromised host. HZ can also result in polyneuropathy and in Guillain-Barré syndrome.[13]

Varicella Zoster Virus Vasculopathy

Population studies indicate that for 3 to 12 months after an episode of HZ, individuals older than 50 years are at higher risk for stroke or myocardial infarction compared with the general population, even after adjusting for other variables. The presence of VZV in intracerebral and coronary arteries of these patients in postmortem studies provides histologic support for this finding.[11,13,35,36] Vasculopathy results from the transaxonal migration of reactivated VZV to the adventia of arteries where infection is established, followed by transmural migration to the media and intima and vascular remodeling.[37] The presence of VZV in the arteries, in conjunction with the increased inflammatory response seen in infected individuals, might result in disruption of atherosclerotic plaques.[7,38] In some instances, VZV vasculopathy may result in cardiac dysfunction without any concomitant neurologic manifestation.[11]

Manifestations of VZV CNS vasculopathy range from transient ischemic attacks, stroke (ischemic or hemorrhagic), aneurysm, subarachnoid and intracerebral hemorrhage, spinal cord infarction, cerebral venous sinus thrombosis, vision loss, giant cell temporal arteritis, or other focal neurologic deficits depending on the location of the infarction.[7,13] The mortality of untreated VZV CNS vasculopathy approaches 25%; treatment with antivirals may be curative.[7,35,39] It is difficult to assess the incidence of stroke secondary to VZV vasculopathy because in most elderly patients, it is presumed to be due to atherosclerotic disease and cerebrospinal fluid (CSF) is not routinely analyzed.[13]

DIAGNOSIS

In most patients, the history and classic dermatomal appearance of the rash permits a clinical diagnosis of HZ. Laboratory-based diagnostic tools can be used for confirmation in patients with atypical clinical presentations for HZ.[40] Of all clinical specimens, the yield from early vesicular lesions is the greatest.[12,41] If vesicular fluid cannot be obtained, other acceptable alternatives include lesion scrapings, crusts, tissue biopsy, saliva, CSF, and blood.[6,12]

VZV DNA PCR has the highest sensitivity and specificity and has become the gold standard for diagnosis. The reverse transcription-PCR assay used in the Shingles

Prevention Study detected as few as 7 copies of the VZV-Wild Type or the VZV-Oka genome and had sensitivity close to 100%.[42] Quantitative PCR is available in most commercial laboratories and provides a rapid and timely diagnostic test. A positive PCR in CSF is indicative of CNS HZ. A positive salivary VZV DNA PCR supports the diagnosis of enteric zoster.[43] Positive VZV DNA PCR from blood or from oropharyngeal samples is useful when the patient has an atypical presentation and/or has zoster sine herpete.[44]

VZV culture is very specific, but the result might take 1 to 2 weeks. Also, the sensitivity ranges from 30% to 75%.[40,45] Serologic tests may show an increase in antibody titers against VZV during an episode of HZ, but it is not a sensitive or specific diagnostic method. Commercial enzyme-linked immunosorbent assay tests for detection of VZV-specific serum antibody have a sensitivity of 66% to 97% and specificity of 82% to 99%.[45,46]

For patients with potential neurologic involvement, serologic studies of CSF may improve diagnostic accuracy. In active CNS HZ, CSF studies show elevated protein level with positive VZV DNA PCR and/or anti-VZV immunoglobulin G (IgG). In VZV CNS vasculopathy, definitive diagnosis depends on detection of anti-VZV IgG in CSF, because VZV DNA PCR from CSF is often negative. A low serum/CSF ratio of anti-VZV IgG can also be supportive of ongoing CNS VZV infection and CNS vasculopathy.[13,39] The presence of an MRI or computed tomographic scan showing evidence of infarction along with supporting CSF studies is essential for a diagnosis of VZV CNS vasculopathy.[45]

The Tzanck smear was one of the earliest diagnostic tools for VZV. Developed by a French dermatologist in 1947, it involves deroofing the vesicle, scraping the base with a sterile blade, and smearing the material onto a clean glass slide. The specimen is then air dried, fixed with methanol, stained with either methylene blue, Giemsa, or Wright's stain, and examined for the presence of multinucleated giant cells and intranuclear inclusions, which might indicate the presence of VZV. However, these cannot be differentiated from herpes simplex virus (HSV).[47] The modified Tzanck technique allows for the staining of the smear with fluorescein-conjugated monoclonal antibodies to differentiate between VZV and HSV. Antigen detection via immunofluorescence has almost entirely been replaced by PCR.[45]

TREATMENT

Treatment can be broken down into treatment of the virus with antivirals and treatment of the sequelae of infection with other agents. **Table 1** lists the various classes of agents used to treat HZ and PHN that are discussed later.

Antiviral Agents

Antiviral therapy for acute HZ[48] is indicated in patients fulfilling any of these criteria: (1) with age greater than 50 years, (2) with moderate to severe rash or pain, (3) with nontruncal involvement, and (4) being immunocompromised.[40] Antivirals initiated within 72 hours of rash onset decrease the duration of viral shedding, new lesion formation, and the severity and duration of acute pain. Experts recommend initiating antiviral therapy more than 72 hours after rash onset if there is evidence of new lesion formation, or when there are motor, neurologic, or ocular complications.[6,40] Hospitalization for closer monitoring and treatment with intravenous acyclovir should be considered in (1) allogenic stem cell transplant recipients, especially those within the first 4 months of transplant; (2) hematopoietic stem cell transplant recipients with moderate to severe graft-versus-host disease; (3) transplant recipients on aggressive antirejection

Table 1
Pharmacologic therapies used in the treatment of herpes zoster and postherpetic neuralgia

Analgesic Agents	HZ	PHN	Recommended Dose
Acyclovir (oral)	+	–	800 mg 5 times daily for 7–10 d
Famciclovir (oral)	+	–	500 mg every 8 h for 7 d
Valacyclovir (oral)	+	–	1 g every 8 h for 7 d
Brivudine (oral)	+	–	125 mg once daily for 7 d. Product licensed in various countries; *not currently available in the United States*
Acyclovir (IV)	+	–	10–15 mg/kg every 8 h until clinical improvement; switch to oral regimen to complete a 10- to 14-d course when formation of new lesions has ceased and signs/symptoms of visceral infection are improving
Foscarnet (intravenous [IV])	+	–	40 mg/kg every 8 h for 7–10 d.[24] *Not approved for this indication by the FDA*
Cidofovir (IV)	+	–	5 mg/kg every week for 2 wk, followed by or 5 mg/kg every other week[76]To be used if patient fails or relapses after therapy with foscarnet. *Not approved for this indication by the FDA*
Anti-inflammatory agents			
Prednisone (oral)	+	–	60 mg daily for 7 d, followed by 30 mg daily for 7 d, then 15 mg daily for 7 d
Intrathecal methylprednisone	–	±	Reserved for intractable PHN due to risk profile. *Not currently available in the United States*
Analgesic agents			
Acetaminophen	+	–	Used for mild pain
NSAIDs	+	–	Used for mild pain
Oxycodone	1st line	3rd line	5 mg every 4 h as needed, carefully titrate upwards by 5 mg 4 times daily every 2 d for pain control. Dosage needs to be converted to a long-acting opioid analgesic and combined with a short-acting medication for breakthrough pain

(continued on next page)

Table 1
(continued)

Analgesic Agents	HZ	PHN	Recommended Dose
Tramadol	±	3rd line	50 mg once or twice daily, increase by 50–100 mg daily in divided doses every 2 d as tolerated. Maximum dose of 400 mg daily or 300 mg daily if older than 75 y
Gabapentin	2nd line	2nd line	300 mg at bedtime or 100–300 mg 3 times daily, increase by 100–300 mg 3 times daily every 2 d as tolerated. Maximum dose of 3600 mg daily
Pregabalin	2nd line	2nd line	75 mg at bedtime or 75 mg twice daily, increase by 75 mg twice daily every 3 d as tolerated. Maximum dose is 600 mg daily
Nortriptyline	3rd line	2nd line	10–25 mg at bedtime, increase by 10–25 mg every 3–7 days as tolerated. Maximum dose 150 mg daily. TCAs have similar efficacy to gabapentin or pregabalin, but cause more serious adverse events[31]
Venlafaxine	±	±	37.5 mg daily, titrate upwards by 75 mg each week over a 4- to 6-wk period. Maximum dose of 225 mg/d. *Used if unable to tolerate TCA side-effect profile; however not as well studied as TCAs. *Not approved for this indication by the FDA[54]*
Duloxetine	±	±	20 mg at bedtime, increase dose by 20 mg every 5 d. Maximum dose 60 mg daily. *Used if unable to tolerate TCA side-effect profile; however not as well studied as TCAs. *Not approved for this indication by the FDA[54]*
Topical analgesic agents			
Lidocaine 5% patch	±	1st line	One patch can be applied to the location of pain. Up to 3 patches can be used at the same time. Current FDA recommendation limits use to 12 h in a 24 h period.
Capsaicin 0.075% cream	−	±	Apply 4 times per day
Capsaicin 8% patch	−	±	Application time of 30–90 min

+, Definitely can be used for this indication; ±, May be used for this indication if no other alternative is present, minimal supportive data present; −, Avoid using for this indication, no supportive data present.

therapy; (4) any individual with suspected visceral dissemination (encephalitis/pneumonitis); and (5) individuals with HZO or VZV retinitis.[13,40,45]

Also, closer monitoring for disease progression and response to therapy should be considered for frail elderly individuals because they have markedly diminished physiologic reserves to deal with stressors and may be noncompliant with the prescribed oral therapy because of a combination of fatigue, pain, confusion, poor appetite, and overall functional decline associated with the acute disease process.[16,40]

Acyclovir, famciclovir, and valacyclovir are guanosine analogues that are phosphorylated by viral thymidine kinase to a triphosphate form that inhibits VZV DNA polymerase. In head-to-head comparisons, there is no difference among acyclovir, famciclovir, and valacyclovir in treatment end points. They also have a similar side-effect profile; however, ease of dosing, bioavailability, and cost need to be factored in when choosing an agent.[40] Valacyclovir has greater oral bioavailability (around 55%) when compared with acyclovir (10%–20%) and is more convenient to dose.[13]

Cases of acyclovir-resistant VZV have been reported in the immunocompromised host, so the possibility of resistance should be considered if the HZ lesions appear to be atypical in nature and are not showing response despite adequate antiviral therapy. If resistance is suspected, testing for mutations in thymidine kinase gene can be sent and the patient switched to intravenous foscarnet or cidofovir.[40]

Corticosteroids

Corticosteroids improve the pain associated with acute HZ and can be used for this purpose after consideration is given to relative contraindications, such as hypertension, diabetes mellitus, glaucoma, osteoporosis, and peptic ulcer disease.[40] However, a meta-analysis indicated that corticosteroids given during acute HZ neither reduce the incidence of PHN after an episode of HZ nor reduce the duration of PHN.[49] Some clinicians use steroids in cases of VZV-induced facial paralysis and cranial polyneuritis to decrease inflammation and swelling and reduce risk of residual peripheral nerve damage, a practice supported by minimal data.[50–52] If used, steroids should always be used in conjunction with antivirals.[6] Intrathecal methylprednisolone was effective in reducing the pain of PHN; however, because of the invasive nature and possible risk of arachnoiditis, it should be considered only after other less invasive options have failed.[53] Methylprednisolone is not approved for intrathecal administration by the US Food and Drug Administration (FDA), and preservative-free methylprednisolone is not currently available in the United States.

Analgesics

Mild pain of HZ can be treated with acetaminophen and nonsteroidal anti-inflammatory drugs (NSAIDs). Acetaminophen and NSAIDs are unlikely to provide pain relief in PHN, although they are first-line agents for pain control in acute HZ. Severe pain of acute HZ might benefit from opioid analgesics. Opioids, although used for PHN, are not approved by the FDA for this indication, and at present, are considered third-line agents for symptom relief in PHN along with tramadol.[6,31] For more severe acute HZ, one should consider initiating control with short-acting opioid agents. Once an effective dose is achieved, then switch to a long-acting opioid agent for more consistent pain relief and dosing convenience. A provision for short-acting agents for breakthrough pain should be in place alongside the long-acting agents. Tramadol is an alternative agent that is a weak μ-opioid antagonist that can be used in the treatment of PHN and HZ. However, it is associated with an increased seizure risk and needs to be avoided in those with a history of seizures and in people who are on medication that lowers their seizure threshold. It also can cause serotonin syndrome in patients on selective serotonin reuptake inhibitor antidepressants.[6,40]

Tricyclic Antidepressants

Tricyclic antidepressants (TCAs) have a role in pain control in both acute HZ and PHN.[24] Although several studies indicate that amitriptyline significantly reduces the pain of PHN, nortriptyline and desipramine are preferred because of their better anticholinergic side effect.[6] Before initiation of therapy with TCAs, an electrocardiogram can screen for prolonged QTc interval.[40] There are some data to suggest that those unable to tolerate the side effects of TCAs could use the selective serotonin and norepinephrine reuptake inhibitor antidepressants, such as venlafaxine and duloxetine, for management of pain and depression that is associated with chronic PHN.[40,54]

Gabapentin/Pregabalin

Classified as anticonvulsants, gabapentin and pregabalin have a role in neuropathic pain relief in both acute HZ and PHN.[40] If acute HZ pain persists even after treatment with antivirals, analgesics, and corticosteroids, gabapentin or pregabalin may help. In PHN, gabapentin or pregabalin is preferred to the use of TCAs or opioids, especially in the elderly. Administering these medications in the evening may reduce some of the side effects, including somnolence, dizziness, and ataxia. The dose can subsequently be increased in frequency and/or amount to achieve pain control. There is the possibility that increasing doses of gabapentin or pregabalin may lead to cognitive impairment among the frail elderly, and in this situation, it is advisable to discontinue the medication.[6] There is currently a randomized placebo-controlled trial to evaluate the effectiveness of gabapentin in the prevention of PHN.[27]

Topical Therapy

Topical lidocaine is one of the best tolerated options for pain control in PHN. It is easily administered and has minimal systemic absorption. Up to 3 patches can be applied locally over a 12-hour period.[6,31] There are few studies on the use of topical lidocaine in the treatment of acute pain of HZ, primarily because of concerns of further local damage to the area with the rash and risk of increased systemic toxicity. A randomized controlled trial has shown that the lidocaine patch can provide significant pain relief in acute HZ, but care should to taken to ensure that it is applied only to the area of intact skin.[24,55] Topical capsaicin is an effective backup alternative in the treatment of PHN.[31] Unfortunately, most patients find the burning sensation from capsaicin intolerable, so it is not recommended for acute pain from HZ.[45]

Regional or Local Anesthetic Nerve Blocks

A meta-analysis by the International Association for the Study of Pain and the Special Interest Group on Neuropathic Pain gave a weak recommendation to use for epidural or paravertebral local anesthetic and steroid nerve blocks as a symptomatic treatment of relief of acute pain associated with HZ.[56] The absence of rigorous randomized controlled trials in the area of interventional management of neuropathic pain associated with HZ and PHN make it difficult to provide a strong evidence-based recommendation. When used to treat PHN, very few elderly patients achieved sustained pain relief.[6,56] Accordingly, nerve blocks tend to be used only when acute HZ pain is not relieved despite the use of antivirals, oral analgesics, steroids, and all adjuvant agents mentioned above.

Herpes Zoster Ophthalmicus Therapy

When HZO is suspected, ophthalmology should be involved in the care of the patient. The standard duration of treatment with antivirals remains 7 to 10 days; however, in elderly patients, VZV DNA persists on the cornea for up to 30 days. Accordingly, older adults and immunocompromised hosts may need a longer course of treatment, although there are no clinical trials done in this regard.[19] If corneal involvement is noted, artificial tears may improve lubrication, and erythromycin ointment may prevent secondary infection. Topical steroids must be used judiciously and only in consultation with an ophthalmologist. Although they have utility in management of stromal keratitis, uveitis, and scleritis/episcleritis, imprudent use of topical steroids can worsen corneal disease and result in corneal ulceration and perforation.[19]

PREVENTION

HZ with vesicular lesions can be contagious, leading to chickenpox in the seronegative, nonimmune persons via direct contact as well as airborne and droplet nuclei. The risk for transmission is greatest when the lesions are still in the maculopapular/vesicular phase and disappears once they have crusted over.[6] Covering the lesions until they have crusted over can be a primary prevention measure to nonimmune or immunocompromised contacts.

Currently, there is one commercially available live attenuated vaccine (Zostavax, Merck) for the prevention of shingles. It is the same strain as the vaccine used for primary prevention of chickenpox but at a 14 times higher dose.[13] In large study of persons over the age of 60, the live-attenuated zoster vaccine reduced the incidence of HZ by 51% and PHN by 66%.[57] Since 2008, the US Advisory Committee on Immunization Practices recommends Zostavax for immunocompetent people older than 60 years. The FDA initially approved the vaccine for those older than 60 years and later licensed it to include those aged 50 and older.[1,5,58] Longitudinal studies of older adults indicate that 7 to 10 years after the vaccine is administered, its efficacy declines to 21% for the prevention of HZ, 35% for the prevention of PHN, and 37% for HZ Burden of Illness. This waning efficacy had led to concerns that if given to early that individuals may not be protected at the age when the incidence of HZ is the highest.[58,59] A booster dose given 10 years after the first dose of Zostavax enhanced VZV-specific cell-mediated immunity.[58,60] There is currently however no recommendation to boost the vaccine. Perhaps there will be a future recommendation after obtaining more data about the timing and potential benefits of boosting.

There has been a poor uptake of this vaccine, with only 24% of US adults older than 60 years having had Zostavax in 2013.[13,57,59,61,62] Although the proportion of the population vaccinated for HZ has increased from 2007, it is still less than the goal of 30% of the target population from Healthy People 2020. Women, those older than 65 years, and non-Hispanic whites were all more likely to be vaccinated for HZ.[63] Also, the chances of being vaccinated were directly proportional to the frequency of outpatient hospital/physician/pharmacy visits and inversely proportional to the number of emergency room and/or inpatient visits. Cost of the vaccine and reimbursement remains one of the top barriers in the uptake of this vaccine.[58,63]

CURRENT DEVELOPMENTS

The herpes zoster subunit vaccine (HZ/su) is under review at the FDA for potential licensure after finishing 2 large phase 3 trials. It contains recombinant VZV glycoprotein E and liposome-based $AS01_B$ adjuvant. The vaccine is a 2-dose series with a booster at 2 months after the primary dose. It was studied in a double-blinded randomized placebo-controlled trial in adults greater than the age of 70 years in 18 different countries. Unlike the currently available live-attenuated vaccine, the efficacy of the HZ/su vaccine was 97% for HZ and 89% for PHN, and it was similar across all age groups, showing no significant decline in protection in those aged 70 and older.[64–66] There are no data available yet for this vaccine on longer-term protection beyond the 3.7-year analysis in those studies. The subunit vaccine is also immunogenic and safe in people that have had a previous episode of HZ.[67]

The subunit vaccine is also showing considerable promise in immunocompromised populations, such as HIV-infected individuals and adults, after autologous hematopoietic stem cell transplant. Before the era of highly active antiretroviral therapy (HAART), HIV-infected people were 10 to 20 times more likely to develop HZ than aged-matched HIV-uninfected cohorts, and even after the introduction of HAART, they continued to be 3 to 4 times more likely to develop HZ.[68–70] In 2013, an estimated 6% of all individuals diagnosed with HIV were older than 65 years, and this number is expected to increase in the future.[71] There are limited data that giving Zostavax to virologically suppressed HIV-infected persons with CD4 greater than 200/μL is safe, but it is still contraindicated in those with CD4 less than 200/μL.[72,73] The HZ/su vaccine has been studied in a phase 1/2, randomized, placebo-controlled study and found to be immunogenic with an acceptable safety profile when given as 3 doses of HZ/su vaccine at months 0, 2, and 6 to 3 separate cohorts of HIV-infected individuals with varying CD4 counts (50–199 while on HAART, >200 while on HAART, >500 but HAART naive). The third dose did not produce any considerable benefit in terms of humoral or cell-mediated immunity.[70]

Similarly, hematopoietic stem cell transplant recipients are at increased risk for developing HZ especially in the first year after transplantation when the rates are at 15% to 30%. At present, patients are placed on prophylaxis with acyclovir or a similar antiviral; however, there are no clear guidelines on dose and duration of therapy. The HZ/su vaccine has been studied in a phase 1/2, randomized, observer-blind, placebo-controlled study in this population of adults with conditions ranging from with multiple myeloma, non-Hodgkin lymphoma (B or T cell), Hodgkin lymphoma, or acute myeloid leukemia who had undergone autologous hematopoietic stem cell transplant 50 to 70 days prior. The study involved 2 different formulations of the HZ/su delivered in 2 different schedules. They were found to be comparable in terms of immunogenicity and safety profile. Again, in those group receiving 3 doses of the vaccine instead of 2, the additional increase in immunity after the third dose was minimal.[74] A phase 3 trial is ongoing evaluating the safety and immunogenicity of HZ/su in adults with hematologic malignancies (ClinicalTrials.gov Identifier: NCT01767467). Understanding the safety and efficacy of this vaccine in oncology patients would be imperative before the vaccine would be used in oncology patients.

Valnivudine hydrochloride (FV-100) is a novel nucleoside analogue now in phase 3 trials that compare it with valacyclovir. The primary endpoint is PHN incidence after 7 days of treatment with valnivudine versus valacyclovir (NCT02412917).[75] In phase 2 trials, although it showed no significant difference when compared with valacyclovir with relation to disease severity at 30 days, it did show decreased burden of illness with a decreased incidence and severity of PHN at 90 days.[26,75] Other novel nucleoside analogues in development include valomaciclovir stearate (EPB-348), N-methanocarbathymidine (N-MCT, NN-001), as well as nonnucleoside helicase-primase inhibitor amenamevir (ASP2151, M5220).[75]

REFERENCES

1. Kawai K, Yawn BP, Wollan P, et al. Increasing incidence of herpes zoster over a 60-year period from a population-based study. Clin Infect Dis 2016;63(2):221–6.
2. Kawai K, Gebremeskel BG, Acosta CJ. Systematic review of incidence and complications of herpes zoster: towards a global perspective. BMJ Open 2014;4(6): e004833.
3. Friesen KJ, Chateau D, Falk J, et al. Cost of shingles: population based burden of disease analysis of herpes zoster and postherpetic neuralgia. BMC Infect Dis 2017;17(1):69.
4. Hales CM, Harpaz R, Joesoef MR, et al. Examination of links between herpes zoster incidence and childhood varicella vaccination. Ann Intern Med 2013;159(11): 739–45.
5. Marra F, Chong M, Najafzadeh M. Increasing incidence associated with herpes zoster infection in British Columbia, Canada. BMC Infect Dis 2016;16(1):589.
6. Schmader K. Herpes zoster. Clin Geriatr Med 2016;32(3):539–53.
7. Mueller NH, Gilden DH, Cohrs RJ, et al. Varicella zoster virus infection: clinical features, molecular pathogenesis of disease, and latency. Neurol Clin 2008; 26(3):675–97, viii.
8. McLaughlin JM, McGinnis JJ, Tan L, et al. Estimated human and economic burden of four major adult vaccine-preventable diseases in the United States, 2013. J Prim Prev 2015;36(4):259–73.
9. Yawn BP, Wollan PC, Kurland MJ, et al. Herpes zoster recurrences more frequent than previously reported. Mayo Clin Proc 2011;86(2):88–93.
10. Shiraki K, Toyama N, Daikoku T, et al, Miyazaki Dermatologist Society. Herpes zoster and recurrent herpes zoster. Open Forum Infect Dis 2017;4(1):ofx007.
11. Nagel MA, Lenggenhager D, White T, et al. Disseminated VZV infection and asymptomatic VZV vasculopathy after steroid abuse. J Clin Virol 2015;66:72–5.
12. Schmader K. Herpes zoster in older adults. Clin Infect Dis 2001;32(10):1481–6.
13. Grahn A, Studahl M. Varicella-zoster virus infections of the central nervous system - prognosis, diagnostics and treatment. J Infect 2015;71(3):281–93.
14. Yawn BP, Gilden D. The global epidemiology of herpes zoster. Neurology 2013; 81(10):928–30.
15. Marin M, Harpaz R, Zhang J, et al. Risk factors for herpes zoster among adults. Open Forum Infect Dis 2016;3(3):ofw119.
16. Sengupta S. Cutaneous herpes zoster. Curr Infect Dis Rep 2013;15(5):432–9.
17. Wareham DW, Breuer J. Herpes zoster. BMJ 2007;334(7605):1211–5.
18. Yawn BP, Wollan PC, St Sauver JL, et al. Herpes zoster eye complications: rates and trends. Mayo Clin Proc 2013;88(6):562–70.
19. Vrcek I, Choudhury E, Durairaj V. Herpes zoster ophthalmicus: a review for the internist. Am J Med 2017;130(1):21–6.
20. Nisa L, Landis BN, Giger R, et al. Pharyngolaryngeal involvement by varicella-zoster virus. J Voice 2013;27(5):636–41.
21. Wang Z, Ye J, Han YH. Acute pancreatitis associated with herpes zoster: case report and literature review. World J Gastroenterol 2014;20(47):18053–6.
22. Bookhout C, Moylan V, Thorne LB. Two fatal herpesvirus cases: treatable but easily missed diagnoses. IDCases 2016;6:65–7.
23. de Jong MD, Weel JFL, van Oers MHJ, et al. Molecular diagnosis of visceral herpes zoster. Lancet 2001;357(9274):2101–2.
24. Cohen JI. Clinical practice: herpes zoster. N Engl J Med 2013;369(3):255–63.
25. Watson P. Postherpetic neuralgia. Am Fam Physician 2011;84(6):690–2.

26. Tyring SK, Lee P, Hill GT Jr, et al. FV-100 versus valacyclovir for the prevention of post-herpetic neuralgia and the treatment of acute herpes zoster-associated pain: a randomized-controlled trial. J Med Virol 2017;89(7):1255–64.
27. Rullan M, Bulilete O, Leiva A, et al. Efficacy of gabapentin for prevention of post-herpetic neuralgia: study protocol for a randomized controlled clinical trial. Trials 2017;18(1):24.
28. Gater A, Uhart M, McCool R, et al. The humanistic, economic and societal burden of herpes zoster in Europe: a critical review. BMC Public Health 2015;15:193.
29. Watson CP, Watt VR, Chipman M, et al. The prognosis with postherpetic neuralgia. Pain 1991;46(2):195–9.
30. Kost RG, Straus SE. Postherpetic neuralgia — Pathogenesis, treatment, and prevention. N Engl J Med 1996;335(1):32–42.
31. Johnson RW, Rice AS. Clinical practice. Postherpetic neuralgia. N Engl J Med 2014;371(16):1526–33.
32. Woznowski M, Quack I, Bolke E, et al. Fulminant staphylococcus lugdunensis septicaemia following a pelvic varicella-zoster virus infection in an immune-deficient patient: a case report. Eur J Med Res 2010;15(9):410–4.
33. Shaikh S, Ta CN. Evaluation and management of herpes zoster ophthalmicus. Am Fam Physician 2002;66(9):1723–30.
34. Ferenczi K, Rosenberg AS, McCalmont TH, et al. Herpes zoster granulomatous dermatitis: histopathologic findings in a case series. J Cutan Pathol 2015; 42(10):739–45.
35. Langan SM, Minassian C, Smeeth L, et al. Risk of stroke following herpes zoster: a self-controlled case-series study. Clin Infect Dis 2014;58(11):1497–503.
36. Breuer J, Pacou M, Gautier A, et al. Herpes zoster as a risk factor for stroke and TIA. Neurology 2014;83(2):e27–33.
37. Nagel M, Gilden D. Editorial commentary: varicella zoster virus infection: generally benign in kids, bad in grown-ups. Clin Infect Dis 2014;58(11):1504–6.
38. Yawn BP, Wollan PC, Nagel MA, et al. Risk of stroke and myocardial infarction after herpes zoster in older adults in a US community population. Mayo Clin Proc 2016;91(1):33–44.
39. Nagel MA, Gilden D. The relationship between herpes zoster and stroke. Curr Neurol Neurosci Rep 2015;15(4):16.
40. Dworkin RH, Johnson RW, Breuer J, et al. Recommendations for the management of herpes zoster. Clin Infect Dis 2007;44(Suppl 1):S1–26.
41. Wilson DA, Yen-Lieberman B, Schindler S, et al. Should varicella-zoster virus culture be eliminated? A comparison of direct immunofluorescence antigen detection, culture, and PCR, with a historical review. J Clin Microbiol 2012;50(12): 4120–2.
42. Harbecke R, Oxman MN, Arnold BA, et al. A real-time PCR assay to identify and discriminate among wild-type and vaccine strains of varicella-zoster virus and herpes simplex virus in clinical specimens, and comparison with the clinical diagnoses. J Med Virol 2009;81(7):1310–22.
43. Gershon AA, Chen J, Gershon MD. Use of saliva to identify varicella zoster virus infection of the gut. Clin Infect Dis 2015;61(4):536–44.
44. Levin MJ. Varicella-zoster virus and virus DNA in the blood and oropharynx of people with latent or active varicella-zoster virus infections. J Clin Virol 2014; 61(4):487–95.
45. Wilson JF. In the clinic. Herpes zoster. Ann Intern Med 2011;154(5). ITC31-15. [quiz: ITC316].

46. Breuer J, Schmid DS, Gershon AA. Use and limitations of varicella-zoster virus-specific serological testing to evaluate breakthrough disease in vaccinees and to screen for susceptibility to varicella. J Infect Dis 2008;197(Suppl 2):S147–51.
47. Oranje AP, Folkers E. The Tzanck smear: old but still of inestimable value. Pediatr Dermatol 1998;5(2):127–9.
48. Arvin AM. Varicella-zoster virus. Clin Microbiol Rev 1996;9(3):361–81.
49. Han Y, Zhang J, Chen N, et al. Corticosteroids for preventing postherpetic neuralgia. Cochrane Database Syst Rev 2013;(3):CD005582.
50. Uscategui T, Doree C, Chamberlain IJ, et al. Corticosteroids as adjuvant to antiviral treatment in Ramsay Hunt syndrome (herpes zoster oticus with facial palsy) in adults. Cochrane Database Syst Rev 2008;(3):CD006852.
51. Gagyor I, Madhok VB, Daly F, et al. Antiviral treatment for Bell's palsy (idiopathic facial paralysis). Cochrane Database Syst Rev 2015;(11):CD001869.
52. Duda JF, Castro JG. Bilateral retrobulbar optic neuritis caused by varicella zoster virus in a patient with AIDS. Br J Med Med Res 2015;5(11):1381–6.
53. Dubinsky RM, Kabbani H, El-Chami Z, et al. Practice parameter: treatment of postherpetic neuralgia: an evidence-based report of the quality standards Subcommittee of the American Academy of Neurology. Neurology 2004;63(6):959–65.
54. Sampathkumar P, Drage LA, Martin DP. Herpes zoster (shingles) and postherpetic neuralgia. Mayo Clin Proc 2009;84(3):274–80.
55. Lin PL, Fan SZ, Huang CH, et al. Analgesic effect of lidocaine patch 5% in the treatment of acute herpes zoster: a double-blind and vehicle-controlled study. Reg Anesth Pain Med 2008;33(4):320–5.
56. Dworkin RH, O'Connor AB, Kent J, et al. Interventional management of neuropathic pain: NeuPSIG recommendations. Pain 2013;154(11):2249–61.
57. Oxman MN, Levin MJ, Johnson GR, et al, Shingles Prevention Study Group. A vaccine to prevent herpes zoster and postherpetic neuralgia in older adults. N Engl J Med 2005;352(22):2271–84.
58. Van Epps PS, Schmader KE, Canaday DH. Herpes zoster vaccination: controversies and common clinical questions. Gerontology 2016;62(2):150–4.
59. Morrison VA, Johnson GR, Schmader KE, et al. Long-term persistence of zoster vaccine efficacy. Clin Infect Dis 2015;60(6):900–9.
60. Levin MJ, Schmader KE, Pang L, et al. Cellular and humoral responses to a second dose of herpes zoster vaccine administered 10 years after the first dose among older adults. J Infect Dis 2016;213(1):14–22.
61. Levin MJ, Oxman MN, Zhang JH, et al. Varicella-zoster virus–specific immune responses in elderly recipients of a herpes zoster vaccine. J Infect Dis 2008;197(6):825–35.
62. Williams WW, Lu PJ, O'Halloran A, et al. Vaccination coverage among adults, excluding influenza vaccination - United States, 2013. MMWR Morb Mortal Wkly Rep 2015;64(4):95–102.
63. Zhang D, Johnson K, Newransky C, et al. Herpes zoster vaccine coverage in older adults in the U.S., 2007-2013. Am J Prev Med 2017;52(1):e17–23.
64. Cunningham AL, Lal H, Kovac M, et al. Efficacy of the herpes zoster subunit vaccine in adults 70 years of age or older. N Engl J Med 2016;375(11):1019–32.
65. Lal H, Cunningham AL, Godeaux O, et al. Efficacy of an adjuvanted herpes zoster subunit vaccine in older adults. N Engl J Med 2015;372(22):2087–96.
66. Sacks HS. In adults ≥ 70 years of age, an adjuvanted herpes zoster subunit vaccine reduced herpes zoster at a mean 3.7 years. Ann Intern Med 2017;166(2):JC5.

67. Godeaux O, Kovac M, Shu D, et al. Immunogenicity and safety of an adjuvanted herpes zoster subunit candidate vaccine in adults ≥ 50 years of age with a prior history of herpes zoster: a phase III, non-randomized, open-label clinical trial. Hum Vaccin Immunother 2017;13(5):1051–8.
68. Moanna A, Rimland D. Decreasing incidence of herpes zoster in the highly active antiretroviral therapy era. Clin Infect Dis 2013;57(1):122–5.
69. Blank LJ, Polydefkis MJ, Moore RD, et al. Herpes zoster among persons living with HIV in the current antiretroviral therapy era. J Acquir Immune Defic Syndr 2012;61(2):203–7.
70. Berkowitz EM, Moyle G, Stellbrink HJ, et al. Safety and immunogenicity of an adjuvanted herpes zoster subunit candidate vaccine in HIV-infected adults: a phase 1/2a randomized, placebo-controlled study. J Infect Dis 2015;211(8):1279–87.
71. Centers for Disease Control and Prevention. HIV/AIDS. 2017. Available at: https://www.cdc.gov/hiv/group/age/olderamericans. Accessed June 03, 2017.
72. Benson CA, Hua L, Jiang JH, et al. ZOSTAVAX is generally safe and immunogenic in HIV+ adults virologically suppressed on ART: results of a phase 2, randomized, double-blind, placebo-controlled trial. The 19th Conference on Retroviruses and Opportunistic Infections. Seattle, Washington, March 5–8, 2012.
73. Centers for Disease Control and Prevention. Immunization schedules. 2017. Available at: https://www.cdc.gov/vaccines/schedules/hcp/imz/adult-conditions.html. Accessed June 03, 2017.
74. Stadtmauer EA, Sullivan KM, Marty FM, et al. A phase 1/2 study of an adjuvanted varicella-zoster virus subunit vaccine in autologous hematopoietic cell transplant recipients. Blood 2014;124(19):2921–9.
75. Birkmann A, Zimmermann H. Drugs in development for herpes simplex and varicella zoster virus. Clin Pharmacol Ther 2017;102(1):30–2.
76. De Clercq E. Clinical potential of the acyclic nucleoside phosphonates cidofovir, adefovir, and tenofovir in treatment of DNA virus and retrovirus infections. Clin Microbiol Rev 2003;16(4):569–96.

Hepatitis C Virus Infection in the Older Patient

Michael Reid, MD, MPH[a], Jennifer C. Price, MD, PhD[a], Phyllis C. Tien, MD, MSc[a,b,*]

KEYWORDS

- HCV • Aging • Comorbidity • Inflammation

KEY POINTS

- Hepatitis C virus (HCV) infection is of concern in older adults, because the proportion of HCV-infected patients that are of older age and that have had infection for a prolonged duration of time has increased.
- Older age has been associated with an increased risk of HCV-associated liver disease including cirrhosis and hepatocellular carcinoma in those with HCV infection likely caused by not only a longer duration of HCV infection but also possibly aging-related mechanisms.
- HCV infection has also been associated with an increased risk of extrahepatic comorbidities common to the aging patient including malignancy, kidney disease, diabetes, cardiovascular disease, and neurocognitive impairment.
- The impact of new direct-acting antiviral agents for the treatment of HCV on HCV-associated comorbidities is unclear.
- Examination of limited published studies of the safety and efficacy of DAAs in the older HCV-infected patient suggests that age should not be a barrier to treatment.

INTRODUCTION

Hepatitis C virus (HCV) infection is the most common blood-borne infection in the United States and is of concern in older adults. Although the rate of new HCV infections has declined over the last two decades because of implementation of HCV screening of donated blood and harm-reduction programs, the proportion of HCV-infected patients that are of older age and that have had infection for a prolonged duration of time has increased. The growing burden of older HCV-infected patients poses challenges for clinicians who care for these patients and for the health care system because of the increased use of health care resources to treat

[a] Department of Medicine, University of California, San Francisco, 513 Parnassus Avenue, San Francisco, CA 94122, USA; [b] Medical Service, Department of Veteran Affairs Medical Center, San Francisco, CA 94121, USA
* Corresponding author. Infectious Disease Section, University of California, San Francisco, VAMC, 111W, 4150 Clement Street, San Francisco, CA 94121.
E-mail address: phyllis.tien@ucsf.edu

Infect Dis Clin N Am 31 (2017) 827–838
http://dx.doi.org/10.1016/j.idc.2017.07.014
0891-5520/17/© 2017 Elsevier Inc. All rights reserved.

id.theclinics.com

the long-term sequelae of HCV-associated liver disease including cirrhosis, hepato-cellular carcinoma (HCC), and liver transplantation.

Before the advent of all oral direct-acting antiviral (DAA) agents, HCV treatment was associated with poor response and increased adverse side effects with some studies showing worse outcomes in the older patient. Since the introduction of DAA agents in 2011 to treat HCV infection, clinicians are now able to successfully treat the growing number of HCV-infected patients of older age. However, information regarding the effect of HCV treatment on short- and long-term clinical outcomes in the older HCV-infected patient is limited.

This article summarizes the literature regarding the epidemiology, natural history, and clinical course of HCV infection; the impact of age on clinical outcomes in persons with HCV infection; and current knowledge regarding the safety and efficacy of newer HCV treatment regimens in the older HCV-infected patient.

EPIDEMIOLOGY AND SCREENING OF HEPATITIS C VIRUS INFECTION IN THE UNITED STATES

An estimated 4.1 million persons in the United States (or 1.6% of the US population) have been exposed to HCV.[1] About 70% of these persons were born between 1945 and 1964, and most were infected between 1970 and 1990 when the incidence of new HCV infections peaked.[2] Since the identification of HCV as the main cause of non-A/non-B chronic hepatitis in 1989, HCV incidence has declined because of the implementation of donor blood screening and increased availability of harm-reduction programs for persons who inject drugs. However, recent data suggest that there may be an emerging epidemic of HCV infection among young nonurban persons mainly of white race; prescription opioid use has been implicated as a factor.[3]

In 2012, the US Centers for Disease Control and Prevention revised their recom-mendations to include one-time HCV serologic testing of all adults born from 1945 through 1965 regardless of HCV risk status.[4] The prevalence of HCV antibodies in per-sons born between 1945 and 1964 (also known as the Baby Boomer cohort in the United States) has been estimated to be about 3.5%, which is more than double the reported HCV prevalence in the US population. The revised recommendations were based on findings from the Chronic Hepatitis Cohort Study of 4689 HCV-infected persons who completed a survey regarding the reason for their HCV testing.[5] That study found that less than 25% of the HCV-infected persons had an identifiable risk factor for HCV infection; rather, 78% were born during the period between 1945 and 1965. With implementation of this new recommendation, an increase in incident HCV infections is expected.

Recent studies[6,7] have also suggested that older patients in long-term care facilities should be targeted for HCV screening and confirmatory HCV RNA screening, and that there should be a shared commitment by all health care facilities to adhere to basic infection control procedures. These studies have largely been borne out of reports of viral hepatitis outbreaks resulting from lapses in infection control practices, partic-ularly in ambulatory care settings. A systematic review and meta-analysis of HCV infection prevalence in long-term care facilities found a pooled prevalence of 3.3% (95% confidence interval, 1.5%–7.2%) compared with the 0.9% to 1.0% prevalence reported in noninstitutionalized elders (generally defined as older than 65 years of age).[6] In that study, it was unclear if adults were previously infected or were exposed to HCV in the long-term care setting. Another case-control study[7] examined the asso-ciation of health care exposures with acute hepatitis B and C from 2006 to 2008 in 71 (mostly acute hepatitis B infection) cases who were 55 years and older and found that

37% of new infections were likely attributable to injections of parenteral medications and 8% to hemodialysis. There is concern that as the Baby Boomer cohort of HCV-infected persons seeks more health care in ambulatory settings and residency in long-term care facilities, there could be a growing reservoir of infected persons who could serve as a source of transmission. Therefore, studies advocate for greater adherence to HCV screening recommendations (particularly in institutionalized settings), basic infection control precautions, and safe injection practices.

NATURAL HISTORY AND CLINICAL COURSE OF HEPATITIS C VIRUS INFECTION AND THE IMPACT OF AGE

Studies estimate that between 55% and 75% of newly infected persons develop chronic HCV infection as determined by detectable HCV RNA in the blood.[8] Patients of older age at time of infection and impaired immune system are at increased risk of developing chronic HCV infection.[8]

A large proportion of chronically HCV-infected persons in the United States are now about 50 to 70 years old and have lived with HCV infection for about 25 to 45 years.[9] The increased duration of HCV infection has been accompanied by an increased incidence of liver disease and related sequelae. Over the natural course of HCV infection, it is expected that at least one-third of HCV-infected persons progress to advanced fibrosis and cirrhosis, and among those with cirrhosis, about 3% to 5% per year develop decompensated cirrhosis (ie, ascites, hepatic encephalopathy, esophageal varices) and/or HCC (**Fig. 1**).[10]

Because several decades can elapse from incident HCV infection until the peak prevalence of cirrhosis, it has been estimated that the proportion of liver-related deaths and patients diagnosed with HCV-related cirrhosis and HCC is fast approaching its peak.[11] This increase is largely driven by the burden of HCV in the Baby Boomer cohort and will be associated with increased health care use and hospitalizations for end-stage liver disease and the subsequent need for liver transplantation.[12]

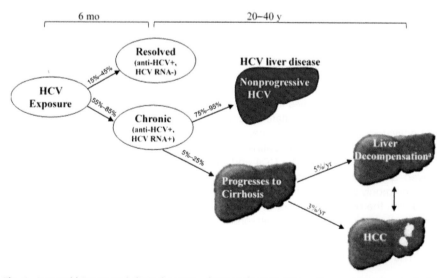

Fig. 1. Natural history and clinical course of HCV infection. [a] Liver Decompensation includes: hepatic encephalopathy, esophageal varies, ascites.

Because the clinical sequelae of HCV disease is expected to increase in the older patient, some studies have specifically examined the association of older age (defined as 65 years or older) with clinical outcomes in HCV-infected persons. One retrospective cohort study[13] of 161,744 HCV-infected patients in the US Veterans Health Administration Hepatitis C Clinical Case Registry compared HCV-infected veterans aged greater than 65 with those aged 20 to 49 years. They found that even after adjusting for several metabolic factors, including diabetes and obesity, age greater than or equal to 65 years remained associated with a 1.14, 2.44, and 2.09 greater risk of cirrhosis, HCC, and death from all causes, respectively. Longer duration of HCV infection is likely a primary reason for the increased risk in older HCV-infected persons. Prolonged duration of HCV infection has been shown to predict faster progression to cirrhosis[14] and has been associated with increased risk of HCC.[15]

However, studies suggest that age-related mechanisms may also play a role. In one study of patients who acquired HCV infection during transfusion, the median time to development of cirrhosis was reported to decrease from 33 years in patients who acquired the infection between the ages of 21 and 30 years to 16 years in patients who acquired the infection when they were 40 years or older.[16] Another study of patients who acquired HCV infection during transfusion found that the mean time to development of HCC was 15 years in persons 50 years or older compared with 32 years in those infected when they were under 50 years of age.[15] Although Poynard and colleagues[14] established that duration of HCV infection predicted faster progression to cirrhosis, they also demonstrated that in those older than 50 years at the time of infection, the progression of fibrosis was substantially greater when compared with those less than 50 years at the time of infection. Finally, recurrent HCV infection after liver transplantation is nearly universal among patients with HCV viremia at the time of transplant, and in this context, older donor age has consistently been associated with accelerated graft loss.[17] These studies indicate that older age independent of duration of HCV infection may also play a role in the progression of HCV-associated liver disease.

Aging-related mechanisms that have been postulated to increase the risk of liver disease outcomes in the setting of HCV infection include a greater vulnerability to environmental factors, such as oxidative stress, with increasing age; reduction in the rate of hepatic flow; reduced mitochondrial capacity; impaired immunity; and increased carcinogenic potential caused by a reduced ability to repair DNA.[18,19] There are also limited data that HCV infection may be associated with increased markers of immune-senescence, which has been shown to occur in the setting of human immunodeficiency virus (HIV) infection and is thought to play a role in the earlier onset of aging-related comorbidities in HIV infection. HCV infection itself might be associated with loss of early differentiated T cells and progressive accumulation of chronically activated, late-differentiated senescent T cells. One small study[20] comparing HCV-infected individuals with healthy control subjects, all of whom were less than 54 years of age, found that the CD4 and CD8 T cells from HCV-infected individuals showed a significant increase in the T-cell immunosenescent phenotype that is more commonly associated with advancing age. Whether or not this increase is associated with the premature onset of not only liver but also nonliver clinical outcomes related to aging in HCV-infected persons is unclear.[21]

HEPATITIS C VIRUS INFECTION AND EXTRAHEPATIC CLINICAL OUTCOMES

HCV infection is also associated with extrahepatic disorders (**Box 1**), likely because in addition to being a hepatotropic virus, it is also lymphotropic leading

---

Box 1
Common extrahepatic outcomes associated with both HCV infection and aging

- Malignancies
  - B-cell non-Hodgkin lymphoma strongly associated with HCV infection
- Chronic kidney disease
  - Glomerulonephritis strongly associated with HCV infection
- Insulin resistance, diabetes
- Cardiovascular disease
- Neuropsychological and cognitive disorders
  - Fatigue, depression, impaired quality of life

---

to immune-system dysregulation. Thus, a variety of autoimmune disorders have been associated with HCV infection including systemic disorders, such as mixed cryoglobulinemia and less commonly arthritis, sicca syndrome, and porphyria cutanea tarda, or organ-specific disorders, such as glomerulonephritis, diabetes, or thyroiditis. Apart from diabetes, these disorders are thought to be uncommon, so few studies have been able to adequately examine the effect of age on these disorders in the HCV-infected patient.

By contrast, HCV infection is a chronic inflammatory process leading to not only hepatic inflammation but also persistent systemic inflammation, which has been associated with extrahepatic outcomes that are also common with aging including extrahepatic malignancies, cardiometabolic complications, and neurocognitive disturbances. The complex interplay between aging outcomes and HCV-induced immune dysregulation and systemic inflammation could partly explain why some but not all studies show an association of HCV infection with these outcomes.

Hepatitis C Virus Infection and Malignancy

Few studies have examined the association of HCV infection with non-HCC malignancy in the older patient. A recent registry-based case-control study[22] using the Surveillance, Epidemiology, and End Results Medicare database in US adults aged greater than or equal to 65 years from 1993 to 2011 found that as expected, HCV infection was strongly associated with cancers of the liver compared with those without HCV infection. However, HCV infection was also associated with higher odds of intrahepatic (adjusted odds ratio [aOR], 3.40) and extrahepatic (aOR, 1.90) bile duct cancer, pancreatic cancer (aOR, 1.23), anal cancer (aOR, 1.97), nonmelanoma nonepithelial skin cancer (aOR, 1.53), myelodysplastic syndrome (aOR, 1.56), and diffuse large B-cell lymphoma (aOR, 1.57).

The increased risk for non-HCC cancers could indicate that HCV infection directly promotes oncogenesis. As a lymphotropic virus, HCV infection is thought to trigger B-cell proliferation and thus, has been associated with a greater risk of lymphoproliferative disorders, such as B-cell lymphoma.[23,24] Alternatively, the increased risk for non-HCC cancers could also be explained as confounding by shared risk factors. Such risk factors as high-risk sexual behaviors and injection drug use could explain the association with anal cancer and skin cancer, but were not accounted for in the analysis. These findings suggest that in addition to HCC, providers should be vigilant to the fact that HCV-infected patients who are 65 years or older could have an increased risk of non-HCC malignancies compared with HCV-uninfected patients who are 65 years or older.

Hepatitis C Virus Infection and Kidney Disease

HCV infection has been associated with an earlier onset of kidney disease and progression to chronic kidney disease (CKD)[25–27] and end-stage renal disease[25,28] when compared with those without HCV infection. Among those with HIV infection, HCV coinfection has also been associated with a greater risk of developing CKD, and increasing age is associated with more advanced CKD in HIV/HCV-coinfected persons compared with HIV-monoinfected persons.[29] Kidney dysfunction is often multifactorial in older HCV-infected patients. Besides the less common immune-mediated renal damage secondary to cryoglobulinemia, lifestyle factors, such as substance abuse,[30,31] and comorbid diseases common with aging, such as diabetes and hypertension,[31] are also important determinants of worsening renal function in HCV-infected persons.

Hepatitis C Virus Infection and Diabetes

An association between HCV infection and diabetes mellitus (DM) has been demonstrated in several studies.[32–35] In one longitudinal study, the development of DM was found to be 11 times more common in HCV-infected than HCV-uninfected persons.[36] In persons older than 39 years of age, HCV infection increased the risk of DM by almost four times.[37] Although a direct effect of HCV on the hepatocyte insulin-signaling cascade[38–40] and pancreatic β-cell function[41] has been postulated as a cause of insulin resistance, the cause of DM is invariably multifactorial. In older HCV-infected persons, DM onset may be a result of the direct effects of HCV and increasing visceral adiposity that occurs with older age.

Hepatitis C Virus Infection and Cardiovascular Disease

Similarly, there is growing evidence that HCV infection is associated with an increased risk of cardiovascular disease (CVD) and heart failure.[42] The mechanisms by which HCV infection might be associated with CVD include an HCV-induced proinflammatory state[43] and possible direct effects of the virus on the myocardium and endothelium.[44] HCV infection is also associated with a higher prevalence of DM, a well-known risk factor for CVD. However, low-density lipoprotein (LDL) cholesterol and total cholesterol are reported to be lower in HCV-infected persons compared with those without HCV infection.[45] Lower circulating levels of LDL cholesterol are commonly observed in primates and humans in response to infection and inflammation, but other changes in LDL cholesterol metabolism (ie, increased small LDL particle size) may occur that could promote atherogenesis.[46] There may also be direct effects of HCV infection that lower LDL levels by lowering very low density lipoprotein (VLDL) secretion independent of liver fibrosis severity,[47] which could potentially decrease the risk of CVD. The contribution of aging to lipid levels and thus CVD in the setting of direct effects of HCV infection and HCV-associated systemic inflammation add some uncertainty as to whether HCV infection is associated with an increased risk of CVD compared with those without HCV infection.

Hepatitis C Virus and Neuropsychological and Neurocognitive Effects

Up to 30% of HCV-infected persons report neuropsychological disorders, not limited to depression, and up to two-thirds complain of fatigue; the older HCV-infected patient may be at particular risk.[48] Although the presence of depressive symptoms might be related to the psychological burden of chronic HCV infection, some studies suggest that HCV infection directly affects the central nervous system (CNS) through alterations in serotoninergic and dopaminergic neurotransmission, with resultant depressive symptoms.[49] This mechanism might also explain other CNS symptoms seen in HCV infection, such as fatigue, although a causal link has not been established.[50,51]

HCV infection is also associated with increased cognitive impairment when compared with those without HCV infection.[52] Between 33% and 50% of all HCV-infected persons report some degree of impaired neurocognition.[53,54] Whether this impairment is directly attributable to HCV infection, advancing age, progressive liver disease, and/or other comorbid conditions is often difficult to elucidate. Studies have demonstrated HCV RNA in brain tissue and cerebrospinal fluid suggesting active HCV replication in the CNS.[55] There is also a growing body of evidence that HCV directly affects the brain and nerves independently of hepatic-mediated processes.[56,57]

HEPATITIS C VIRUS TREATMENT IN THE OLDER PATIENT WITH HEPATITIS C VIRUS INFECTION

Because patients between the ages of 50 and 70 will constitute a large proportion of the patients being treated in the next decade, understanding the impact of age on HCV treatment outcomes in the era of all-oral DAA regimens is important. Before the advent of DAA agents, some[58,59] but not all studies[13,60] found that HCV-infected patients that were of older age had worse sustained virologic response (SVR) rates than those that were of younger age. Some attributed the worse response to the more frequent treatment discontinuation and/or dose reductions in the older patient resulting from treatment with an interferon-based regimen plus ribavirin, which are often accompanied by adverse effects including cytopenia, flu-like symptoms, and CNS effects.

Few studies have examined the association of older age with SVR rates using all oral DAA regimens partly because elderly patients are often excluded from clinical trials. A recent study of four open-label phase 3 clinical trials was able to examine the safety and efficacy of ledipasvir/sofosbuvir for the treatment of genotype 1 HCV in subjects 65 years or older.[61] Of the 2293 subjects in the four trials, 264 (12%) were greater than or equal to 65 years of age (and 24 of those were ≥75). That study found little difference in SVR rates (97% in those <65 years vs 98% in those ≥65 years) despite subjects greater than 65 years being more likely to have cirrhosis. Furthermore, there was little difference by age in the proportion reporting at least one adverse effect (78% in those <65 years vs 80% in those ≥65 years).

The most common adverse effects were fatigue and headache in both groups, but in subjects who were also on ribavirin, the rate of study drug modification or interruption was double in the older group (6% in those <65 years vs 13% in those ≥65 years). That study suggests that age is not a barrier to achieving SVR in patients taking ledipasvir/sofosbuvir, but ribavirin-free regimens should be considered for the treatment of elderly patients. If ribavirin must be used, then close monitoring is needed for the development of anemia.

Furthermore, because sofosbuvir and ribavirin are renally eliminated, safe and effective doses of sofosbuvir in those with an estimated glomerular filtration rate less than 30 mL/min have not been established. In the HCV-infected patient with severely compromised renal function, other HCV regimens, such as grazoprevir plus elbasvir, have been shown to be safe and effective.

Another cohort-based retrospective study[62] of 17,487 HCV-infected patients grouped into six age categories (<55 years, 55–59, 60–64, 65–69, 70–74, and ≥75 years) in the Veterans Affairs Healthcare System who started an all-oral HCV regimen between 2014 and 2015 also found that DAAs were associated with high

SVR rates (from 90% to 94%) even in the oldest age cohort (≥75 years) and that advanced age was not a negative predictor for SVR. Although the SVR rates were lower in those with cirrhosis compared with those without cirrhosis, the SVR rates were similar between age groups among those with cirrhosis. Similarly, SVR rates were lower in treatment-experienced patients compared with treatment-naive patients but similar between age groups among those who were treatment-experienced.

Another question of tremendous interest to clinicians is whether HCV treatment will be associated with improvement in long-term outcomes, especially in the older patient. A study of US veterans[13] before the advent of DAA therapy found that successful HCV treatment is associated with significant reductions in HCC and overall mortality. That study found mortality benefit in all age categories including those 65 to 85 years. The same group also reported in another publication[63] that although achievement of SVR was associated with decreased HCC risk, the annual risk of HCC among those who cleared the virus was not negligible ranging from 0.1% to 1.55% (overall 0.33%) with the highest residual risk in those diagnosed with cirrhosis followed by those who achieved SVR after age 65 irrespective of cirrhosis. They concluded that there remains a risk of HCC post-SVR, and the risk may be greater in those with cirrhosis or in the elderly, supporting HCV treatment before the development of cirrhosis and continued surveillance even after SVR in those who already developed cirrhosis.

Finally, whether HCV treatment improves long-term nonliver disease outcomes is unclear. A recent small study of HIV/HCV-coinfected persons demonstrated that even after SVR, older patients treated with DAA agents did not experience any change in neuropsychological assessments.[64] By contrast, a small study from the interferon era of 34 HCV-infected adults with a median age less than 40 years found that successful HCV eradication can lead to improvements in cognitive function, at least for individuals with mild deficits.[65] These apparently contradictory findings from the pre- and post-DAA area may reflect how older patients with more advanced neurocognitive deficits who may not have been candidates for treatment are now being treated more readily. Additional studies examining the impact of HCV cure in the era of DAA agents on long-term outcomes are needed.

SUMMARY

Understanding the impact of older age and HCV infection on liver and nonliver outcomes is critical. The advent of potent all-oral DAA agents for HCV infection has ushered in a new era where declines in HCV-associated liver disease are tangible; yet whether there will be an effect on longer-term outcomes in other organ tissues besides the liver is unclear and needs study. Examination of limited published studies of the safety and efficacy of DAAs in the older HCV-infected patient suggests that age should not be a barrier to treatment. Given that the proportion of older patients with HCV is increasing, clinical trials of DAA agents should include older HCV-infected patients.

REFERENCES

1. Armstrong GL, Wasley A, Simard EP, et al. The prevalence of hepatitis C virus infection in the United States, 1999 through 2002. Ann Intern Med 2006; 144(10):705–14.
2. Rein DB, Smith BD, Wittenborn JS, et al. The cost-effectiveness of birth-cohort screening for hepatitis C antibody in U.S. primary care settings. Ann Intern Med 2012;156(4):263–70.

3. Suryaprasad AG, White JZ, Xu F, et al. Emerging epidemic of hepatitis C virus infections among young nonurban persons who inject drugs in the United States, 2006-2012. Clin Infect Dis 2014;59(10):1411–9.

4. Smith BD, Morgan RL, Beckett GA, et al. Recommendations for the identification of chronic hepatitis C virus infection among persons born during 1945-1965. MMWR Recomm Rep 2012;61(RR-4):1–32.

5. Smith BD, Beckett GA, Yartel A, et al. Previous exposure to HCV among persons born during 1945-1965: prevalence and predictors, United States, 1999-2008. Am J Public Health 2014;104(3):474–81.

6. Alvarez KJ, Smaldone A, Larson EL. Burden of hepatitis C virus infection among older adults in long-term care settings: a systematic review of the literature and meta-analysis. Curr Infect Dis Rep 2016;18(4):13.

7. Perz JF, Grytdal S, Beck S, et al. Case-control study of hepatitis B and hepatitis C in older adults: do healthcare exposures contribute to burden of new infections? Hepatology 2013;57(3):917–24.

8. Wasley A, Alter MJ. Epidemiology of hepatitis C: geographic differences and temporal trends. Semin Liver Dis 2000;20(1):1–16.

9. Denniston MM, Jiles RB, Drobeniuc J, et al. Chronic hepatitis C virus infection in the United States, National Health and Nutrition Examination Survey 2003 to 2010. Ann Intern Med 2014;160(5):293–300.

10. Alter HJ, Seeff LB. Recovery, persistence, and sequelae in hepatitis C virus infection: a perspective on long-term outcome. Semin Liver Dis 2000;20(1):17–35.

11. Davis GL, Albright JE, Cook SF, et al. Projecting future complications of chronic hepatitis C in the United States. Liver Transpl 2003;9(4):331–8.

12. Pessoa MG, Wright TL. Hepatitis C infection in transplantation. Clin Liver Dis 1997;1(3):663–90.

13. El-Serag HB, Kramer J, Duan Z, et al. Epidemiology and outcomes of hepatitis C infection in elderly US Veterans. J Viral Hepat 2016;23(9):687–96.

14. Pradat P, Voirin N, Tillmann HL, et al. Progression to cirrhosis in hepatitis C patients: an age-dependent process. Liver Int 2007;27(3):335–9.

15. Tong MJ, el-Farra NS, Reikes AR, et al. Clinical outcomes after transfusion-associated hepatitis C. N Engl J Med 1995;332(22):1463–6.

16. Minola E, Prati D, Suter F, et al. Age at infection affects the long-term outcome of transfusion-associated chronic hepatitis C. Blood 2002;99(12):4588–91.

17. Lake JR, Shorr JS, Steffen BJ, et al. Differential effects of donor age in liver transplant recipients infected with hepatitis B, hepatitis C and without viral hepatitis. Am J Transplant 2005;5(3):549–57.

18. Poynard T, Ratziu V, Charlotte F, et al. Rates and risk factors of liver fibrosis progression in patients with chronic hepatitis c. J Hepatol 2001;34(5):730–9.

19. Horiike N, Masumoto T, Nakanishi K, et al. Interferon therapy for patients more than 60 years of age with chronic hepatitis C. J Gastroenterol Hepatol 1995; 10(3):246–9.

20. Barathan M, Mohamed R, Saeidi A, et al. Increased frequency of late-senescent T cells lacking CD127 in chronic hepatitis C disease. Eur J Clin Invest 2015;45(5): 466–74.

21. Chou JP, Effros RB. T cell replicative senescence in human aging. Curr Pharm Des 2013;19(9):1680–98.

22. Mahale P, Torres HA, Kramer JR, et al. Hepatitis C virus infection and the risk of cancer among elderly US adults: a registry-based case-control study. Cancer 2017;123(7):1202–11.

23. Zignego AL, Macchia D, Monti M, et al. Infection of peripheral mononuclear blood cells by hepatitis C virus. J Hepatol 1992;15(3):382–6.

24. Zignego AL, Giannini C, Gragnani L. HCV and lymphoproliferation. Clin Dev Immunol 2012;2012:980942.

25. Molnar MZ, Alhourani HM, Wall BM, et al. Association of hepatitis C viral infection with incidence and progression of chronic kidney disease in a large cohort of US veterans. Hepatology 2015;61(5):1495–502.

26. Park H, Adeyemi A, Henry L, et al. A meta-analytic assessment of the risk of chronic kidney disease in patients with chronic hepatitis C virus infection. J Viral Hepat 2015;22(11):897–905.

27. Perico N, Cattaneo D, Bikbov B, et al. Hepatitis C infection and chronic renal diseases. Clin J Am Soc Nephrol 2009;4(1):207–20.

28. Chen YC, Lin HY, Li CY, et al. A nationwide cohort study suggests that hepatitis C virus infection is associated with increased risk of chronic kidney disease. Kidney Int 2014;85(5):1200–7.

29. Fischer MJ, Wyatt CM, Gordon K, et al. Hepatitis C and the risk of kidney disease and mortality in veterans with HIV. J Acquir Immune Defic Syndr 2010;53(2):222–6.

30. Buettner M, Toennes SW, Buettner S, et al. Nephropathy in illicit drug abusers: a postmortem analysis. Am J Kidney Dis 2014;63(6):945–53.

31. Abraham AG, Althoff KN, Jing Y, et al. End-stage renal disease among HIV-infected adults in North America. Clin Infect Dis 2015;60(6):941–9.

32. Stepanova M, Lam B, Younossi Y, et al. Association of hepatitis C with insulin resistance and type 2 diabetes in US general population: the impact of the epidemic of obesity. J Viral Hepat 2012;19(5):341–5.

33. Mangia A, Ripoli M. Insulin resistance, steatosis and hepatitis C virus. Hepatol Int 2013;7(Suppl 2):782–9.

34. Younossi ZM, Stepanova M, Nader F, et al. Associations of chronic hepatitis C with metabolic and cardiac outcomes. Aliment Pharmacol Ther 2013;37(6):647–52.

35. Mehta SH, Brancati FL, Sulkowski MS, et al. Prevalence of type 2 diabetes mellitus among persons with hepatitis C virus infection in the United States. Hepatology 2001;33(6):1554.

36. Mehta SH, Brancati FL, Strathdee SA, et al. Hepatitis C virus infection and incident type 2 diabetes. Hepatology 2003;38(1):50–6.

37. Mehta SH, Strathdee SA, Thomas DL. Association between hepatitis C virus infection and diabetes mellitus. Epidemiol Rev 2001;23(2):302–12.

38. Kawaguchi Y, Mizuta T. Interaction between hepatitis C virus and metabolic factors. World J Gastroenterol 2014;20(11):2888–901.

39. Aytug S, Reich D, Sapiro LE, et al. Impaired IRS-1/PI3-kinase signaling in patients with HCV: a mechanism for increased prevalence of type 2 diabetes. Hepatology 2003;38(6):1384–92.

40. Kawaguchi T, Yoshida T, Harada M, et al. Hepatitis C virus down-regulates insulin receptor substrates 1 and 2 through up-regulation of suppressor of cytokine signaling 3. Am J Pathol 2004;165(5):1499–508.

41. Kawaguchi T, Ide T, Taniguchi E, et al. Clearance of HCV improves insulin resistance, beta-cell function, and hepatic expression of insulin receptor substrate 1 and 2. Am J Gastroenterol 2007;102(3):570–6.

42. Fibach E, Gatt S, Rachmilewitz EA. Selective photosensitization of human leukemic cells by a pyrene-containing fatty acid. Exp Hematol 1990;18(2):89–93.

43. Oliveira CP, Kappel CR, Siqueira ER, et al. Effects of hepatitis C virus on cardio-vascular risk in infected patients: a comparative study. Int J Cardiol 2013;164(2): 221–6.

44. Boddi M, Abbate R, Chellini B, et al. Hepatitis C virus RNA localization in human carotid plaques. J Clin Virol 2010;47(1):72–5.

45. Fabris C, Federico E, Soardo G, et al. Blood lipids of patients with chronic hepatitis: differences related to viral etiology. Clin Chim Acta 1997;261(2):159–65.

46. Khovidhunkit W, Kim MS, Memon RA, et al. Effects of infection and inflammation on lipid and lipoprotein metabolism: mechanisms and consequences to the host. J Lipid Res 2004;45(7):1169–96.

47. Siagris D, Christofidou M, Theocharis GJ, et al. Serum lipid pattern in chronic hepatitis C: histological and virological correlations. J Viral Hepat 2006;13(1): 56–61.

48. Hassoun Z, Willems B, Deslauriers J, et al. Assessment of fatigue in patients with chronic hepatitis C using the Fatigue Impact Scale. Dig Dis Sci 2002;47(12): 2674–81.

49. Forton DM. Altered monoaminergic transporter binding in hepatitis C related cerebral dysfunction: a neuroimmunologial condition? Gut 2006;55(11):1535–7.

50. Casato M, Saadoun D, Marchetti A, et al. Central nervous system involvement in hepatitis C virus cryoglobulinemia vasculitis: a multicenter case-control study using magnetic resonance imaging and neuropsychological tests. J Rheumatol 2005;32(3):484–8.

51. Weissenborn K, Ennen JC, Bokemeyer M, et al. Monoaminergic neurotransmission is altered in hepatitis C virus infected patients with chronic fatigue and cognitive impairment. Gut 2006;55(11):1624–30.

52. Perry W, Hilsabeck RC, Hassanein TI. Cognitive dysfunction in chronic hepatitis C: a review. Dig Dis Sci 2008;53(2):307–21.

53. Kramer L, Bauer E, Funk G, et al. Subclinical impairment of brain function in chronic hepatitis C infection. J Hepatol 2002;37(3):349–54.

54. Fontana RJ, Bieliauskas LA, Back-Madruga C, et al. Cognitive function in hepatitis C patients with advanced fibrosis enrolled in the HALT-C trial. J Hepatol 2005; 43(4):614–22.

55. Laskus T, Radkowski M, Bednarska A, et al. Detection and analysis of hepatitis C virus sequences in cerebrospinal fluid. J Virol 2002;76(19):10064–8.

56. Paulino AD, Ubhi K, Rockenstein E, et al. Neurotoxic effects of the HCV core protein are mediated by sustained activation of ERK via TLR2 signaling. J Neurovirol 2011;17(4):327–40.

57. Letendre S, Paulino AD, Rockenstein E, et al. Pathogenesis of hepatitis C virus coinfection in the brains of patients infected with HIV. J Infect Dis 2007;196(3): 361–70.

58. Sato I, Shimbo T, Kawasaki Y, et al. Efficacy and safety of interferon treatment in elderly patients with chronic hepatitis C in Japan: a retrospective study using the Japanese Interferon Database. Hepatol Res 2015;45(8):829–36.

59. Tsui JI, Currie S, Shen H, et al. Treatment eligibility and outcomes in elderly patients with chronic hepatitis C: results from the VA HCV-001 Study. Dig Dis Sci 2008;53(3):809–14.

60. Ioannou GN, Beste LA, Chang MF, et al. Effectiveness of sofosbuvir, ledipasvir/ sofosbuvir, or paritaprevir/ritonavir/ombitasvir and dasabuvir regimens for treatment of patients with hepatitis C in the Veterans Affairs National Health Care System. Gastroenterology 2016;151(3):457–71.e5.

61. Saab S, Park SH, Mizokami M, et al. Safety and efficacy of ledipasvir/sofosbuvir for the treatment of genotype 1 hepatitis C in subjects aged 65 years or older. Hepatology 2016;63(4):1112–9.

62. Su F, Beste LA, Green PK, et al. Direct-acting antivirals are effective for chronic hepatitis C treatment in elderly patients: a real-world study of 17 487 patients. Eur J Gastroenterol Hepatol 2017;29(6):686–93.

63. El-Serag HB, Kanwal F, Richardson P, et al. Risk of hepatocellular carcinoma after sustained virological response in Veterans with hepatitis C virus infection. Hepatology 2016;64(1):130–7.

64. Mastrorosa I, Lorenzini P, Ricottini M, et al. DAAs improve VACS but do not influence cognitive impairment in HIV/HCV coinfected. Seattle (WA): CROI; 2017.

65. Thein HH, Maruff P, Krahn MD, et al. Improved cognitive function as a consequence of hepatitis C virus treatment. HIV Med 2007;8(8):520–8.

Norovirus Infection in Older Adults

Epidemiology, Risk Factors, and Opportunities for Prevention and Control

Cristina V. Cardemil, MD, MPH*, Umesh D. Parashar, MBBS, MPH,
Aron J. Hall, DVM, MSPH

KEYWORDS

• Norovirus • Gastroenteritis • Long-term care • Vaccine • Older adults

KEY POINTS

- Estimates indicate that a vast majority (90%) of norovirus-associated deaths in the United States occur among persons greater than or equal to 65 years of age.
- In the United States, long-term care facilities are the most commonly reported setting for norovirus outbreaks.
- Norovirus can spread through many routes, including person-to-person contact, contact with contaminated surfaces, and airborne dissemination of vomitus.
- Transmission-based precautions are among the most effective means of interrupting transmission.
- Antiviral therapy is not yet available for norovirus gastroenteritis, but research to identify antiviral treatment strategies for norovirus is in progress.

BACKGROUND

Norovirus is the leading cause of acute gastroenteritis across all age groups in the United States.[1] It is also a frequent cause of outbreaks in health care settings, including long-term care facilities (LTCFs) and acute care hospitals.[2] The total burden of disease is high; norovirus is estimated to cause approximately 21 million total illnesses annually across all age groups in the United States.[1] Certain populations

Disclaimer: The findings and conclusions in this report are those of the authors and do not necessarily represent the official position of the Centers for Disease Control and Prevention.
Funding: This work was carried out with usual funds from the Centers for Disease Control and Prevention.
Disclosures: No commercial or financial conflicts of interest exist for any of the authors.
Viral Gastroenteritis Branch (proposed), Division of Viral Diseases, Centers for Disease Control and Prevention, Atlanta, GA, USA
* Corresponding author. 1600 Clifton Road, MS A-34, Atlanta, GA 30329.
E-mail address: iyk8@cdc.gov

Infect Dis Clin N Am 31 (2017) 839–870
http://dx.doi.org/10.1016/j.idc.2017.07.012
0891-5520/17/Published by Elsevier Inc.

id.theclinics.com

are at higher risk of infection and severe illness, including those at the extremes of age. In high-income and upper-middle–income (HI/UMI) countries, between 2000 and 13,000 norovirus-associated deaths occur in older adults greater than 65 years of age.[3] Infection with norovirus is also costly to society. Annual hospitalization costs in the United States are estimated at $493 million[4] and outpatient and emergency department visits at $284 million.[5] For patients greater than 65 years of age, total hospitalization costs for norovirus and gastroenteritis are higher compared with younger age groups.[4] Additionally, all foodborne norovirus illness, including productivity losses, are estimated at $2 billion per year in the United States.[6] This review summarizes knowledge on norovirus infection in older adults.

VIROLOGY AND VIRAL DIVERSITY

The norovirus genome is composed of a linear, positive-sense RNA that is approximately 7.6 kb in length.[7] The 3 open reading frames (ORFs), ORF-1, ORF-2, and ORF-3, encode 8 viral proteins (VPs); ORF-2 and ORF-3 encode the structural components of the virion, VP1 and VP2. ORF-1 encodes nonstructural proteins, including the norovirus protease and RNA-dependent RNA polymerase.[8]

Noroviruses belong to the family *Caliciviridae* and are divided into 7 genogroups based on the viral capsid gene. Three of these genogroups, GI, GII, and GIV, include strains that infect humans. Noroviruses are classified further into genotypes, and there are at least 21 genotypes in GII and 8 genotypes in GI.[9] Globally, GII.4 viruses are the predominant pathogen, include new variants that emerge every 2 to 4 years, and are associated with greater symptom severity in the young and elderly, resulting in more hospitalizations and deaths.[10,11] In the most recent United States norovirus season, from September 1, 2016, to April 21, 2017, of 502 samples tested, the predominant strain was GII.P16-GII.4 Sydney, accounting for 60% of outbreaks; other strains included GII.2 (14% of outbreaks), GI.3 (7% of outbreaks), GII.6 (4% of outbreaks), and GII.Pe-GII.4 Sydney (3% of outbreaks); other genotypes accounted for the remaining 12%.[12]

CLINICAL PRESENTATION AND DISEASE COURSE

After an incubation period of 12 hours to 48 hours,[13] the classic symptoms of norovirus disease include sudden onset of vomiting, abdominal cramps, and watery diarrhea.[14,15] Constitutional symptoms, including low-grade fever, generalized myalgias, malaise, headache, and chills, frequently accompany the gastroenteritis.[13] Vomiting and diarrhea are usually present together, but either can be seen alone.[16] Most patients experience a brief, self-limited infection with symptoms resolving within 2 days to 3 days. The clinical spectrum of illness is varied, however, and up to one-third of those infected are asymptomatic.[17] On the other end of the spectrum, the most vulnerable include those with underlying medical conditions, the very young, the elderly, and the immunocompromised, who are at greater risk for severe symptoms and complications,[18] such as acute renal failure leading to hemodialysis, cardiac complications including arrhythmias, acute graft organ rejection in transplant recipients, and death.[19,20]

Complications among healthy adults are less common. Transient postinfectious inflammatory bowel syndrome has been reported up to 3 months postonset of symptoms compared with controls[21] as well as long-term sequelae among US military recruits who experienced gastroenteritis during norovirus outbreaks, including dyspepsia, constipation, and gastrointestinal reflux disease.[22] Neurologic symptoms are rare but have been observed. Headache, neck stiffness, photophobia, and obtundation were observed together with gastrointestinal symptoms in 3 British military personnel; 1 of these patients also had disseminated intravascular coagulation, and 2 patients required ventilator support.[23] Other infrequent complications have been reported among healthy people, including necrotizing enterocolitis, seizures, and postinfectious arthritis in the pediatric population[24-26] as well as individual case reports among adults of ischemic colitis, transient hepatocellular injury, and hemolytic uremic syndrome.[27-29]

Clinical Symptoms and Severity of Norovirus in Older Adults (Greater Than or Equal to 65 Years of Age)

Older adults form a high-risk group for severe symptoms and clinical outcomes.[20] Norovirus outbreak investigations have reported a longer duration of diarrhea, from 3 days to 9 days, in older adults[20,30] and even slower recovery from illness in patients greater than or equal to 85 years of age, with almost half of those affected still symptomatic after 4 days.[31] Clinical symptoms other than diarrhea may also be prolonged in this age group; 1 study reported persistent headache, thirst, and vertigo as long as 19 days postonset of illness in 10 individuals 79 years old to 94 years old in an aged-care facility, although the diarrhea and vomiting had resolved by day 4 postonset.[30]

If they are hospitalized with norovirus infection, older adults are more frequently admitted to an ICU.[32] Also, compared with younger hospitalized patients, older adults who are hospitalized for other conditions are more likely to acquire a nosocomial norovirus infection.[33,34] This propensity for ICU care–acquired and hospital-acquired infections could be due to longer hospital stays and increased exposures, but it could also be secondary to increased susceptibility to the virus due to age-related changes in B-cell and T-cell function and immunosenescence or underlying chronic conditions and comorbidities.

These age-related factors are also likely contributors to the high mortality rate in this age group from norovirus-associated illness.[35] It is estimated that a vast majority (90%) of norovirus-associated deaths in the United States occur among persons greater than or equal to 65 years of age (**Fig. 1**). In a study of norovirus outbreaks in nursing homes, all-cause mortality was higher in outbreak periods compared with nonoutbreak periods.[36] When norovirus-associated deaths do occur, most infections are acquired in LTCFs and hospitals; a global review in developed countries found that immediate causes of death in these scenarios included sepsis, aspiration pneumonia, and cardiac complications.[37]

Prolonged Infection and Complications in the Immunocompromised

Immunocompromised hosts, including those who are immunosuppressed due to congenital or acquired immunodeficiencies, transplant, receipt of immunosuppressive therapy, and cancer, are at increased risk for prolonged and more severe norovirus illness.[38] Several studies have demonstrated chronic infection and prolonged shedding of norovirus for months to years after solid or liquid organ transplant and prolonged illness in individuals with leukemia and lymphoma.[39-43] Duration of symptoms and viral excretion in immunocompromised hosts has ranged from 6 days to 420 days and 11 days to 420 days in hematopoietic stem cell transplant recipients, respectively, and 24 days to 1004 days and 6 days to 898 days in renal transplant recipients.[44] Immunocompromised patients who are chronically infected with norovirus potentially transmit the infection to immunocompetent adults, although nosocomial outbreaks stemming from immunocompromised patients are rare.[18]

Norovirus infections in renal transplant patients have also been shown to result in more severe symptoms compared with gastroenteritis due to bacteria or parasites,

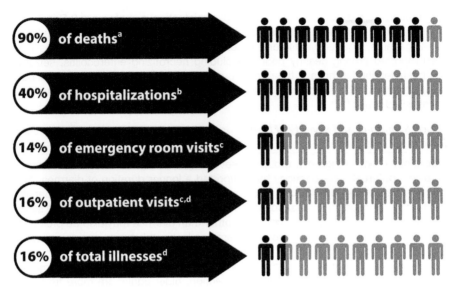

Fig. 1. Proportion of annual norovirus burden in the United States that occurs in older adults greater than or equal to 65 years old, by outcome. [a]Hall and colleagues,[35] 2012; [b]Lopman and colleagues,[4] 2011; [c]Gastañaduy and colleagues,[5] 2013; and [d]Grytdal and colleagues,[102] 2015.

including greater weight loss, 8.7-fold longer duration of symptoms, more frequent medication adjustments, prolonged viral shedding, and post-transplant chronic diarrhea potentially complicated by severe kidney graft impairment.[40] In some cases, immunosuppressive therapy has been temporarily suspended in renal transplant patients because of the severity of clinical symptoms, including severe dehydration and cardiovascular instability.[20] Further complicating the care of norovirus-infected immunocompromised patients is a potential delay in diagnosis that can result from overlapping clinical symptoms experienced by oncologic patients undergoing therapy with those typical for acute norovirus infection.[41] Norovirus-associated deaths in patients with varying degrees of immunosuppression have been reported[37] as well as deaths directly attributable to norovirus in immunocompromised patients.[18,45]

VIRAL SHEDDING AND TRANSMISSION

Norovirus is highly contagious, and the infectious dose can be small (18–2800 viral particles).[46,47] The most common route for transmission is person to person, either directly through the fecal-oral route, by ingestion of aerosolized vomitus, or by indirect exposure via fomites or contaminated environmental surfaces.[9] Foodborne transmission is also common and can occur by contamination from infected food handlers or directly from contaminated foods. Foods often implicated in norovirus outbreaks include leafy greens, fresh fruits (such as raspberries), and shellfish (such as oysters), but any food that is served raw or handled after being cooked can be contaminated.[48–52] Waterborne transmission is also possible, particularly when drinking or recreational water are not chlorinated. In health care settings, the most common mode of transmission is through direct contact with infected persons or contaminated equipment.

The characteristics of norovirus shedding also play a role in transmission dynamics, although the infectivity of the virus beyond the symptomatic period is not well established.[9,53] Shedding occurs primarily in stool but can also be present in vomitus. Although peak viral shedding occurs 2 days to 5 days after infection,[9] viral RNA has been detected in stool samples for up to 4 weeks to 8 weeks in otherwise healthy individuals.[53] Higher viral loads have been reported in symptomatic patients compared with those who have been asymptomatic for at least 3 weeks,[54] but other studies have shown timing of onset, peak, and resolution of shedding was similar for inoculated participants whether or not they developed clinical gastroenteritis.[53] Because the highest period of infectivity is believed to coincide with clinical symptoms and the period shortly thereafter, the Centers for Disease Control and Prevention recommends excluding sick health care personnel, food workers, and caregivers for 48 hours to 72 hours after symptoms resolve.[9]

IMMUNITY

Immunity to norovirus is complex and an ongoing field of research; both acquired immunity and innate host factors and are thought to contribute to susceptibility to infection. Data from volunteer challenge studies indicate a pattern of short-term, acquired immunity, with protection against the same norovirus strain lasting for weeks up to 2 years.[55–57] Modeling studies suggest a slightly longer duration of protection (4–9 years).[58] As a result, immunity to norovirus is thought to be of limited duration, with most individuals experiencing several infections throughout their lifetime.

Antibodies from natural infection have been studied as possible markers of immunity. Antibody prevalence correlates with increasing age; 1 study of hospitalized patients with acute gastroenteritis demonstrated that infants had the lowest GII.4-specific IgG and IgA prevalence, increasing with age up to 100% prevalence in adults.[59] Although antibody seroprevalence to norovirus in adulthood is high, this does not necessarily correlate with protection from disease.[55,60] At the same time, other studies have indicated high blocking ability of antibodies is correlated with protection against infection.[61–63]

Immunity to norovirus seems to be homotypic, with greater protection to strains within genogroups compared with between genogroups[57,59] and could be one reason why high seroprevalence to norovirus does not necessarily equate with protection from disease. Challenge studies have indicated protection against homologous strains but lack of cross-protection to heterologous strains.[57] Even within a genogroup, protection might be incomplete; studies have shown that although repeat infections by the same genotype are rare, repeat infections by the same genogroup occur commonly.[64,65]

In addition to acquired immunity, innate host factors play an important role in immunologic protection. Intrinsic susceptibility to norovirus infection is mediated by histo-blood group antigens (HBGAs), including ABO, secretor, and Lewis types. HBGAs have been demonstrated to serve as a docking site or receptor for noroviruses and are believed to play a role in virus entry to the gut mucosal epithelial cells.[62] The expression of HBGAs is regulated in part by the FUT2 gene, which encodes an alpha(1,2) fucosyltransferase to generate H-antigens, which are catalyzed to produce A or B blood group antigens. Those individuals who possess a functional FUT2 gene, which results in ABH glycans secreted into bodily fluids, are known as secretor-positive individuals and have been found to have a higher risk of norovirus infection.[66] Conversely, individuals with polymorphisms in FUT2 that can result in a homozygous nonsense mutation are known as nonsecretors; these mutations vary by ethnicity and occur in approximately 5% to 50% of different populations worldwide.[67] Protection may not be complete, however, based on FUT2 status alone, because secretor-negative individuals can be infected with norovirus, with some demonstrated differences in susceptibility to certain genotypes.[67–69]

DIAGNOSIS

Individual cases of norovirus gastroenteritis can be suspected on the basis of clinical manifestations. Routine laboratory tests in affected individuals are generally nonspecific, although peripheral white blood cell counts can be slightly elevated with increased polymorphonuclear cells and relative lymphopenia.[16] Renal and hepatic function is generally normal unless dehydration ensues.

Confirmation of norovirus as an infectious agent in patients requires laboratory testing of stool specimens. Whole-stool samples are the preferred clinical specimen for detection of norovirus and ideally are collected during the acute phase of illness, but norovirus can also be detected from rectal swabs and vomitus. Serum specimens are not recommended for routine diagnostics[9]; although several serologic markers, including norovirus-specific IgA and IgG titers, HBGA-blocking antibodies, and mucosal and fecal IgA, are being explored in the context of research and vaccine trials,[10] correlates of protection for use in the clinical setting are still under development.

Molecular tests, including conventional reverse transcription (RT)–polymerase chain reaction (PCR) and real-time RT-PCR are most sensitive and currently the gold standard for norovirus detection but are usually only available in public health laboratories and research facilities (**Table 1**). RT-quantitative (q)PCR afford several advantages, because it is the most sensitive assay available, can detect GI, GII, and GIV strains simultaneously and in several types of specimens (stool, vomitus, food, water, and environmental) and through use of an internal extraction control can reduce false-negative results.[70,71] It can also provide an estimate of viral load based on the cycle threshold value; some data suggest that patients with higher viral loads excrete virus longer.[71] One consideration when using RT-qPCR is that norovirus is frequently detected in stool samples of healthy and asymptomatic individuals, which can complicate interpretation of results; however, detection of norovirus in asymptomatic controls seems more common in developing countries.[72] Laboratory diagnostics in the clinical setting have only recently become more widely available. Molecular-based assays for multiple enteric pathogens, such as xTAG GPP (Luminex, Toronto, Canada), FilmArray gastrointestinal panel (BioFire Diagnostics, Salt Lake City, Utah), and Verigene Enteric Pathogens Test (Nanosphere, Northbrook, Illinois), can detect multiple viral, bacterial, and parasitic pathogens simultaneously within a few hours.[71] The equipment and testing can be expensive, however, and interpretation of positive results with mixed infections can pose challenges for appropriate treatment and management of patients.

Other diagnostic tests include electron microscopy assays, enzyme immunoassay, and immunochromatographic lateral flow assays. Electron microscopy can detect multiple viral pathogens but is expensive and insensitive and generally only used in reference laboratories.[71] Enzyme immunoassay and immunochromatographic assays are commercially available, allow for rapid results and have high specificity, but, because of large genetic and antigenic variation among noroviruses and variable viral loads in stool samples, they have low sensitivity (35%–76%) and are not recommended for individual patients.[71,73–75] They can be useful, however, for rapid screening of multiple samples, such as in an outbreak setting.[75] Negative tests should still be confirmed by a second technique in an outbreak setting, such as RT-qPCR.

In an outbreak setting, and in situations where stool samples are not available for testing but rapid diagnosis is paramount, norovirus infections can be suspected

Table 1
Laboratory methods for detection of norovirus

Method	Characteristics	Availability	Use in Clinical Setting?	Use in Outbreak Setting?
Conventional RT-PCR, real-time RT-PCR	• Gold standard test • High sensitivity • Frequently detects specimen in asymptomatic and healthy patients	Public health and reference laboratories	Not widely[a]	Yes
Multiple enteric pathogen tests (xTAG GPP, FilmArray gastrointestinal panel, and Verigen Enteric Pathogens Test)	• Detects multiple viral, bacterial, and parasitic pathogens simultaneously • High sensitivity • Expensive	Public health and clinical laboratories	Yes	Yes
Enzyme immunoassay, immunochromatographic	• Low sensitivity, high specificity	Public health and clinical laboratories	Not recommended for individual patients	Yes, for rapid screening of multiple samples
Electron microscopy	• Detect multiple viral pathogens • Low sensitivity • Expensive	Reference laboratories	No	No

[a] Individual patient specimens can be tested such as in an outbreak at a reference laboratory and positive specimens genotyped, but due to lack of availability in the clinical setting is unlikely to provide results back to the patient in a timely fashion. Some commercial diagnostic laboratories, however, offer their own in-house RT-PCR as do some tertiary care hospitals.

based on the clinical and epidemiologic profile. The Kaplan criteria provide the means to discriminate between outbreaks due to norovirus and due to bacterial agents and include (1) vomiting in more than half of affected persons, (2) mean (or median) incubation period of 24 hours to 48 hours, (3) mean (or median) duration of illness of 12 hours to 60 hours, and (4) no bacterial pathogen in stool culture.[76,77] These criteria are highly specific (99%) but less sensitive (68%) in discriminating between outbreaks due to bacteria versus norovirus.[78] Other clinical and epidemiologic profiles have been suggested to help discriminate norovirus outbreaks from non-norovirus gastroenteritis outbreaks, including an increased vomiting to fever ratio and decreased diarrhea-to-vomiting ratio.[79,80] These clinical definitions are of particular importance in nursing homes and assisted living facilities, where diagnostic testing might not be obtained and could lead to delays in diagnosis and implementation of control measures.

TREATMENT

As with other causes of viral gastroenteritis, treatment is primarily supportive with replenishment of intravascular depletion of volume and electrolytes as well as unrestricted nutrition.[13,16] Oral rehydration remains the first-line therapy for uncomplicated illness and intravenous fluids for severe vomiting and dehydration.[15] Older adults with signs of hypovolemia are at greatest risk for complications and are more likely to require hospitalization. Symptomatic treatment with analgesics, antimotility, antiemetic, and antisecretory agents can be used as adjuncts in adults, depending on the type and severity of symptoms and necessity of continued performance, such as work and travel. One study demonstrated that bismuth salicylate improved symptoms from gastroenteritis in Norwalk virus–infected volunteers but had no effect on the number or consistency of stools or rates of viral shedding.[81] A more recent study found that in vitro, bismuth subsalicylate and bismuth oxychloride slightly reduced the level of Norwalk replicon-bearing cells.[82] Loperamide has been shown to reduce the duration of diarrhea from a variety of causes compared with placebo and has few side effects,[83] although constipation was reported in 1 study in adults greater than 70 years old.[84] In adults with diarrhea for less than 24 hours, diphenoxylate-atropine [Lomotil] was superior to placebo in reducing the rate of bowel movements in the 24 hours after treatment, but there was no statistically significant difference in median time to last loose or watery stool.[85]

Antibiotics are not recommended for the treatment of uncomplicated viral gastroenteritis, and no Food and Drug Administration–approved antiviral therapies are available for norovirus gastroenteritis, but research to identify antiviral treatment strategies for norovirus is in progress.[86,87] Nitazoxanide, a broad-spectrum thiazolide anti-infective licensed for use against Cryptosporidium spp and Giardia lamblia, has been used off-label as a treatment of norovirus infection in transplant recipients and immunocompromised patients,[88–90] and a small clinical trial demonstrated significant reductions in time to resolution of symptoms of norovirus diarrhea in immunocompetent adults and adolescents treated with nitazoxanide.[91] Other investigational agents, including the antiviral favipiravir, under development for influenza treatment, have shown modest potency against norovirus replication.[92] Human alpha-interferon and ribavirin also reduced replication of a human norovirus replicon in cell culture.[93] Probiotics and vitamin A are also being explored for their antiviral effects[94]; reductions in incidence and shorter duration of diarrhea and viral shedding have been demonstrated with probiotic regimens in pigs inoculated with human norovirus.[95] Until recently, lack of a robust and reproducible in vitro cultivation system hampered research and development for therapeutics, but a human intestinal enteroid culture system has been described to support human norovirus replication in vitro[96] and is expected to yield new insights for antivirals as well as in diagnostics and vaccine development.

ENDEMIC DISEASE

Studies of endemic norovirus gastroenteritis have elucidated some important trends. In the United States, norovirus is the leading cause of gastroenteritis in the community, outpatient setting, and emergency departments in all age groups, accounting for 19 million to 21 million cases annually.[1] Estimates of the total number of cases in adults greater than or equal to 65 years of age in the United States have not previously been reported; extracting a recently reported community incidence rate in this age group and multiplying by the total number of persons greater than or equal to age 65 in 2015[97] results in an estimated 3.7 million total cases of norovirus annually in the United States in older adults (**Fig. 2**). Additionally, norovirus cases in older adults account for an estimated 320,000 outpatient visits; 69,000 emergency department visits; 39,000

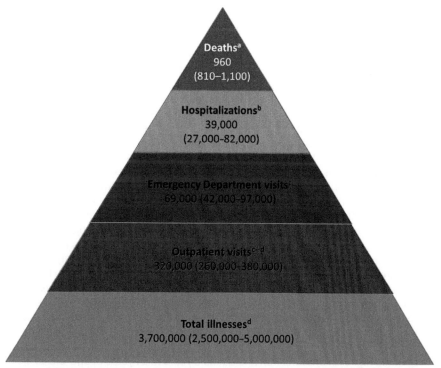

Fig. 2. Estimated annual norovirus cases in older adults (≥65 years old) in the United States in 2015, by outcome. To generate case counts, incidence rates by outcome were obtained or calculated from existing literature ([a]Hall and colleagues,[35] 2012; [b]Lopman and colleagues,[4] 2011; [c]Gastañaduy and colleagues,[5] 2013; and [d]Grytdal and colleagues,[102] 2015) and multiplied by the US population estimate for older adults in 2015 (47.8 million). For deaths and emergency department visits, 95% CIs are shown in parentheses; for outpatient visits, the average from 2 studies is shown; for hospitalizations, high and low seasonal estimates from 1996 to 2007 are shown; for total illnesses, 95% credible intervals are shown. All numbers are rounded to 2 significant digits. Data collected at the community level are used as proxy for determining total illnesses.

hospitalizations; and 960 deaths annually in the United States. These estimates are in line with a recent systematic review of older adults in HI/UMI countries, which reported 1.2 million to 4.8 million illnesses;723,000 million to 2.2 million outpatient visits; 40,000 million to 763,000 inpatient visits; and 2000 to 13,000 norovirus-associated deaths annually in these countries.[3] Putting these counts together with the overall population of 402 million older adults in HI/UMI countries, norovirus incidence rates can be calculated for these countries, which are similar to incidence rates previously reported from the United States (total cases: 12 vs 77 per 1000; outpatient visits: 5.5 vs 5.4–7.9 per 1000; inpatient visits: 190 vs 81 per 100,000; deaths: and 32 vs 20 per 1,000,000; rates are in HI/UMI vs United States, respectively). As the world population continues to grow and age, these numbers will correspondingly increase.

Studies from the United States, the United Kingdom, Canada, and Germany have reported age-specific norovirus incidence rates that have included adult populations (**Table 2**). Estimates vary by outcome, country, and estimation methods, but a U-shaped pattern of illness with the youngest and eldest most highly affected was evident among several studies that examined all age groups. For example, a study of patients submitting stool specimens for routine clinical diagnostics from a health maintenance organization in 2 regions of the United States reported highest incidence rates in children less than 5 years of age in the community (1521 per 10,000), followed by adults 46 years to 65 years of age (1012 per 10,000) and greater than 65 years of age (771 per 10,000); similarly, children less than 5 years of age had the highest outpatient incidence rate (256 per 10,000), followed by adults greater than 65 of age (79 per 10,000).[98] Another US modeling study estimated norovirus associated hospitalization discharges that likewise followed the U-shaped distribution, with the oldest age groups most affected.[4] When examining hospitalization, emergency department, and outpatient visit rates among adults only, higher incidence is observed among adults greater than 65 compared with adults less than or equal to 65 years old.[4,99–105] Among adults greater than 65 years, the hospitalization rate appears to be even greater with increasing age, because the greater than 84-year-old group exhibited rates at least twice as high.[4,101] Unlike the studies discussed previously, 2 studies reported rates in adults that were much lower than the others (0.61 per 10,000 in >59 year olds and 0.0041 per 10,000 in 65–85 year olds), but these were the only estimates that relied entirely on *International Classification of Diseases, Ninth Revision*, and *International Classification of Diseases, Tenth Revision*, codes, and the investigators noted that a substantial proportion of undiagnosed viral gastroenteritis cases were likely.[103,106]

Adults greater than or equal to 65 years of age are at highest risk for death from norovirus; a study in the Netherlands reported a case fatality rate 21 times higher in this age group compared with adults 18 years old to 64 years old.[107] Among studies estimating the incidence of norovirus-associated mortality, death rates were much higher in older adults compared with other age groups (see **Table 2**). In 2012, Hall and colleagues[35] reported a death rate in adults greater than or equal to 65 that was 2 orders of magnitude higher than in children and adults 5 years to 64 years of age (0.2 vs 0.002 per 10,000, respectively) and in 2013 Werber and colleagues[105] reported a similarly high rate in older adults greater than or equal to 70 compared with less than 70 years of age (0.32 vs <0.01 per 10,000).

Prevalence studies in patients with acute gastroenteritis have also demonstrated a high burden of norovirus disease. Globally, noroviruses account for 18% of all patients with acute gastroenteritis, with slightly lower rates in the inpatient (17%) compared with outpatient (20%) and community (24%) setting.[72] Studies from Canada, China, the Netherlands, Portugal, Spain, Qatar, the United States, and the United Kingdom have demonstrated that norovirus accounted for 6% to 27% of acute gastroenteritis

Table 2
Studies estimating endemic norovirus incidence in adults greater than or equal to18 y of age, by outcome

	Country	Data Period Studied	Study Design	Population	Reported Incidence by Age Group (per 10,000 Population)
Deaths					
Werber et al,[105] 2013	Germany	2004–2008	Retrospective analysis surveillance	National surveillance system for notifiable diseases, Federal Statistical Office	≥70 y: 0.32 <70 y: <0.01
Hall et al,[35] 2012	US	1999–2007	Retrospective analysis using time-series regression models	Gastroenteritis-associated deaths from National Center for Health Statistics multiple cause-of-death mortality data	≥65 y: 0.20 5–64 y: 0.0022
Hospitalizations					
Chan et al,[101] 2015	China	2012–2014	Prospective cohort	Inpatients admitted with AGE at 1 hospital in Hong Kong	0–4 y: 148[b] 5–9 y: 12 10–14: 4.4 15–19: 2.9 20–24: 1.0 25–29: 0.7 30–34: 1.1 35–39: 0.8 40–44: 0.8 45–49: 1.1 50–54: 1.1 55–59: 1.5 60–64: 4.3 65–69: 9.3 70–74: 10.5 75–79: 17.7 80–84: 34.5 ≥84 y: 58.1

(continued on next page)

Table 2
(continued)

	Country	Data Period Studied	Study Design	Population	Reported Incidence by Age Group (per 10,000 Population)
Lopman et al,[4] 2011	US	1996–2007	Retrospective analysis using time-series regression models	Gastroenteritis-associated hospital discharges from National Inpatient Sample	<5 y: 9.4 5–17 y: 1.1 18–64 y: 1.0 65–74 y: 4.7 75–84 y: 9.2 85+ y: 18.5
Grytdal et al,[102] 2015	US	2011–2012	Prospective passive surveillance	AGE cases at 4 Veterans Affairs hospitals	<65 y: 0.8 community-acquired inpatient; 4.5 for hospital-acquired inpatient ≥65 y: 1.4 for community-acquired inpatient; 6.6 per 10,000 for hospital-acquired inpatient
Haustein et al,[100] 2009	UK	2000–2006	Retrospective analysis using linear regression models	Gastroenteritis-associated hospital discharges from national statistical data warehouse and national laboratory database	18–64 y: 0.23–0.48 ≥65 y: 1.0–4.3 (range, low to high season)
Chui et al,[106] 2011	US	1991–2004	Retrospective database review	Norwalk virus hospital discharge codes and US Census	65–85 y: 0.0041
Ruzante et al,[103] 2011	Canada	2001–2004	Retrospective database review	Norovirus hospital discharge codes and Canadian Institute for Health Information, Vital Statistics Registry, National Notifiable Diseases database	<1 y: 0.59 1–59 y: range 0.06–0.2 >59 y: 0.61

Emergency department visits

Study	Country	Years	Design	Setting/population	Age (y): n
Gastañaduy et al,[5] 2013	US	2001–2009	Retrospective analysis using time-series regression models	Gastroenteritis-associated health care encounters from MarketScan Commercial Claims and Encounters database	0–4 y: 38 5–17 y: 10 18–64 y: 12 65+ y: 15

Outpatient visits

Study	Country	Years	Design	Setting/population	Age (y): n
Grytdal et al,[98] 2016	US	2012–2013	Retrospective laboratory-based cohort	AGE specimens submitted for routine clinical diagnostics from health maintenance organization in 2 US locations	<5 y: 256 5–15 y: 37 16–25 y: 29 26–45 y: 43 45–65 y: 55 >65 y: 79 Total: 56
O'Brien et al,[99] 2016	UK	2008–2009	Prospective cohort (IID2 study)	AGE patients presenting for primary-health care consultations nationwide	<5 y: 144 5–15 y: 15 15–64 y: 11 ≥65 y: 21
Grytdal et al,[102] 2015	US	2011–2012	Prospective laboratory-based passive surveillance	AGE cases using at 4 Veterans Affairs hospitals	<65 y: 17.2 ≥65 y: 20

(continued on next page)

Table 2
(continued)

	Country	Data Period Studied	Study Design	Population	Reported Incidence by Age Group (per 10,000 Population)
Gastañaduy et al,[5] 2013	US	2001–2009	Retrospective analysis using time-series regression models	Gastroenteritis-associated health care encounters from MarketScan Commercial Claims and Encounters database	0–4 y: 233 5–17 y: 85 18–64 y: 35 ≥65 y: 54
Phillips et al,[104] 2010	UK	1993–1996	Prospective cohort	AGE cases presenting to 70 general practitioner clinics nationwide	<5 y: 320 5–14 y: 44 15–44 y: 38 45–64 y: 26 >65 y: 37
Bernard et al,[108] 2014[a]	Germany	2001–2009	Retrospective analysis surveillance	National surveillance system for notifiable diseases, Federal Statistical Office, includes sporadic and outbreak cases	<5 y: 40–45[b] 5–9 y: 10–11 10–14 y: 3.5–4.1 15–19 y: 3.5–5.9 20–24 y: 5.0–9.4 25–29 y: 4.4–8.2 30–34 y: 4.7–6.8 35–39 y: 4.1–7.1 40–44 y: 3.8–7.4 45–49 y: 4.1–8.2 50–54 y: 4.7–8.5 55–59 y: 6.5–8.5 60–64 y: 7.1–7.4 65–69 y: 9.1–10.0 70–74 y: 16–17 75–79 y: 26–30 80–84 y: 43–62 ≥85 y: 79–134

Study	Country	Years	Study design	Setting	Incidence
Werber et al,[105] 2013[a]	Germany	2004–2008	Retrospective analysis surveillance	National surveillance system for notifiable diseases, Federal Statistical Office	0–4 y: 54[b] 5–9 y: 13 10–19 y: 5.1 20–29 y: 8.0 30–39 y: 6.7 40–49 y: 7.2 50–59 y: 8.1 60–69 y: 9.5 ≥70 y: 49
Community					
Grytdal et al,[98] 2016	US	2012–2013	Retrospective laboratory-based cohort	AGE specimens submitted for routine clinical diagnostics from health maintenance organization in 2 US locations	<5 y: 1522 >65 y: 758
O'Brien et al,[99] 2016	UK	2008–2009	Prospective cohort (IID2 study)	AGE cases in community nationwide	15–64 y: 390 ≥65 y: 277
Phillips et al,[104] 2010	UK	1993–1996	Prospective cohort (IID study)	AGE cases in community nationwide	14–44 y: 410 ≥45 y: 170

Abbreviations: AGE, acute gastroenteritis; IID, infectious intestinal disease.

[a] In Germany, norovirus is nationally notifiable, and many cases are captured through the acute gastroenteritis surveillance system when patients present to providers, which may include laboratory testing. Thus, these estimates include medically-attended cases and, therefore, likely extend beyond the outpatient setting.

[b] If point estimate was not reported in text or table, data points were extracted by digitizing plots.

cases in adults of all ages, and 8% to 41% of acute gastroenteritis in adults greater than or equal to 65 years old (**Table 3**).

OUTBREAKS

Globally, norovirus is the predominant cause of gastroenteritis outbreaks and accounts for approximately half of all outbreaks in developed countries.[122] In the United States, norovirus is also the leading cause of foodborne disease outbreaks[123] and a frequent cause of outbreaks in institutional settings, such as LTCFs and child care centers.[122] Other common norovirus outbreak settings include restaurants, catered events, cruise ships, schools, prisons, and military encampments.

These outbreaks occur year-round but are more frequent during the winter, with more than half occurring in the December-February timeframe.[9,124] Although multiple routes of transmission can occur within a single outbreak, norovirus is the most frequently reported cause of acute gastroenteritis outbreaks transmitted through person-to-person contact, environmental contamination, and unknown mode of transmission.[125] Most norovirus outbreaks globally and in the United States are caused by GII noroviruses, and GII.4 is the most common genotype identified in norovirus outbreaks in the United States.[12,126]

Long-term Care Facility Outbreaks

Older adults living in LTCFs might be at additional risk for norovirus infection and complications.[127] In the United States, LTCFs, which generally refer to facilities that provide prolonged care for individuals who require daily living and/or nursing care support, are the most commonly reported setting for norovirus outbreaks.[125,128,129] In the United States and Australia, 6 to 17 norovirus outbreaks per 100 LTCFs are estimated annually.[130,131]

The unique setting of LTCFs can promote norovirus transmission, such as in shared rooms and common areas, where norovirus can spread through many routes, including person-to-person contact, contact with contaminated surfaces, and airborne dissemination of vomitus.[132] Most norovirus outbreaks in LTCF settings have high levels of person-to-person transmission, likely due to the caregiving and close contact required between staff and residents with limited mobility.[130,131,133,134] Shared dining facilities in some LTCFs might also increase the risk for foodborne exposures and transmission.

Attack rates and deaths are also higher in norovirus outbreaks in LTCF compared with other causes of acute gastroenteritis outbreaks.[36,105,130,131,133] A systematic review of norovirus disease risk among older adults in HI/UMI countries found that attack rates ranged from 3% to 45%, case hospitalization rates 0.5% to 4.3%, and case fatality rates 0.3% to 1.6% in norovirus-associated LTCF outbreaks.[3] Once infected, LTCF residents are more likely to suffer severe outcomes due to nutritional status, immunosenescence, chronic inflammation, microbiome alterations, and use of certain medications.[135] Outbreaks in LTCFs have been reported to recur within the same facility despite implementation of control measures; can last for prolonged periods, up to months in some cases[136]; and result in increased hospitalizations and mortality rates for residents.[36,125]

Hospital Outbreaks

Norovirus outbreaks are common in hospitals, with attack rates ranging from 5% to 60%.[31,108,133,137,138] These outbreaks tend to occur seasonally, more commonly occurring in the 6 months from November to April and peaking in January, February,

Table 3
Studies of endemic norovirus disease in adult populations estimating prevalence of norovirus among cases with gastroenteritis

Study	Country	Data Period Studied	Study Design	Population	Prevalence of Norovirus Among Gastroenteritis Cases (n/N), Unless Otherwise Specified
Deaths					
Hall et al,[35] 2012	US	1999–2007	Retrospective analysis using time-series regression models	Gastroenteritis-associated deaths from National Center for Health Statistics multiple cause-of-death mortality data	0–4 y: 4.5% (27/599) 5–64 y: 3.9% (52/1347) ≥65 y: 7.7% (718/9310)
Harris et al,[19] 2008	UK	2001–2006	Retrospective regression analysis	Mortality statistics of gastrointestinal pathogens from Health Protection Agency, Office of National Statistics/ England and Wales	≥65 y: 20% of deaths caused by IID other than C difficile were associated with norovirus infection; 13% of deaths from noninfectious IID were associated with norovirus
Hospitalizations					
Grytdal et al,[102] 2015	US	2011–2012	Prospective laboratory-based passive surveillance	AGE cases presenting to 4 Veterans Affairs hospitals	<65 y: 4.6% (10/217) ≥65 y: 8.2% (13/158)
Rovida et al,[109] 2013	Italy	2011–2012	Retrospective laboratory based	GE inpatients at 1 hospital	>65 y: 13.6% (20/147)
Verhoef et al,[107] 2013	Netherlands	2008–2009	Retrospective regression analysis	AGE patients admitted to 6 hospitals	≥18 y: 6.7% (905/13,598) noroviruses cases/AGE hospitalizations; 4/41 samples = 9.8%
Fernandez et al,[110] 2011	Spain	2000–2007	Retrospective laboratory based	GE specimens submitted from inpatients at 1 hospital	6–16 y: 7.2% 16–64 y: 8.6% ≥65 y: 11.1%

(continued on next page)

Table 3
(continued)

Study	Country	Data Period Studied	Study Design	Population	Prevalence of Norovirus Among Gastroenteritis Cases (n/N), Unless Otherwise Specified
Hospital and emergency department					
Yi et al,[32] 2016	US	2013	Retrospective laboratory based	Residual specimens sent for culture from emergency department or inpatients at 2 hospitals	≥65 y: 11%
Tang et al,[111] 2013	Taiwan	2011–12	Prospective cohort	AGE patients at 1 hospital (53 outpatients, 6 emergency unit, 19 inpatients)	<10 y: 28.1% (9/32) 10–40 y: 9.6% (3/31) >40 y: 5.4% (5/92)
Emergency department					
Al-Thani,[155] 2013	Qatar	2009	Prospective cohort	AGE patients presenting to emergency department in 1 hospital	<1 y: 26.3% (10/38) 1–10 y: 20.5% (17/83) 11–20 y: 31.0% (9/29) 21–50 y: 38.7% (29/75) 51–60 y: 29.1% (7/24) >60 y: 34.5% (10/29)
Gastañaduy et al,[5] 2013	US	2001–2009	Retrospective analysis using time-series regression models	Gastroenteritis-associated health care encounters from MarketScan Commercial Claims and Encounters database	18–64 y: 17% (15,013/87,417) ≥65 y: 17% (10,744/133,007)
Outpatient					
Yu et al,[112] 2017	China	2012–2013	Prospective cohort surveillance	AGE cases presenting to 10 outpatient clinics at sentinel hospitals	5–24 y: 18% 25–44 y: 21% 45–64 y: 24% ≥65 y: 20%

Study	Country	Years	Study type	Setting	Results
Leblanc et al,[113] 2017	Canada	2008–2009	Prospective laboratory based	Diarrheic and nondiarrheic cases receiving medical care	<1 y: 11%[a] 2–5 y: 54% 6–10 y: 3% 10–20 y: 18% 20–30 y: 20% 30–40 y: 25% 40–50 y: 21% 50–60 y: 16% 60–70 y: 12% >70 y: 19%
Costa et al,[114] 2015	Portugal	2011–2013	Prospective cohort surveillance	National surveillance of hospitalized acute diarrhea cases	≥19 y: 6.4% (16/250)
Wu et al,[115] 2015	China	2013–2014	Prospective laboratory based	AGE patients presenting as outpatients at 1 hospital	≥16 y: 26.5% (211/796) >60 y: 15.2% (32/211)
Gao et al,[116] 2015	China	2011–2013	Prospective laboratory based	AGE patients presenting as outpatients to 17 hospitals	≥18 y: 17.9% detection of Human Calicivirus (overall of 287 HuCV-positive samples, including from kids, 8% were sapovirus, 83% norovirus GII, and 7.3% norovirus GI) 18–29 y: 16.2% (191/1179) 30–39 y: 19.2% (129/672) 40–49 y: 19.7% (92/467) 50–59 y: 19.0% (96/504) 60–69 y: 18.8% (53/282) 70–79 y: 15.5% (42/271)

(continued on next page)

Table 3
(continued)

Study	Country	Data Period Studied	Study Design	Population	Prevalence of Norovirus Among Gastroenteritis Cases (n/N), Unless Otherwise Specified
Grytdal et al,[102] 2015	US	2011–2012	Prospective laboratory based passive surveillance	AGE cases using at 4 Veterans Affairs hospitals	≥65 y: 9.2% <65 y: 5.5%
Tian et al,[117] 2014	China	2008–2009	Prospective cohort	AGE patients presenting to gastroenterology department of 1 hospital	14–19 y: 23% (9/40)[a] 20–29 y: 25% (43/174) 30–39 y: 26% (24/90) 40–49 y: 25% (16/65) 50–59 y: 22% (15/69) ≥14 y: 26.2% (136/519) ≥60 y: 36.7% (28/36)
Manso et al,[118] 2013	Spain	2010–2011	Prospective laboratory based	GE cases presenting as outpatients (90%) or inpatients (10%) at 1 hospital	0–2 y: 31.4% (281/895) 3–5 y: 20.7% (41/198) 6–12 y: 31.3% (76/243) 13–18 y: 28.6% (20/70) 19–59 y: 28.2% (180/637) >60 y: 24.6% (146/593)
Gao et al,[119] 2011	China	2007–2008	Prospective laboratory based	AGE patients presenting as outpatients at 1 hospital	18–83 y: 11.9% (48/403)
Jin et al,[120] 2011	China	2007–2008	Prospective laboratory based	AGE patients presenting as outpatients at 1 hospital	15–83 y: 19.6% (106/547) 15–24 y: 16.2% (20/123) 25–34 y: 18.4% (29/158) 35–44 y: 16.7% (19/114) 45–83 y: 26.9% (41/152)
Gastañaduy et al,[5] 2013	US	2001–2009	Retrospective analysis using time-series regression models	Gastroenteritis-associated health care encounters from MarketScan Commercial Claims and Encounters database	18–64 y: 8% (43,709/533,224) ≥65 y: 8% (10,744/133,007)

Lau,[156] 2004	China	2001–2002	Retrospective laboratory based	1. Patients at outpatient clinics in the Acute Diarrheal Disease Surveillance Program 2. Patients with AGE at public hospitals	1. 14-24 y: 4.7% (4/85) 25–59 y: 7.6% (38/497) >60 y: 10.3% (26/252) 2. 14-24 y: 9.7% (3/31) 25–59 y: 8.9% (5/56) ≥60 y: 7.7% (2/26)
Huhulescu et al,[121] 2009	Austria	2007	Prospective cohort	AGE cases to 3 general practitioners	>60 y: 2/59 = 4.1%
Community					
deWit,[157] 2001	Netherlands	1998–1999	Prospective cohort study (Sensor)	AGE in community cases	18-64 y: 7.0% >65 y: 12.9%
Amar et al,[54] 2007	UK	1993–1996	Retrospective analysis of prospective cohort (IID study)	AGE in community cases initially drawn from the catchment of 70 general practices and followed over time	10-19 y: 26% (30/117) 20-29 y: 33% (100/303) 30-39 y: 36% (137/382) 40-49 y: 24% (70/295) 50-59 y: 22% (47/209) 60-69 y: 25% (48/194) ≥70 y: 41% (57/138)

Abbreviations: AGE, acute gastroenteritis; GE, gastroenteritis; HuCV, human calicivirus; IID, infectious intestinal disease.
[a] If point estimate was not reported in text or table, data points were extracted by digitizing plots.

and March.[108,133] Transmission is most likely to be person to person, and the outbreak length can range from 1 day to months.[133] Hospital outbreaks are more commonly reported from several developed countries, at times leading to closure of wards or hospitals compared with the United States, where outbreaks in LTCFs predominate.[9,137–141] The reason for these differences in norovirus hospital outbreak setting and control measures by country is not well understood but could be due to differences in reporting, testing, infection control, or epidemiology.[142,143]

Few studies have examined norovirus genotypes affecting older adults, but available evidence suggests that GII.4 viruses predominate as a cause of norovirus disease in both LTCFs and health care–associated outbreaks as well as among older adults hospitalized for acute gastroenteritis.[32,101,135] GII.4 outbreaks have been associated with more severe illness, hospitalizations, and deaths.[10,11,144]

PREVENTION AND CONTROL OF NOROVIRUS OUTBREAKS IN HEALTH CARE SETTINGS

Health care facilities, including LTCFs and hospitals, are the most commonly reported settings for norovirus outbreaks in the United States and other industrialized countries.[9] These outbreaks pose risks to patients, health care personnel, facility staff, and visitors and can affect the provision of care extending beyond an affected ward or unit.

Patient Cohorting and Isolation Precautions

In health care settings where the risk of transmission is high, transmission-based precautions can be the most effective means of interrupting transmission. Patients with symptoms of norovirus gastroenteritis should be separated from asymptomatic patients, and placed in a single occupancy room whenever possible.[77] In absence of available private rooms, facilities should cohort symptomatic patients to reduce ongoing transmission. The patients should be managed with standard and contact precautions. Contact precautions should be maintained until at least 48 hours after resolution of symptoms; longer periods of time can be considered for those with complex medical problems who may experience prolonged diarrhea, viral shedding, and symptom relapse. Patient movement within a ward or unit should be minimized, and symptomatic and recovering patients should not leave the patient care area unless it is medically necessary. Nonessential visitors should be restricted from affected areas.[77]

Staff Precautions, Hand Hygiene, and Personal Protective Equipment

Ill staff members should be excluded during their illness and for 48 hours to 72 hours after symptom resolution.[77] To minimize the spread of infection, staff who have worked on affected areas should not be transferred to or work on unaffected areas for 48 hours after exposure.[9] Nonessential staff should be excluded from working in areas experiencing a norovirus outbreak.

During outbreaks, washing hands with plain or antiseptic soap and running water for 20 seconds is paramount before and after providing care for patients with suspected or confirmed norovirus gastroenteritis. The use of alcohol-based hand sanitizers might additionally provide protection in between handwashing; however, studies have shown mixed effectiveness of alcohol-based hand sanitizers against norovirus and their use for norovirus remains controversial.[9]

Personal protective equipment with contact and standard precautions (ie, gown and gloves) is recommended for persons entering the patient care area.[77] If there are anticipated risks of splashing to the face, such as with patients who are vomiting, use of a surgical or procedure mask and eye protection or a full face shield can be considered.

Patient Transfer and Ward Closure

Consideration to the closure of wards to new admissions or transfers should be given to help reduce the size of the outbreak. Individuals recovering from symptoms can be discharged to their residence. Ward closure can be a costly measure and disruptive to the provision of care; the threshold for ward closure depends on the size of the outbreak and risk assessments by infection control personnel and facility leadership.[2,77]

Environmental Cleaning

Routine cleaning and disinfection of frequently touched environmental surfaces are key to interrupting norovirus spread; high-contact areas include toilets, faucets, hand/bed railings, phones, door handles, computer equipment, and kitchen preparation surfaces. In health care settings, Environmental and Protection Agency–registered products with label claims for use in health care settings should be used according to manufacturer's recommendations (https://www.epa.gov/pesticide-registration/list-g-epa-registered-hospital-disinfectants-effective-against-norovirus). Sodium hypochlorite (chlorine bleach) is the preferred agent to disinfect human norovirus from surfaces and should be applied at a concentration of 1000 ppm to 5000 ppm (5–25 tablespoons household bleach per gallon of water).[9]

VACCINE PROSPECTS

A norovirus vaccine has the potential to reap enormous benefits to society, through reduction in morbidity and mortality as well as cost savings. In the United States, vaccination could avert 1.0 million to 2.2 million cases annually, assuming 50% efficacy and 12 months of protection; a vaccine with longer duration of protection up to 48 months and 75% efficacy at a cost of $50 could prevent 21,000 to 47,000 hospitalizations and 240 to 550 deaths and save $100 million to $2.1 billion dollars annually.[145] Norovirus vaccines in development have been based on virus-like particles (VLPs), which contain the major capsid antigen but lack genetic material for viral replication.[146] VLPs have been shown to be morphologically and antigenically similar to native viruses and cause humoral, mucosal, and cellular immune responses after oral and intranasal administration.[147–149]

There are several norovirus vaccines that are under development in preclinical and clinical trials using VLPs and involving intranasal, oral, and intramuscular routes of administration. One of the earlier candidates was a monovalent intranasal GI.1 VLP vaccine that demonstrated a serologic response in 70% of healthy adults who received 2 doses of the vaccine.[150] This candidate vaccine was also efficacious against homologous challenge, and reduced the risk of gastroenteritis by 47% (95% CI, 15%-67%) and infection by 26% (95%CI, 1%-45%) and was well tolerated and immunogenic.[150] The vaccine was subsequently modified from an intranasal to an intramuscular route of administration and from a monovalent to a bivalent formulation. It is currently in phase II clinical trials, contains GI.1 and GII.4 VLPs, and is the vaccine furthest along in clinical development.[151] Serologic responses were demonstrated for both GI.1 and GII.4 as well as protection against severe clinical symptoms; however, vaccine efficacy was only 13.6% (95%CI, −21.0%-38.3%) for human norovirus infection. The only other vaccine in clinical trials is an adenoviral-vector based vaccine in a tablet formulation that encodes for a full length VP1 gene from GI.1; this vaccine recently met primary and secondary endpoints for safety and immunogenicity in an adult population in a phase I trial.[152]

Because norovirus affects multiple age groups, and unique populations have specific risk factors, including travelers, health care workers, individuals in LTCFs, and food handlers, developing a research agenda and clinical development plan has been challenging. The vaccine candidates discussed previously have been studied in healthy adults, but the greatest burden of disease is in young children and older adults, and a vaccine is likely to yield greatest impact in these age groups.[145] Ongoing clinical trials in these groups include the intramuscular GI.1/GII.4 vaccine candidate with aluminum hydroxide adjuvant in the pediatric population as well as safety and immunogenicity studies of the bivalent formulation in adult and elderly participants.[153]

Several considerations remain for the development of a norovirus vaccine. First, due to limited duration of immunity after natural infection and challenge studies, as well as the continual emergence of new strains, any vaccine candidate will warrant close attention to the duration of protection, need for booster doses, and reformulation. Second, the diversity between and within genogroups will necessitate development of a vaccine that affords broad heterotypic protection; a multivalent vaccine could offer such protection.[154] Third, given prior exposure and underlying conditions, the immune response is likely to differ in children, adults, the elderly, and the immunocompromised; consideration of different vaccines for these populations might be explored. Fourth, uptake of vaccines in the elderly has proved challenging. Incorporation into the childhood immunization schedule might be more feasible and could have important indirect benefits by limiting transmission in the general population, but the complexity of the pediatric schedule necessitates careful consideration of many factors, including acceptability and level of vaccine effectiveness. Combination vaccines could improve acceptability across different age groups; products in the preclinical phase include a trivalent norovirus/rotavirus combination vaccine, and a norovirus P particle dual vaccine that includes norovirus with influenza, hepatitis E, and rotavirus.[10] Additionally, targeting high-risk groups for vaccine receipt, such as vaccination of older adults who are living in LTCFs as well as staff and employees who work there, could be an attractive option for this particularly vulnerable population.

SUMMARY

The burden of norovirus disease is vast, and older adults are particularly at risk for severe outcomes, including prolonged symptoms and death. LTCFs and hospitals are the most commonly reported settings for norovirus outbreaks in developed countries, and older adults in these settings are more likely to experience health care–associated infection with more severe infections and poor outcomes. Although the current treatment of norovirus infection is primarily supportive, with the recent description of a human enteroid culture system, renewed interest in development of antivirals is anticipated. In addition, the future holds promise for prevention of disease, because several norovirus vaccines in clinical trials have the potential to reap enormous benefits for multiple age groups and populations.

REFERENCES

1. Hall AJ, Lopman BA, Payne DC, et al. Norovirus disease in the United States. Emerg Infect Dis 2013;19(8):1198–205.

2. Kambhampati A, Koopmans M, Lopman BA. Burden of norovirus in healthcare facilities and strategies for outbreak control. J Hosp Infect 2015;89(4): 296–301.

3. Lindsay L, Wolter J, De Coster I, et al. A decade of norovirus disease risk among older adults in upper-middle and high income countries: a systematic review. BMC Infect Dis 2015;15:425.

4. Lopman BA, Hall AJ, Curns AT, et al. Increasing rates of gastroenteritis hospital discharges in US adults and the contribution of norovirus, 1996-2007. Clin Infect Dis 2011;52(4):466–74.

5. Gastañaduy PA, Hall AJ, Curns AT, et al. Burden of norovirus gastroenteritis in the ambulatory setting–United States, 2001-2009. J Infect Dis 2013;207(7): 1058–65.

6. Batz MB, Hoffman S, Morris JG Jr. Ranking the disease burden of 14 pathogens in food sources in the United States using attribution data from outbreak investigations and expert elicitation. J Food Prot 2012;75(7):1278–91.

7. Jian X, Wang M, Wang K, et al. Sequence and genomic organization of Norwalk virus. Virology 1993;195:51–61.

8. Thorne LG, Goodfellow IG. Norovirus gene expression and replication. J Gen Virol 2014;95:278–91.

9. Hall AJ, Vinje J, Lopman B, et al. Updated norovirus outbreak management and disease prevention guidelines. MMWR Recomm Rep 2011;60(RR-03):1–18.

10. Lopman B. Global burden of norovirus and prospects for vaccine development. Centers for Disease Control and Prevention. Available at: https://www.cdc.gov/norovirus/downloads/global-burden-report.pdf. Accessed January 11, 2017.

11. Desai R, Hembree CD, Handel A, et al. Severe outcomes are associated with genogroup 2 genotype 4 norovirus outbreaks: a systematic literature review. Clin Infect Dis 2012;55(2):189–93.

12. Centers for Disease Control and Prevention. Outbreaks to calicinet by genotype data. Available at: https://www.cdc.gov/norovirus/reporting/calicinet/data.html. Accessed January 27, 2017.

13. Hall AJ, Patel M, Lopman B, et al. Norovirus. In: Magill AJ, Ryan E, Soloman T, et al, editors. Hunter's tropical medicine and emerging infectious disease. 9th edition; 2012.

14. Atmar RL, Estes MK. The epidemiologic and clinical importance of norovirus infection. Gastroenterol Clin North Am 2006;35(2):275–90.

15. Glass RI, Parashar UD, Estes MK. Norovirus gastroenteritis. N Engl J Med 2009; 361(18):1776–85.

16. Dolin R, Treanor JJ. Noroviruses and sapoviruses (caliciviruses). Chapter 178. In: Bennett JE, Dolin R, Blaser MJ, editors. Mandell, Douglas, and Bennett's principles and practice of infectious diseases. 8th edition. Saunders; 2015. p. 2122–7.

17. Gallimore CI, Cubitt D, du Plessis N, et al. Asymptomatic and symptomatic excretion of noroviruses during a hospital outbreak of gastroenteritis. J Clin Microbiol 2004;42(5):2271–4.

18. Schwartz S, Vergoulidou M, Schreier E, et al. Norovirus gastroenteritis causes severe and lethal complications after chemotherapy and hematopoietic stem cell transplantation. Blood 2011;117(22):5850–6.

19. Harris JP, Edmunds WJ, Peabody R, et al. Deaths from norovirus among the elderly, England and Wales. Emerg Infect Dis 2008;14(10):1546–52.

20. Mattner F, Sohr D, Heim A, et al. Risk groups for clinical complications of norovirus infections: an outbreak investigation. Clin Microbiol Infect 2006;12(1):69–74.

21. Marshall JK, Thabane M, Borgaonkar MR, et al. Postinfectious irritable bowel syndrome after a food-borne outbreak of acute gastroenteritis attributed to a viral pathogen. Clin Gastroenterol Hepatol 2007;5(4):457–60.

22. Porter CK, Faix DJ, Shiau D, et al. Postinfectious gastrointestinal disorders following norovirus outbreaks. Clin Infect Dis 2012;55(7):915.

23. Centers for Disease Control and Prevention (CDC). Outbreak of acute gastroenteritis associated with Norwalk-like viruses among British military personnel–Afghanistan, May 2002. MMWR Morb Mortal Wkly Rep 2002;51(22):477.
24. Stuart RL, Tan K, Mahar JE, et al. An outbreak of necrotizing enterocolitis associated with norovirus genotype GII.3. Pediatr Infect Dis J 2010;29:644–7.
25. Bartolini L, Mardari R, Toldo I, et al. Norovirus gastroenteritis and seizures: an atypical case with neuroradiological abnormalities. Neuropediatrics 2011; 42(4):167–9.
26. Gemulla G, Pessler F. Can norovirus infection lead to a postinfectious arthritis? Report of 2 possible cases. Klin Padiatr 2011;223:43–4.
27. Sugimoto T, Ogawa N, Aoyama M, et al. Haemolytic uraemic syndrome complicated with norovirus-associated gastroenteritis. Nephrol Dial Transplant 2007; 22:2098–9.
28. Zenda T, Kaneko S, Noriki S. Norovirus gastroenteritis accompanied by ischemic colitis: a case report. Hiroshima J Med Sci 2010;59(4):83–5.
29. Zenda T, Miyamoto M, Kaneko S. Norovirus gastroenteritis accompanied by marked elevation of transaminases. Hiroshima J Med Sci 2011;60(2):41–3.
30. Goller JL, Dimitriadis A, Tan A, et al. Long-term features of norovirus gastroenteritis in the elderly. J Hosp Infect 2004;58(4):286.
31. Lopman BA, Reacher MH, Vipond IB, et al. Clinical manifestation of norovirus gastroenteritis in health care settings. Clin Infect Dis 2004;39(3):318–24.
32. Yi J, Wahl K, Sederdahl BK, et al. Molecular epidemiology of norovirus in children and the elderly in Atlanta, Georgia, United States. J Med Virol 2016;88: 961–70.
33. Spackova M, Altmann D, Eckmanns T, et al. High level of gastrointestinal nosocomial infections in the German surveillance system, 2002–2008. Infect Control Hosp Epidemiol 2010;31:1273–8.
34. Franck KT, Nielsen RT, Holzknecht BJ, et al. Norovirus genotypes in hospital settings: differences between nosocomial and community-acquired infections. J Infect Dis 2015;212(6):881–8.
35. Hall AJ, Curns AT, McDonald LC, et al. The roles of clostridium difficile and norovirus among gastroenteritis-associated deaths in the United States, 1999–2007. Clin Infect Dis 2012;55(2):216–23.
36. Trivedi TK, DeSalvo T, Lee L, et al. Hospitalizations and mortality associated with norovirus outbreaks in nursing homes, 2009-2010. JAMA 2012;308(16): 1668–75.
37. Trivedi TK, Desai R, Hall AJ, et al. Clinical characteristics of norovirus-associated deaths: a systematic literature review. Am J Infect Control 2013; 41(7):654–7.
38. Bok K, Green KY. Norovirus gastroenteritis in immunocompromised patients. N Engl J Med 2012;367(22):2126–32.
39. Schorn R, Höhne M, Meerbach A, et al. Chronic norovirus infection after kidney transplantation: molecular evidence for immune-driven viral evolution. Clin Infect Dis 2010;51:307–14.
40. Roos-Weil D, Ambert-Balay K, Lanternier F. Impact of norovirus/sapovirus-related diarrhea in renal transplant recipients hospitalized for diarrhea. Transplantation 2011;92:61–9.
41. Ludwig A, Adams O, Laws HJ, et al. Quantitative detection of norovirus excretion in pediatric patients with cancer and prolonged gastroenteritis and shedding of norovirus. J Med Virol 2008;80:1461–7.

42. Ueda R, Fuji S, Mori S, et al. Characteristics and outcomes of patients diagnosed with norovirus gastroenteritis after allogeneic hematopoietic stem cell transplantation based on immunochromatography. Int J Hematol 2015;102(1): 121–8.

43. Ghosh N, Malik FA, Daver RG, et al. Viral associated diarrhea in immunocompromised and cancer patients at a large comprehensive cancer center: a 10-year retrospective study. Infect Dis (Lond) 2017;49(2):113.

44. Robilotti E, Deresinski S, Pinsky BA. Norovirus. Clin Microbiol Rev 2015;28(1): 134–64.

45. Roddie C, Paul JP, Benjamin R, et al. Allogeneic hematopoietic stem cell transplantation and norovirus gastroenteritis: a previously unrecognized cause of morbidity. Clin Infect Dis 2009;49:1061–8.

46. Teunis PF, Moe CL, Liu P, et al. Norwalk virus: how infectious is it? J Med Virol 2008;80:1468–76.

47. Atmar RL, Opekun AR, Gilger MA, et al. Determination of the 50% human infectious dose for Norwalk virus. J Infect Dis 2014;209(7):1016–22.

48. Dowell SF, Groves C, Kirkland KB, et al. A multistate outbreak of oyster-associated gastroenteritis: implications for interstate tracing of contaminated shellfish. J Infect Dis 1995;171:1497–503.

49. Morse DL, Guzewich JJ, Hanrahan JP, et al. Widespread outbreaks of clam- and oyster-associated gastroenteritis. Role of Norwalk virus. N Engl J Med 1986;314: 678–81.

50. Falkenhorst G, Krusell L, Lisby M, et al. Imported frozen raspberries cause a series of norovirus outbreaks in Denmark, 2005. Euro Surveill 2005;10: E050922.2.

51. Gaulin CD, Ramsay D, Cardinal P, et al. Epidemic of gastroenteritis of viral origin associated with eating imported raspberries. Can J Public Health 1999;90: 37–40 [in French].

52. Le Guyader FS, Mittelholzer C, Haugarreau L, et al. Detection of noroviruses in raspberries associated with a gastroenteritis outbreak. Int J Food Microbiol 2004;97:179–86.

53. Atmar RL, Opekun AR, Gilger MA, et al. Norwalk virus shedding after experimental human infection. Emerg Infect Dis 2008;14:1553–7.

54. Amar CFL, East CL, Gray J, et al. Detection by PCR of eight groups of enteric pathogens in 4,627 faecal samples: re-examination of the English case-control Infectious Intestinal Disease Study (1993–1996). Eur J Clin Microbiol Infect Dis 2007;26:311–23.

55. Johnson PC, Mathewson JJ, DuPont HL, et al. Multiple-challenge study of host susceptibility to Norwalk gastroenteritis in US adults. J Infect Dis 1990;161(1): 18–21.

56. Parrino TA, Schreiber DS, Trier JS, et al. Clinical immunity in acute gastroenteritis caused by Norwalk agent. N Engl J Med 1977;297(2):86–9.

57. Wyatt RG, Dolin R, Blacklow NR, et al. Comparison of three agents of acute infectious nonbacterial gastroenteritis by cross-challenge in volunteers. J Infect Dis 1974;129(6):709–14.

58. Simmons K, Gambhir M, Leon J, et al. Duration of immunity to norovirus gastroenteritis. Emerg Infect Dis 2013;19(8):1260–7.

59. Nurminen K, Blazevic V, Huhti L, et al. Prevalence of norovirus GII-4 antibodies in Finnish children. J Med Virol 2011;83(3):525–31.

60. Baron RC, Greenberg HB, Cukor G, et al. Serological responses among teenagers after natural exposure to Norwalk virus. J Infect Dis 1984;150(4):531–4.

61. Reeck A, Kavanagh O, Estes MK, et al. Serological correlate of protection against norovirus-induced gastroenteritis. J Infect Dis 2010;202(8):1212–8.
62. Harrington PR, Lindesmith L, Yount B, et al. Binding of Norwalk virus-like particles to ABH histo-blood group antigens is blocked by antisera from infected human volunteers or experimentally vaccinated mice. J Virol 2002;76(23): 12335–43.
63. Lindesmith L, Moe C, Marionneau S, et al. Human susceptibility and resistance to Norwalk virus infection. Nat Med 2003;9(5):548–53.
64. Saito M, Goel-Apaza S, Espetia S, et al. Multiple norovirus infections in a birth cohort in a Peruvian Periurban community. Clin Infect Dis 2014;58(4): 483–91.
65. Malm M, Uusi-Kerttula H, Vesikari T, et al. High serum levels of norovirus genotype-specific blocking antibodies correlate with protection from infection in children. J Infect Dis 2014;210(11):1755–62.
66. Currier R, Payne DC, Staat MA, et al. Innate susceptibility to norovirus infections influenced by FUT2 genotype in a United States pediaric population. Clin Infect Dis 2015;60(11):1631–8.
67. Nordgren J, Sharma S, Kambhampati A, et al. Innate resistance and susceptibility to Norovirus infection. PLoS Pathog 2016;12(4):e1005385.
68. Lopman BA, Trivedi T, Vicuna Y, et al. Norovirus infection and disease in an Ecuadorian birth cohort: association of certain norovirus genotypes with host FUT2 secretor status. J Infect Dis 2015;211(11):1813–21.
69. Kambhampati A, Payne DC, Costantini V, et al. Host genetic susceptibility to enteric viruses: a systematic review and metaanalysis. Clin Infect Dis 2016; 62(1):11–8.
70. Lopman BA, Steele D, Kirkwood CD, et al. The vast and varied global burden of norovirus: prospects for prevention and control. PLoS Med 2006;13(4): e1001999.
71. Vinje J. Advances in laboratory methods for detection and typing of norovirus. J Clin Microbiol 2015;53(2):373–81.
72. Ahmed SM, Hall AJ, Robinson AE, et al. Global prevalence of norovirus in cases of gastroenteritis: a systematic review and meta-analysis. Lancet Infect Dis 2014;14(8):725–30.
73. Bruggink LD, Catton MG, Marshall JA. Evaluation of the bioline standard diagnostics SD immunochromatographic norovirus detection kit using fecal specimens from Australian gastroenteritis incidents. Diagn Microbiol Infect Dis 2013;76(2):147–52.
74. Gray JJ, Kohli E, Ruggeri FM, et al. European multicenter evaluation of commercial enzyme immunoassays for detecting norovirus antigen in fecal samples. Clin Vaccine Immunol 2007;14(10):1349–55.
75. Costantini V, Grenz L, Fritzinger A, et al. Diagnostic accuracy and analytical sensitivity of IDEIA Norovirus assay for routine screening of human norovirus. J Clin Microbiol 2010;48(8):2770–8.
76. Kaplan JE, Feldman R, Campbell DS, et al. The frequency of a Norwalk-like pattern of illness in outbreaks of acute gastroenteritis. Am J Public Health 1982;72(12):1329–32.
77. MacCannell T, Umscheid CA, Agarwal RK, et al. Guideline for the prevetion and control of norovirus gastroenteritis outbreaks in healthcare settings. Available at: https://www.cdc.gov/hicpac/pdf/norovirus/Norovirus-Guideline-2011.pdf. Accessed January 13, 2017.

78. Turcios RM, Widdowson MA, Sulka AC, et al. Reevaluation of epidemiological criteria for identifying outbreaks of acute gastroenteritis due to norovirus: United States, 1998-2000. Clin Infect Dis 2006;42(7):964–9.

79. Hedberg CW, Osterholm MT. Outbreaks of food-borne and waterborne viral gastroenteritis. Clin Microbiol Rev 1993;6(3):199–210.

80. Dalton C, Mintz E, Wells J, et al. Outbreaks of enterotoxigenic Escherichia coli infection in American adults: a clinical and epidemiologic profile. Epidemiol Infect 1999;123(01):9–16.

81. Steinhoff MC, Douglas RG Jr, Greenberg HB, et al. Bismuth subsalicylate therapy of viral gastroenteritis. Gastroenterology 1980;78(6):1495–9.

82. Pitz AM, Park GW, Lee D, et al. Antimicrobial activity of bismuth subsalicylate on Clostridium difficile, Escherichia coli O157:H7, norovirus, and other common enteric pathogens. Gut Microbes 2015;6(2):93–100.

83. de Bruyn G. Diarrhoea in adults (acute). BMJ Clin Evid 2008;2008 [pii:0901].

84. Gallelli L, Colosimo M, Tolotta GA, et al. Prospective randomized double-blind trial of racecadotril compared with loperamide in elderly people with gastroenteritis living in nursing homes. Eur J Clin Pharmacol 2010;66(2):137–44.

85. Lustman F, Walters EG, Shroff NE, et al. Diphenoxylate hydrochloride (Lomotil) in the treatment of acute diarrhoea. Br J Clin Pract 1987;41(3):648–51.

86. Rocha-Pereira J, Neyts J, Jochmans D. Norovirus: targets and tools in antiviral drug discovery. Biochem Pharmacol 2014;91(1):1–11.

87. Kaufman SS, Green KY, Korba BE. Treatment of norovirus infections: moving antivirals from the bench to the bedside. Antiviral Res 2014;105:80–91.

88. Jurgens PT, Allen LA, Ambardekar AV, et al. Chronic norovirus infections in cardiac transplant patients. Prog Transplant 2017;27(1):69–72.

89. Siddiq DM, Koo HL, Adachi JA, et al. Norovirus gastroenteritis successfully treated with nitazoxanide. J Infect 2011;63(5):394–7.

90. Avery RK, Lonze BE, Krause ES, et al. Severe chronic norovirus diarrheal disease in transplant recipients: clinical features of an under-recognized syndrome. Transpl Infect Dis 2017;19:e12674.

91. Rossignol JF, El-Gohary YM. Nitazoxanide in the treatment of viral gastroenteritis: a randomized double-blind placebo-controlled clinical trial. Aliment Pharmacol Ther 2006;24(10):1423–30.

92. Furuta Y, Gowen BB, Takahashi K, et al. Favipiravir (T-705), a novel viral RNA polymerase inhibitor. Antiviral Res 2013;100:446–54.

93. Chang KO, George DW. Interferons and ribavirin effectively inhibit Norwalk virus replication in replicon-bearing cells. J Virol 2007;81:12111–8.

94. Lee H, Ko G. Antiviral effect of vitamin A on norovirus infection via modulation of the gut microbiome. Sci Rep 2016;6:25835.

95. Lei S, Ramesh A, Twitchell E, et al. High protective efficacy of probiotics and rice bran against human norovirus infection and diarrhea in gnotobiotic pigs. Front Microbiol 2016;7:1699.

96. Ettayebi K, Crawford SE, Murakami K, et al. Replication of human noroviruses in stem cell-derived human enteroids. Science 2016;353(6306):1387–93.

97. U.S. Census Bureau, Population Division. Annual estimates of the civilian population by single year of age and sex for the United States and States: April 1, 2010 to July 1, 2015. Available at: https://www2.census.gov/programs-surveys/popest/datasets/2010-2015/state/asrh/. Accessed March 31, 2017.

98. Grytdal SP, DeBess E, Lee LE, et al. Incidence of norovirus and other viral pathogens that cause acute gastroenteritis (AGE) among Kaiser Permanente Member Populations in the United States, 2012–2013. PLoS One 2016;11(4):e0148395.

99. O'Brien SJ, Donaldson AL, Iturriza-Gomara M, et al. Age-specific incidence rates for norovirus in the community and presenting to primary healthcare facilities in the United Kingdom. J Infect Dis 2016;213(Suppl 1):S15–8.

100. Haustein T, Harris JP, Pebody R, et al. Hospital admissions due to norovirus in adult and elderly patiens in England. Clin Infect Dis 2009;49(12):1890–2.

101. Chan MCW, Leung TF, Chung TWS, et al. Virus genotype distribution and virus burden in children and adults hospitalized for norovirus gastroenteritis, 2012–2014, Hong Kong. Sci Rep 2015;5:11507.

102. Grytdal SP, Rimland D, Shirley SH, et al. Incidence of medically-attended norovirus-associated acute gastroenteritis in four veteran's affairs medical center populations in the United States, 2011-2012. PLoS One 2015;10(5):e0126733.

103. Ruzante JM, Majowicz SE, Fazil A, et al. Hospitalization and deaths for select enteric illnesses and associated sequelae in Canada, 2001-2004. Epidemiol Infect 2011;139(6):937–45.

104. Phillips G, Tam CC, Conti S, et al. Community incidence of norovirus-associated infectious intestinal disease in England: improved estimates using viral load for norovirus diagnosis. Am J Epidemiol 2010;171(9):1014–22.

105. Werber D, Hille K, Frank C, et al. Years of potential life lost for six major enteric pathogens, Germany, 2004-2008. Epidemiol Infect 2013;141(5):961–8.

106. Chui KKH, Jagai JS, Griffiths JK, et al. Hospitalization of the elderly in the United States for nonspecific gastrointestinal diseases: a search for etiological clues. Am J Public Health 2011;101(11):2082–6.

107. Verhoef L, Koopmans M, Van Pelt W, et al. The estimated disease burden of norovirus in The Netherlands. Epidemiol Infect 2013;141:496–506.

108. Bernard H, Höhne M, Niendorf S, et al. Epidemiology of norovirus gastroenteritis in Germany 2001-2009: eight seasons of routine surveillance. Epidemiol Infect 2014;142(1):63–74.

109. Rovida F, Campanini G, Piralla A, et al. Molecular detection of gastrointestinal viral infections in hospitalized patients. Diagn Microbiol Infect Dis 2013;77(3):231–5.

110. Fernandez J, de Ona M, Melon S, et al. Noroviruses as cause of gastroenteritis in elderly patients. Aging Clin Exp Res 2011;23:145–7.

111. Tang MB, Chen CH, Chen SC, et al. Epidemiological and molecular analysis of human norovirus infections in Taiwan during 2011 and 2012. BMC Infect Dis 2013;13:338.

112. Yu J, Ye C, Lai S, et al. Incidence of norovirus-associated diarrhea, Shanghai, China, 2012-2013. Emerg Infect Dis 2017;23(2):312–5.

113. Leblanc D, Inglish GD, Boras VF, et al. The prevalence of enteric RNA viruses in stools from diarrheic and non-diarrheic people in southwestern Alberta, Canada. Arch Virol 2017;162(1):117–28.

114. Costa I, Mesquita JR, Veiga E, et al. Surveillance of norovirus in Portugal and the emergence of the Sydney variant, 2011–2013. J Clin Virol 2015;70:26–8.

115. Wu X, Han J, Chen L, et al. Prevalence and genetic diversity of noroviruses in adults with acute gastroenteritis in Huzhou, China, 2013–2014. Arch Virol 2015;160:1705–13.

116. Gao Z, Li X, Yan H, et al. Human calicivirus occurrence among outpatients with diarrhea in Beijing, China, between April 2011 and March 2013. J Med Virol 2015;87(12):2040–7.

117. Tian G, Jin M, Li H, et al. Clinical charactersitics and genetic diversity of noroviruses in adults with acute gastroenteritis in Beijin, China in 208-2009. J Med Virol 2014;86:1235–42.

118. Manso CF, Torres E, Bou G, et al. Role of norovirus in acute gastroenteritis in the Northwest of Spain during 2010–2011. J Med Virol 2013;85:2009–15.

119. Gao Y, Jin M, Cong X, et al. Clinical and molecular epidemiologic analyses of norovirus-associated sporadic gastroenteritis in adults from Beijing, China. J Med Virol 2011;83:1078–85.
120. Jin M, Chen J, Zhang XH, et al. Genetic diversity of noroviruses in Chinese adults: potential recombination hotspots and GII-4/Den Haag-specific mutations at a putative epitope. Infect Genet Evol 2011;11:1716–26.
121. Huhulescu S, Kiss R, Brettlecker M, et al. Etiology of acute gastroenteritis in three sentinel general practices, Austria 2007. Infection 2009;37(2):103–8.
122. Patel MM, Hall AJ, Vinje J, et al. Noroviruses: a comprehensive review. J Clin Virol 2009;44(1):1–8.
123. Hall AJ, Wikswo ME, Pringle K, et al. Vital signs: foodborne norovirus outbreaks — United States, 2009–2012. MMWR Morb Mortal Wkly Rep 2014;63(22):491–5.
124. Centers for Disease Control and Prevention. Outbreaks reported to NoroSTAT. Available at: https://www.cdc.gov/norovirus/reporting/norostat/data.html. Accessed May 15, 2017.
125. Wikswo M, Kambhampati A, Shioda K, et al. Outbreaks of acute gastroenteritis transmitted by person-to-person contact, environmental contamination, and unknown modes of transmission — United States, 2009–2013. MMWR Surveill Summ 2015;64(12):1–16.
126. Zheng DP, Widdowson MA, Glass RI, et al. Molecular epidemiology of genogroup II-genotype 4 noroviruses in the United States between 1994 and 2006. J Clin Microbiol 2010;48:168–77.
127. Chen Y, Hall AJ, Kirk MD. Norovirus disease in older adults living in long-term care facilities: strategies for management. Curr Geri Rep 2017;1(1):26–33.
128. Vega E, Barclay L, Gregoricus N, et al. Genotypic and epidemiologic trends of norovirus outbreaks in the United States, 2009 to 2013. J Clin Microbiol 2014; 52(1):147–55.
129. Hall AJ, Wikswo ME, Manikonda K, et al. Acute gastroenteritis surveillance through the national outbreak reporting system, United States. Emerg Infect Dis 2013;19(8):1305–9.
130. Rosenthal NA, Lee LE, Vermeulen BA, et al. Epidemiological and genetic characteristics of norovirus outbreaks in long-term care facilities, 2003-2006. Epidemiol Infect 2011;139(2):286–94.
131. Kirk MD, Fullerton KE, Hall GV, et al. Surveillance for outbreaks of gastroenteritis in long-term care facilities, Australia, 2002-2008. Clin Infect Dis 2010;51(8):907–14.
132. Rajagopalan S, Yoshikawa TT. Norovirus infections in long-term care facilities. J Am Geriatr Soc 2016;64(5):1097–103.
133. Lopman BA, Adak GK, Reacher MH, et al. Two epidemiologic patterns of norovirus outbreaks: surveillance in England and Wales, 1992-2000. Emerg Infect Dis 2003;9(1):71–7.
134. Greig JD, Lee MB. Enteric outbreaks in long-term care facilities and recommendations for prevention: a review. Epidemiol Infect 2009;137(2):145–55.
135. Iturriza-Gómara M, Lopman B. Norovirus in healthcare settings. Curr Opin Infect Dis 2014;27(5):437–43.
136. Centers for Disease Control and Prevention (CDC). Recurring norovirus outbreaks in a long-term residential treatment facility—Oregon, 2007. MMWR Morb Mortal Wkly Rep 2009;58:694–8.
137. Lynn S, Toop J, Hanger C, et al. Norovirus outbreaks in a hospital setting: the role of infection control. N Z Med J 2004;117(1189):U771.
138. Johnston CP, Qiu H, Ticehurst JR, et al. Outbreak management and implications of a nosocomial norovirus outbreak. Clin Infect Dis 2007;45(5):534–40.

139. Hansen S, Stamm-Balderjahn S, Zuschneid I, et al. Closure of medical departments during nosocomial outbreaks: data from a systematic analysis of the literature. J Hosp Infect 2007;65(4):348–53.

140. Danial J, Cepeda JA, Cameron F, et al. Epidemiology and costs associated with norovirus outbreaks in NHS Lothian, Scotland 2007-2009. J Hosp Infect 2011; 79(4):354–8.

141. Barclay L, Park GW, Vega E, et al. Infection control for norovirus. Clin Microbiol Infect 2014;20(8):731–40.

142. Balter S, Weiss D, Hanson H, et al. Three years of emergency department gastrointestinal syndromic surveillance in New York City: what have we found? MMWR Suppl 2005;54:175–80.

143. Centers for Disease Control and Prevention. Norovirus activity—United States, 2002. JAMA 2003;289(6):693–6.

144. Kumazaki M, Usuku S. Norovirus genotype distribution in outbreaks of acute gastroenteritis among children and older people: an 8-year study. BMC Infect Dis 2016;16(1):643.

145. Bartsch SM, Lopman BA, Hall AJ, et al. The potential economic value of a human norovirus vaccine for the United States. Vaccine 2012;30(49):7097–104.

146. Jiang X, Wang M, Graham DY, et al. Expression, self-assembly, and antigenicity of the Norwalk virus capsid protein. J Virol 1992;66(11):6527–32.

147. Herbst-Kralovetz M, Mason HS, Chen Q. Norwalk virus-like particles as vaccines. Expert Rev Vaccines 2010;9(3):299–307.

148. Ball JM, Graham DY, Opekun AR, et al. Recombinant Norwalk virus-like particles given orally to volunteers: phase I study. Gastroenterology 1999;117(1):40–8.

149. Tacket CO, Sztein MB, Losonsky GA, et al. Humoral, mucosal, and cellular immune responses to oral Norwalk virus-like particles in volunteers. Clin Immunol 2003;108(3):241–7.

150. Atmar RL, Bernstein DI, Harro CD, et al. Norovirus vaccine against experimental human Norwalk virus illness. N Engl J Med 2011;365(23):2178–87.

151. Efficacy and immunogenicity of norovirus GI.1/GII.4 bivalent virus-like particle vaccine in adults. Available at: https://clinicaltrials.gov/ct2/show/NCT02669121? term=norovirus+vaccine&rank=7. Accessed May 15, 2017.

152. Phase I placebo-controlled, randomized trial of an adenoviral-vector based norovirus vaccine. Available at: https://clinicaltrials.gov/ct2/show/NCT02868073? term=norovirus+vaccine&rank=1. Accessed May 15, 2017.

153. Safety and immunogenicity of norovirus GI.1/GII.4 bivalent VLP vaccine in children. Available at: https://clinicaltrials.gov/ct2/show/NCT02153112?term= norovirus+vaccine&rank=4. Accessed May 15, 2017.

154. LoBue AD, Lindesmith L, Yount B, et al. Multivalent norovirus vaccines induce strong mucosal and systemic blocking antibodies against multiple strains. Vaccine 2006;24(24):5220–34.

155. Al-Thani A, Baris M, Al-Lawati N, et al. Characterising the aetiology of severe acute gastroenteritis among patients visiting a hospital in Qatar using real-time polymerase chain reaction. BMC Infectious Diseases 2013;13:329.

156. Lau C-S, Wong DA, Tong LKL, et al. High rate and changing molecular epidemiology pattern of norovirus infections in sporadic cases and outbreaks of gastroenteritis in Hong Kong. Journal of Medical Virology 2004;73:113–7.

157. de Wit MAS, Koopmans MPG, Kortbeek LM, et al. Sensor, a population-based cohort study on gastroenteritis in the Netherlands: incidence and etiology. American Journal of Epidemiology 2001;154(7):666–74.

UNITED STATES POSTAL SERVICE®

Statement of Ownership, Management, and Circulation
(All Periodicals Publications Except Requester Publications)

1. Publication Title	2. Publication Number	3. Filing Date
INFECTIOUS DISEASE CLINICS OF NORTH AMERICA	001 – 556	9/18/2017

4. Issue Frequency	5. Number of Issues Published Annually	6. Annual Subscription Price
MAR, JUN, SEP, DEC	4	$301.00

7. Complete Mailing Address of Known Office of Publication (Not printer) (Street, city, county, state, and ZIP+4®)

ELSEVIER INC.
230 Park Avenue, Suite 800
New York, NY 10169

Contact Person
STEPHEN R. BUSHING

Telephone (Include area code)
215-239-3688

8. Complete Mailing Address of Headquarters or General Business Office of Publisher (Not printer)

ELSEVIER INC.
230 Park Avenue, Suite 800
New York, NY 10169

9. Full Names and Complete Mailing Addresses of Publisher, Editor, and Managing Editor (Do not leave blank)

Publisher (Name and complete mailing address)

ADRIANNE BRIGIDO, ELSEVIER INC.
1600 JOHN F KENNEDY BLVD. SUITE 1800
PHILADELPHIA, PA 19103-2899

Editor (Name and complete mailing address)

KERRY HOLLAND, ELSEVIER INC.
1600 JOHN F KENNEDY BLVD. SUITE 1800
PHILADELPHIA, PA 19103-2899

Managing Editor (Name and complete mailing address)

PATRICK MANLEY, ELSEVIER INC.
1600 JOHN F KENNEDY BLVD. SUITE 1800
PHILADELPHIA, PA 19103-2899

10. Owner (Do not leave blank. If the publication is owned by a corporation, give the name and address of the corporation immediately followed by the names and addresses of all stockholders owning or holding 1 percent or more of the total amount of stock. If not owned by a corporation, give the names and addresses of the individual owners. If owned by a partnership or other unincorporated firm, give its name and address as well as those of each individual owner. If the publication is published by a nonprofit organization, give its name and address.)

Full Name	Complete Mailing Address
WHOLLY OWNED SUBSIDIARY OF REED/ELSEVIER, US HOLDINGS	1600 JOHN F KENNEDY BLVD. SUITE 1800 PHILADELPHIA, PA 19103-2899

11. Known Bondholders, Mortgagees, and Other Security Holders Owning or Holding 1 Percent or More of Total Amount of Bonds, Mortgages, or Other Securities. If none, check box ▶ ☒ None

Full Name	Complete Mailing Address
N/A	

12. Tax Status (For completion by nonprofit organizations authorized to mail at nonprofit rates) (Check one)
The purpose, function, and nonprofit status of this organization and the exempt status for federal income tax purposes:
☒ Has Not Changed During Preceding 12 Months
☐ Has Changed During Preceding 12 Months (Publisher must submit explanation of change with this statement)

13. Publication Title	14. Issue Date for Circulation Data Below
INFECTIOUS DISEASE CLINICS OF NORTH AMERICA	JUNE 2017

15. Extent and Nature of Circulation		Average No. Copies Each Issue During Preceding 12 Months	No. Copies of Single Issue Published Nearest to Filing Date
a. Total Number of Copies (Net press run)		410	327
b. Paid Circulation (By Mail and Outside the Mail)	(1) Mailed Outside-County Paid Subscriptions Stated on PS Form 3541 (Include paid distribution above nominal rate, advertiser's proof copies, and exchange copies)	246	205
	(2) Mailed In-County Paid Subscriptions Stated on PS Form 3541 (Include paid distribution above nominal rate, advertiser's proof copies, and exchange copies)	0	0
	(3) Paid Distribution Outside the Mails Including Sales Through Dealers and Carriers, Street Vendors, Counter Sales, and Other Paid Distribution Outside USPS®	78	67
	(4) Paid Distribution by Other Classes of Mail Through the USPS (e.g. First-Class Mail®)	0	0
c. Total Paid Distribution (Sum of 15b (1), (2), (3), and (4))		324	272
d. Free or Nominal Rate Distribution (By Mail and Outside the Mail)	(1) Free or Nominal Rate Outside-County Copies included on PS Form 3541	41	55
	(2) Free or Nominal Rate In-County Copies Included on PS Form 3541	0	0
	(3) Free or Nominal Rate Copies Mailed at Other Classes Through the USPS (e.g. First-Class Mail)	0	0
	(4) Free or Nominal Rate Distribution Outside the Mail (Carriers or other means)	0	0
e. Total Free or Nominal Rate Distribution (Sum of 15d (1), (2), (3) and (4))		41	55
f. Total Distribution (Sum of 15c and 15e)		365	327
g. Copies not Distributed (See Instructions to Publishers #4 (page #3))		45	0
h. Total (Sum of 15f and g)		410	327
i. Percent Paid (15c divided by 15f times 100)		88.77%	83.18%

* If you are claiming electronic copies, go to line 16 on page 3. If you are not claiming electronic copies, skip to line 17 on page 3.

16. Electronic Copy Circulation	Average No. Copies Each Issue During Preceding 12 Months	No. Copies of Single Issue Published Nearest to Filing Date
a. Paid Electronic Copies ▶	0	0
b. Total Paid Print Copies (Line 15c) + Paid Electronic Copies (Line 16a) ▶	324	272
c. Total Print Distribution (Line 15f) + Paid Electronic Copies (Line 16a) ▶	365	327
d. Percent Paid (Both Print & Electronic Copies) (16b divided by 16c × 100) ▶	88.77%	83.18%

☒ I certify that 50% of all my distributed copies (electronic and print) are paid above a nominal price.

17. Publication of Statement of Ownership

☒ If the publication is a general publication, publication of this statement is required. Will be printed in the DECEMBER 2017 issue of this publication. ☐ Publication not required.

18. Signature and Title of Editor, Publisher, Business Manager, or Owner

STEPHEN R. BUSHING - INVENTORY DISTRIBUTION CONTROL MANAGER

Date 9/18/2017

I certify that all information furnished on this form is true and complete. I understand that anyone who furnishes false or misleading information on this form or who omits material or information requested on the form may be subject to criminal sanctions (including fines and imprisonment) and/or civil sanctions (including civil penalties).

PS Form 3526, July 2014 (Page 3 of 4)   PRIVACY NOTICE: See our privacy policy on www.usps.com

PS Form 3526, July 2014 (Page 1 of 4 (see instructions page 4)) PSN 7530-01-000-9931   PRIVACY NOTICE: See our privacy policy on www.usps.com

Printed and bound by CPI Group (UK) Ltd, Croydon, CR0 4YY

08/05/2025

01864703-0004